PATIENT-CENTERED CURE ASSESSMENT

A Methodology to Assess Whether Medical Interventions
Succeed in Curing Individual Patients

JAMES R. MILLER III, PHD
MOHAMMED KASHANI-SABET, MD
AND
RICHARD W. SAGEBIEL, MD

iUniverse®

PATIENT-CENTERED CURE ASSESSMENT
A METHODOLOGY TO ASSESS WHETHER MEDICAL INTERVENTIONS
SUCCEED IN CURING INDIVIDUAL PATIENTS

iUniverse books may be ordered through booksellers or by contacting:

iUniverse
1663 Liberty Drive
Bloomington, IN 47403
www.iuniverse.com
1-800-Authors (1-800-288-4677)

ISBN: 978-1-5320-2969-1 (sc)
ISBN: 978-1-5320-2967-7 (e)

Library of Congress Control Number: 2017912506

Print information available on the last page.

iUniverse rev. date: 12/16/2017

CONTENTS

Page

PREFACE v

ACKNOWLEDGMENTS x

1.0   INTRODUCTION 1

      1.1   Interpreting the Concept of Cure Probabilistically: A Bayesian
            Framework 4
      1.2   Consequences of the Altered and Selective Focus of PCM 5

2.0   THE RESULTS OF 469 KIDNEY TRANSPLANTS 9

      2.1   A Bayesian Kidney Transplant Model 15
      2.2   How Can a Table Be Constructed to Implement Such a Model? 19
      2.3   By How Much Did PCM Improve the Accuracy of Predicting Early
            Success? 23
      2.4   What Do the Tailored Bayesian Posterior Success Probabilities
            Look Like? 33
      2.5   What Probabilities Apply to the Subsequent Time Period? 37
      2.6   A Brief Summary of Some Useful Statistical Concepts and
            Procedures 39

3.0   THE CONCEPT OF CURE 40

      3.1   What Constitutes a Focal Event in the Cure Context? 40

4.0   A FIRST ILLUSTRATIVE ANALYSIS 42

      4.1   Selecting the Target Intervention 42
      4.2   Additional Steps to Homogenize the Analysis 43
      4.3   The First Intervention Sample 44
      4.4   Verifying No Differences Between Radical and Modified Radical
            Mastectomy 44
      4.5   Executing an Initial Kaplan-Meier Survival Analysis 45
      4.6   A Preliminary Interpretation of the Kaplan-Meier Survival
            Analysis 53
      4.7   The RISKTEST Simulator 55
      4.8   A Systematic Search for Evidence of Cure 60
      4.9   Executing the CURE Option of the KAPM Procedure 62
      4.10 Fine-Tuning the Initial Estimate of the Actual Proportion
            Cured 68
      4.11 Convincing Confirmation of the Existence of Cure 73

5.0   THE MINIMAL RISK PARTITIONING ALGORITHM (MRPA) 74

      5.1   A Bayesian Cure Model 74
      5.2   Logistic Regression Analysis (Logit): Obtaining Individually
            Tailored Prior Cure Probabilities from the Fine-Tuned Initial
            Partitioning of Patients into MR and SR Subsamples 77
      5.3   By How Much Did PCM Improve the Consistency of the Initial
            Prior Cure Probabilities with the Initial Partitioning of
            Patients into MR and SR Subsamples? 80

5.4 Converting PCM-Generated UIRIs ·into Dummy Variables to Drive MRPA 82

5.5 Cox Regression Analysis (Cox): Survival Given the Initial Partitioning 87

5.6 By How Much Did Bayesian Revision Based on Cox Regression Further Improve the Consistency of Cure Probabilities with the Initial Partitioning by Reducing Misclassifications? 96

5.7 Further Reducing Misclassifications: MRPA's Next Iteration 99

5.8 Eliminating All Misclassifications: MRPA's Final Iteration 103

5.9 Checking the Final Partitioning for Reasonableness 107

5.10 A Dramatically Revised Kaplan-Meier Survival Curve: The Apparent Disappearance of a Declining Hazard Rate over Time ... 111

5.11 Constructing an Individually Tailored Cure Curve and a Substitutable Survival Curve for a "Typical" Patient, for a High-Risk Patient, and for a Low-Risk Patient 119

5.11.1 Constructing Tailored Curves for the "Typical" Patient 119

5.11.2 Constructing Tailored Curves for High-Risk and Low-Risk Patients 123

6.0 A SECOND ILLUSTRATIVE ANALYSIS 128

6.1 Selecting a Comparable Target Intervention 128

6.2 Additional Steps to Homogenize the Second Analysis 128

6.3 The Second Intervention Sample 129

6.4 Executing an Initial Kaplan-Meier Survival Analysis 129

6.5 A Preliminary Interpretation of the Kaplan-Meier Survival Analysis 137

6.6 The RISKTEST Simulator 138

6.7 A Systematic Search for Evidence of Cure 142

6.8 Executing the CURE Option of the KAPM Procedure 144

6.9 Fine-Tuning the Initial Estimate of the Actual Proportion Cured 149

6.10 Convincing Confirmation of the Existence of Cure 154

7.0 APPLYING MRPA TO THE SECOND ILLUSTRATIVE ANALYSIS 155

7.1 Replicating the Bayesian Cure Model 155

7.2 Logistic Regression Analysis (Logit): Obtaining Individually Tailored Prior Cure Probabilities from the Fine-Tuned Initial Partitioning of Patients into MR and SR Subsamples 155

7.3 By How Much Did PCM Improve the Consistency of the Initial Prior Cure Probabilities with the Initial Partitioning of Patients into MR and SR Subsamples? 158

7.4 Converting PCM-Generated UIRIs into Dummy Variables to Drive MRPA 161

7.5 Cox Regression Analysis (Cox): Survival Given the Initial Partitioning 164

7.6 By How Much Did Bayesian Revision Based on Cox Regression Further Improve the Consistency of Cure Probabilities with the Initial Partitioning by Reducing Misclassifications? 173

7.7 Further Reducing Misclassifications: MRPA's Second Iteration .. 176

7.8 Further Reducing Misclassifications: MRPA's Third Iteration ... 180

7.9 Eliminating All Misclassifications: MRPA's Final Iteration 184

7.10 Checking the Final Partitioning for Reasonableness 187

7.11 A Dramatically Revised Kaplan-Meier Survival Curve: The Apparent Disappearance of a Declining Hazard Rate over Time ... 191

7.12 Constructing an Individually Tailored Cure Curve and a Substitutable Survival Curve for a "Typical" Patient, for a High-Risk Patient, and for a Low-Risk Patient 200

    7.12.1 Constructing Tailored Curves for the "Typical" Patient 200

    7.12.2 Constructing Tailored Curves for High-Risk and Low-Risk Patients 204

8.0 CONCLUDING COMMENTS 209

Appendix A - Initial (SP) Early Success Probabilities and Succeeding Monthly Posterior Early Success RSP(t) Probabilities (POSTPR1, POSTPR2, ..., POSTPR6) for 469 Patients Who Underwent Kidney Transplants 215

Appendix B - Some Concepts Underlying Probabilistic Medical Models 224

Appendix C - Four Probabilistic Models 231

Appendix D - Logistic Regression Analysis 238

Appendix E - The Kaplan-Meier Survival Model 240

Appendix F - The Proportional Hazards Model and Cox Regression Analysis .. 243

Appendix G - Variable Characteristics of the First Illustrative 550-Patient Intervention Sample of Breast Cancer Patients from Turku, Finland 246

Appendix H - The RISKTEST Simulator 250

Appendix I - Variable Characteristics of the Second Illustrative 578-Patient Intervention Sample of Breast Cancer Patients from Guy's Hospital in London, England 255

ANNOTATED REFERENCES 259

AUTHOR BIOGRAPHIES 262

INDEX 263

This is the third in a series of books about making more accurate predictions of individual patient outcomes in particular medical situations.

Our first book introduced the concept of a Patient-Centered Methodology (PCM). It described several selective modifications to analytical procedures regularly applied to medical problems that facilitate greater prognostic utility. It demonstrated how these modifications separately and in combination improve predictive accuracy at the individual patient level. PCM'S accuracy-improving modifications are summarized in section 2.3 of this, our third book.

PCM was inspired by a comment published in 2006 by a leading biostatistician. The essence of the comment was that merely demonstrating the statistical significance of some influencing factor in accounting for medical outcomes in a population of patients does not, by itself, guarantee adequate prognostic accuracy for any of the patients in that population when they are viewed and treated as separate individuals.

Statistical significance as typically reported in medical journals is a collective property of a population of patients. It characterizes the relationship between some influencing factor and a set of salient patient outcomes. However, it is not an individual attribute of any particular patient.

Focusing attention on and reporting such population relationships is a most appropriate goal of ongoing clinical research. Among other things it serves to identify which influencing factors are likely to affect which particular patient outcomes in which situations. Yet something more seems required to translate knowledge of general relationships in a population to the selection of specific treatments for particular patients in given circumstances.

PCM was originally designed to address and to explain what might underlie the biostatistician's disappointing observation and then to alleviate it. Medical records of more than two thousand patients diagnosed with two separate forms of cancer were analyzed. PCM's selective modifications achieved greater predictive accuracy at the individual patient level in both analyses.

So what is different about PCM? It begins by redefining its overall methodological objective. Much clinical research is factor centered. It seeks to explain whether, through what mechanisms, and by how much certain influencing factors can bring about desirable patient outcomes and avoid undesirable ones. Testing the efficacy of a newly developed drug via a clinical trial is a quintessential illustration of the factor-centered orientation.

In contrast, PCM does not focus primarily on influencing factors. It focuses on individual patients and specific outcomes. Whereas the concept of statistical significance and the calculation of p values support probabilistic statements about separate factors in traditional clinical research, PCM makes probabilistic statements about separate patients. How likely will a particular patient experience a specified outcome in a certain situation? Answering that variety of question is PCM's central task.

Also different are PCM's appeals to statistical significance and the kind of p values it calculates. PCM draws probabilistic conclusions not about influencing factors, such as drug efficacy, but rather about increasing the accuracy of individual patient assessments, such as which ones did the drug actually cure.

Astronomy is about galaxies, stars, planets, asteroids, comets, and other celestial bodies. It seeks to explain and predict their relative motions and other interrelationships through gravity and radiation. It is an essentially factor-centered science. Newton's law of gravitation was originally conceived as universally applicable to all objects possessing physical mass, including celestial bodies. Einstein altered our fundamental concept of gravity, but all masses are still regarded as interacting gravitationally in a uniform manner. Our concept of the universe has also been expanded to include much more than just our Milky Way galaxy, but Maxwell's equations concerning electromagnetic radiation are still regarded as similarly operative in other galaxies.

Medicine is like astronomy in that a factor-centered orientation is most appropriate. Since medicine deals with biological entities, the widely shared aspects of biological factors and mechanisms are useful in explaining and predicting individual patient outcomes. A firm grasp of underlying anatomy and physiology is essential to effective patient management.

Yet medicine is different in other important respects. Central to the practice of medicine is a requirement to care for individual patients. It is not enough just to understand and to explain the general factors influencing patient well-being. For one thing, the impact of biology and other factors on patient health is far less uniform than the impact of gravity and radiation on separate astronomical objects. Patients are far less homogeneous in this respect. For another thing, obtaining a license to practice medicine normally involves a commitment to care separately and independently for individual patients. One can become an astronomer without pledging to care for any particular asteroid or comet.

The patient-centered orientation is not offered as a substitute for the factor-centered orientation. It is offered as an adjunct or extension. PCM explicitly requires that predictive factors be prequalified via convincing factor-centered research before being declared admissible as patient-centered predictors. In other words, PCM does not seek to replace traditional analytical methodology. It invites traditional analyses to expand in certain specific ways to accommodate medicine's additional and individually tailored requirements.

Our second book sought immediately actionable and practically useful applications of the PCM methodology. Medical diagnosis appeared to offer many fruitful opportunities.

It is not unusual for patients to be recommended to undergo specific diagnostic procedures on the basis of established guidelines. Guidelines are agreed upon and promulgated by prominent professional groups. The American Joint Committee on Cancer (AJCC) is such a group. The AJCC issues and regularly updates staging guidelines in both breast cancer and melanoma. These guidelines are widely followed throughout the United States.

Diagnostic guidelines are typically stated in simple and obvious terms. They are easy to understand and easy to follow. That is their virtue. In breast cancer, for example, when a woman should begin to undergo regular mammograms is generally stated in terms of her age. At various times the recommended starting date has been at fifty, at forty, and (most recently) at age forty-five. In both breast cancer and melanoma whether or not a patient is recommended to undergo a sentinel lymph node biopsy (SLNB) as part of the diagnostic workup is frequently based on the size and grade (breast cancer) or depth (melanoma) of the patient's primary tumor.

In our second book we reasoned that PCM could both reduce the cost and improve the triage efficiency of diagnostic procedures. The diagnostic test outcome (positive or negative) was chosen as the specific end point to be predicted.

Anything known about a patient at the time of diagnosis that has prognostic utility in predicting the test outcome can serve as a PCM prognostic factor. PCM then produces an individually tailored probability that each patient who is contemplating undergoing the diagnostic test would experience a positive test outcome. The patient's outcome probability predicted by PCM becomes the guideline for recommending whether or not the patient should undergo the procedure. A patient is recommended to undergo a diagnostic test when the likelihood of a positive test result is "high enough." By using this as a triage criterion we anticipated that PCM's greater predictive accuracy would contribute to both cost reduction and efficiency improvement.

The information conveyed in existing guidelines (e.g., whether a patient is old enough to begin having regular mammograms) is easy to incorporate into the set of PCM's predictive factors. When so incorporated, it seems obvious that substituting PCM's individually tailored test outcome probabilities for the component guideline information, taken just by itself, should constitute a more effective triage criterion. It does. Utilizing all available prognostically useful information instead of just part of it is generally a good idea, and it proved to be in this case.

The anticipated improvement was demonstrated in two separate diagnostic procedures for melanoma. More than thirteen hundred patient records were collected to investigate whether or not and according to which criteria undergoing a SLNB should be recommended. Close to three hundred patient records were similarly analyzed to investigate the criteria for undergoing positron emission tomography (PET) scans. The two analyses showed that cost reductions in excess of 40 percent were attainable by substituting PCM-generated probabilities for traditional guidelines. By forgoing the procedure in some patients who underwent it, but probably did not need to, and by giving it to other patients overlooked by traditional guidelines, but who probably would have benefited from it, the same number of positive test outcomes appeared realizable from administering, on balance, fewer tests. That is how the more than 40 percent cost reduction was achieved. Equivalently, this can be regarded as more than 66 percent improvement in triage efficiency.

These encouraging results suggested that many medical institutions offering diagnostic tests could benefit from an institutional audit. How to conduct such an audit was outlined in our second book. Substituting "high enough" PCM-generated positive mammogram probabilities for patient age as the official guideline for undergoing one's initial mammogram would seem to offer an especially profitable opportunity for improvement. Hundreds of thousands of mammograms are conducted every year. Uniformly adopting the "one shoe fits all" approach of recommending mammograms (almost) solely on the basis of patient age may not be the best triage procedure. An institutional audit that reviewed available historical data and actual mammogram results would indicate whether or not and how much room for improvement existed at any given medical center.

Our second book also demonstrated how PCM can improve the sensitivity, the specificity, and the correct discrimination rate in the differential diagnosis of malignant melanomas versus benign nevi (ordinary moles). Once again PCM performed quite well in the diagnosis of nearly seven hundred lesions. All three success measures were elevated to more than 95 percent. Furthermore, the diagnostic algorithm originally generated by a different technique and improved by PCM was validated in two independent data sets. This ruled out attributing the unusually good diagnostic performance to statistical overfitting.

PCM is applied in this third book to another type of medical situation. Some medical interventions have the capacity to bring about a favorable change in the patient's fundamental state of health. The intervention may not always be successful. It may benefit some, but not all patients.

The success or failure of an organ transplant is one such example. Whether or not a potentially curative intervention succeeds in permanently curing a cancer patient is another example.

These two examples differ in one important respect. Whether or not a fundamental change in patient state has actually occurred is not always clear. There may be some ambiguity, especially in drawing an appropriate long-term conclusion.

The short-term success of an organ transplant is generally unambiguous. Whether or not a patient survives the initial accommodation period with a properly functioning transplanted organ can usually be determined within a year or so. Even given short-term survival, however, the long-term survival of the transplanted organ remains difficult to predict with certainty. Yet despite this long-term uncertainty, initial accommodation is usually unambiguous.

Whether or not a surgical intervention or some type of drug therapy succeeds in bringing about a permanent cure of cancer is an entirely different matter. Its determination can sometimes be quite ambiguous.

That the intervention has failed may become obvious. When a patient subsequently experiences further disease progression, it is safe to conclude that no permanent cure was achieved. Even if potentially curative, the intervention appears to have failed with respect to that particular patient.

The opposite conclusion is more difficult to draw with confidence. Even after a lengthy time period has elapsed with no evidence of further disease progression, there still remains some ambiguity. The cancer may be in temporary remission, or it may not be. It may just be one of those cancers or one of those patients where relapse or recurrence takes a long time to materialize. Alternatively, a lengthy disease-free experience may actually signify permanent cure. The point is that one can never be completely certain.

Whether ambiguously or unambiguously discernible, conceiving of the impact of a medical intervention as potentially inducing a fundamental change in the patient's state of health enables an expanded form of statistical analysis. Conventional procedures, such as logistic regression and Cox (proportional hazards) regression analysis, can then be reformulated in a Bayesian framework. Logistic regression can be adapted to produce a (Bayesian prior) probability that some target intervention does or does not actually succeed in transforming a patient at risk of further disease progression into the cured state, where little or no such risk remains. Cox regression can be applied selectively (conditionally) only to those patients who remain at risk (not cured), despite the intervention.

These modifications permit the conclusions generated by both forms of regression analysis to become logically integrated and mutually reinforcing. Their combined result is a (Bayesian posterior) probability that the intervention was successful in curing the patient, depending on how much time elapsed following the intervention with no evidence of further disease progression. Individually tailored cure assessment probabilities (time-phased cure curves) can then be produced separately for each patient.

Situations with only ambiguously discernible outcome states require additional analytical procedures. The additional procedures stipulate, provisionally, in which state each patient exists. Only then can Cox regression, Kaplan-Meier analysis, and other survival-related statistical techniques be properly conditioned to fit comfortably within the expanded Bayesian framework.

The important question to ask in cure assessment is whether any patients were actually cured by some medical intervention. A special modification of Kaplan-Meier survival analysis specifically designed to detect evidence of cure has been devised to answer this question.

Only after clear evidence of cure has been detected by the modified Kaplan-Meier analysis is Monte Carlo simulation invoked to estimate the proportion of a cohort of patients receiving the intervention who were thereby cured. Simulation provides an initial estimate of this cure rate. It also provides an initial partitioning of patients into two states. The initial partitioning is a first guess. It is a guess concerning which patients were cured and which patients were not cured (i.e., remained at risk of further disease progression) despite the intervention.

Fine-tuning of the initial Monte Carlo partitioning is then carried out by the minimal risk partitioning algorithm (MRPA). It is an iterative procedure designed to refine the initial guess by reclassifying selected patients between the cured and still-at-risk states in a manner most consistent with all the data collected over a long period of time from all the patients.

Predictive accuracy of the individually tailored Bayesian posterior state probabilities recalculated during successive iterations is the consistency criterion driving MRPA. The algorithm is said to have converged to a successful solution when additional patient reclassifications between the two states can no longer improve consistency with the collected data.

The three books in our series are based on faith in a single proposition. There exists today throughout the world a wealth of medical information that has been only partially exploited. Already collected patient records constitute a still largely untapped resource, even though recent advances in data mining applied to collections of "big data" have for some time been bearing fruit.

During the late 1990s, one of the authors was a member of a civilian advisory group convened to help the US government formulate and execute measures to deal with cancer. The most appropriate allocation of limited resources was a frequent focus of the group's ongoing discussions. Designing and conducting clinical trials was then and still remains a well-developed and effective way to do so. It continues to deserve substantial resources.

What is new since the 1990s is the growing success of data mining techniques and improvements in storing, accessing, and analyzing "big data." It may now be appropriate to restructure our priorities. Additional resources devoted to dealing more effectively with existing patient records may now earn handsome dividends. Truly evidence-based and precision-directed medicine may no longer be just two pleasant thoughts, like motherhood and apple pie. The practice of medicine may actually begin to achieve both. The methodologies described in all three of our books were specifically designed to be helpful in this regard.

ACKNOWLEDGMENTS

All analyses reported in section 2 were derived from the raw data describing 469 patients receiving kidney transplants. The raw data appeared as appendix A of Chap T. Le's 1997 book describing applied survival analysis (entry 8, "ANNOTATED REFERENCES"). We are grateful for the opportunity to illustrate with these data the initial formulation of our Bayesian framework.

The cure assessment model outlined in section 3 was originally conceived in 2000. Initial formulation was carried out in close collaboration with Dr. Laura J. Esserman, then Associate Professor of Surgery and Director of the Breast Care Center, University of California at San Francisco (UCSF). Actual development of the model was carried out in 2001 through 2003.

At the suggestion of Dr. Debu Tripathy, Dr. Esserman sought to obtain the data set describing more than two thousand breast cancer patients from Turku, Finland. Dr. Tripathy's hope was that the Turku data would provide a vehicle to study the natural course of breast cancer development. Only about fifty patients in the Turku data set remained untreated, so these data were never used for their original purpose.

Dr. Harry B. Burke, then Associate Professor of Medicine, George Washington University School of Medicine, Washington, DC, was a consultant to the UCSF Breast Care Center. It was he who actually procured the Turku data through his association with two doctors in Finland. The two doctors were Dr. Johan Lundin and Dr. Michael Lundin, then both at the HUCH Clinical Research Institute, Helsinki, Finland.

The Turku data analyzed in sections 4 and 5 were obtained with the understanding that no patients would be identified, that data would be used only for research purposes, and that those providing the data would be properly recognized.

The Turku data were carefully collected, regularly checked, and painstakingly updated over a fifty-one-year period between 1945 and 1996. It is only because of the cleanliness of the data and the duration and thoroughness of patient follow-up that the analyses reported in sections 4 and 5 were successful.

Drs. Heikki Joensuu and Sakari Toikkanen deserve the credit for producing the Turku data. Their 1995 analysis of the same data (entry 4, "ANNOTATED REFERENCES") suggested that a number of the Turku patients had been cured.

Dr. David Miles provided the Guy's Hospital data set analyzed in sections 6 and 7. It included records of more than thirty-three hundred breast cancer patients collected between 1975 and 2003 in London, England. The Guy's Hospital data were obtained in 2003.

Again, no Guy's Hospital patients were individually identifiable, the data were extremely clean, and patient follow-up was quite thorough. Thanks are due both to David Miles and to Ken Ryder for providing us with a second vehicle to illustrate successfully our cure assessment procedure.

Finally, special thanks are due to Mehdi Nosrati, currently at the California Pacific Medical Center Research Institute, for producing the twenty-two figures presented in this book.

1.0   INTRODUCTION

Suppose that a patient has just been diagnosed with a progressive disease. Heart disease and cancer are two serious and sometimes fatal examples. The patient is then at risk of continuing disease progression, possibly resulting in death. The patient remains at risk until some intervention (medical or otherwise) succeeds in changing the patient's state back to no longer being at risk or until the same change occurs spontaneously.

When a patient is at risk of disease progression, the following three kinds of questions become salient.

1. In the absence of any intervention, what is the likely prognosis? That is, how is the disease likely to progress in this particular patient?

    A. Which events signifying disease progression is the patient likely to experience, in what sequence, and when?
    B. How debilitating could these experiences become, and how could they affect the patient's quality of life?
    C. If the disease is potentially fatal, how likely is the patient to die as a direct consequence of the disease, how, and when?

2. How might some particular intervention alter the patient's prognosis? How, if at all, will the intervention likely alter the way the disease progresses in that patient?

    A. What changes will the intervention likely bring about in the sequence and timing of events signifying disease progression?
    B. After taking into account its unavoidable side effects, what would be the intervention's net impact on the patient's quality of life?
    C. What chance is there that the intervention will avoid or at least postpone death due to the disease and with what quality of remaining life?

3. Is there any chance that some particular intervention can actually change the patient's state back to no longer being at risk? That is, does the intervention have the capacity to cure patients?

    A. If so, what is the likelihood that a particular intervention will turn out to be curative for a particular patient? Specifically, what fraction of patients who were in a condition similar to that of the patient in question and who then experienced that intervention were transformed to a state of very low or no risk of further disease progression?
    B. In the case of a disease such as cancer, whose underlying mechanisms are not yet fully understood, for how long must one wait with no evidence of further disease progression before concluding that such an intervention was successful; that the disease has actually been overcome; and, therefore, that the patient "won the battle" (i.e., became effectively cured)?

Medical records are generally collected on people who are sick. There are numerous exceptions. Medical records also include the results of routine medical examinations that uncover no medical problems and that require no special follow-up. They also include studies drawn from populations of healthy people to compare with patients who suffer from some particular illness. Despite these and other exceptions, however, a substantial portion of today's medical records concern patients who are known to be sick or who are suspected of being at risk of something.

Such medical records are quite useful in answering the first two kinds of prognostic questions posed on the previous page. Both of these assume an underlying state of risk. Both are about patients who are at risk and who remain at risk, even following a variety of interventions.

Only the third kind of question embraces the concept of an explicit change in underlying state. It asks whether or not some intervention can have a curative impact. Can it transform a patient from a state of being at substantial risk of further disease progression to a state of very low or no such risk?

We shall refer to untransformed patients who remain at substantial risk as SR patients. We shall refer to patients who are successfully transformed to a state of minimal risk as MR patients. MR patients are at very low or no risk of further disease progression. They are effectively cured.

Answering this third kind of question becomes challenging when most of the available data have been collected on patients who are and who remain sick. Once a patient is deemed cured, the data collection process frequently subsides. Medical data useful in identifying transformations to the cured state are thereby rendered less abundant.

Fortuitously, the manner of posing this third kind of question suggests a way to extend and to recharacterize some of the probabilistic models and prognostic tools traditionally used in medicine. To the extent that observations are drawn from patients who are sick and who remain at risk of something, probabilistic inferences derived therefrom may then be regarded as conditional rather than as unconditional conclusions. Conditional means as long as the patient remains in a sick state; only then does the patient remain at risk of further disease progression. This, in turn, permits making selective modifications to the traditional statistical models and prognostic tools themselves to accommodate such an extended recharacterization.

For example, to say that some particular intervention has the potential to cure patients suffering from a progressive disease is to say that it can transform at least some of them from a state of being at substantial risk (SR) of further disease progression to a state of minimal risk (MR, very low or no such risk).

The intervention need not be 100 percent successful. As long as it can transform an appreciable proportion of SR patients to MR patients, it has curative potential. The successful transformation of patients constitutes its curative impact.

Patients who have experienced a potentially curative intervention should then be partitioned into two distinct groups for diagnostic and prognostic purposes.

Untransformed patients remain in the SR state. They are still at substantial risk of further disease progression. Applying traditional Kaplan-Meier analysis and Cox (proportional hazards) regression analysis to them is therefore appropriate, but only with the stipulation that all probabilistic inferences drawn therefrom are conditional upon their having remained in the SR state.

In contrast, patients effectively cured by the intervention are transformed into the MR state. Traditional Kaplan-Meier and Cox regression analyses are no longer appropriate for them. They are no longer at risk of further disease progression. They are effectively cured.

Recharacterization in this manner has important implications. Mechanically applying traditional statistical models and prognostic tools to an undifferentiated population of patients who have experienced a potentially curative medical intervention may be inappropriate. Since SR patients remain at substantial risk of further disease progression, while MR patients do not, indiscriminately combining both groups in a single analysis may generate quite misleading conclusions.

What does it mean to generate a misleading conclusion? Can this have serious practical consequences? A purely hypothetical example will illustrate answers to both questions.

1. Imagine that a survival analysis is to be performed on patients diagnosed with ovarian cancer.
2. Since ovarian cancer is potentially fatal, suppose that disease-specific death is selected as the end point of the analysis.
3. Now imagine that a clerical accident occurs. Many records gathered on male patients diagnosed with a variety of cancers are inadvertently mixed in with the female records of ovarian cancer.
4. Because males cannot possibly die of ovarian cancer the survival curve estimated from this contaminated sample cannot possibly fall to zero as the duration of follow-up increases.
5. Extending the duration of follow-up observations will not help. The larger the proportion of males in the contaminated sample, the more positive (further from zero) will be the apparent horizontal limit on the graph that the survival curve appears to be approaching as follow-up times increase.
6. Perhaps more insidious, statistical techniques regularly used to fit survival curves to patient data, such as Kaplan-Meier analysis and Cox regression, will indicate a declining hazard rate over time to a greater extent than would be appropriate without the inadvertent contamination, and just because of that contamination.
7. The exaggerated rate of decline in hazard rate has no biological or medical interpretation. It is a statistical artifact. It is the result of a clerical accident. However, it will increase with the proportion of males in the contaminated sample and the consequent upward shift in the level of the horizontal limit to which the survival curve appears to approach. The higher the horizontal limit, the more the curve-fitting statistical algorithms must force a survival curve to "twist around" to accommodate it. Survival curves are expected to fall asymptotically to zero over time, but they cannot in this situation.

An obvious lesson can be drawn from this example. A survival curve fitted statistically by standard techniques that appears to approach a decidedly positive horizontal limit may indicate at least one inappropriate framing assumption. The inappropriate assumption in the hypothetical example was that all data to which the survival curve was fitted were obtained from female ovarian cancer patients.

By analogy, incorrectly assuming that a particular cancer is incurable could blind one to the possibility that MR patients exist. If they exist, they could be inadvertently mixed with SR patients in a sample from which a survival curve is estimated. The consequence would be just like contaminating a sample of ovarian cancer patients with males who do not possess ovaries. MR patients might be recommended to undergo unnecessary procedures. SR patients and their physicians might relax too soon in terms of both diligent diagnosis and appropriate therapy under the happy illusion of a spuriously declining hazard rate over time.

Conceiving of cure as a change in underlying patient state enables a certain degree of conceptual fluidity that might not otherwise exist. Such does not guarantee avoiding the problems just illustrated. One could embrace the concept of different underlying states, but still deny the possibility of moving back from the SR to the MR state. It does, however, encourage one to consider a wider range of possibilities. It also opens the door to an extended form of statistical analysis that is about to be introduced.

This book is about both the curative potential and the successful curative impact of medical interventions. More precisely, it introduces and outlines an assessment procedure through which the curative impact of some particular medical intervention against a progressive and potentially fatal disease may be ascertained. The intervention's curative efficacy is what is being assessed.

Conclusions from the assessment procedure are probabilistic in nature. They are generated on an individually tailored, patient-by-patient basis. The intervention's separate curative efficacy for each individual patient is what is being assessed.

This book is the third in our series describing patient-centered methodologies (PCM). Various devices have been incorporated within PCM to improve the predictive accuracy of individually tailored probabilistic conclusions. Cure assessment, along with prognosis and diagnosis, serves as a third context in which the medical benefits of improved predictive accuracy can be exploited.

Focusing on medical interventions is not intended to suggest that nonmedical interventions lack impact. Deciding not to become a lifetime cigarette smoker can reduce substantially the likelihood of developing lung cancer. Neither is our focus intended to suggest that spontaneous cures are either infrequent or insubstantial. The human body is quite capable of healing itself in many ways and in many different contexts without the aid of medical intervention. It is because the efficacy of medical interventions is of such compelling interest to so many people and because so much medical data are available to support evidence-based conclusions concerning their efficacy that we have chosen this focus.

Our central thesis is that expanding prognostic models traditionally used in medicine and their accompanying analytical procedures to encompass the explicit possibility of achieving a cure is more than just conceptually broadening. When appropriate, such analytical enhancements can also generate dramatically different conclusions that are useful in the actual treatment of patients.

1.1   Interpreting the Concept of Cure Probabilistically: A Bayesian Framework

Interpreting cure as a fundamental change in underlying patient state opens the door to utilizing a branch of statistical analysis not all that frequently applied to medical problems. It enables recasting medical data in a Bayesian framework. If a patient can be in either the SR or the MR state following a medical intervention, probabilistic statements describing patient experiences can then be described as and analyzed in terms of conditional probabilities. The conditioning factor is which state a patient falls into following the intervention. This, in turn, permits interpreting the concept of cure in terms of a Bayesian posterior state probability, conditional upon the direct observation of further disease progression or lack thereof.

Specifically, it permits answering the all-too-familiar question, "Hey, Doc, I just underwent a treatment designed to cure my cancer. Was it successful? Did I beat the cancer?" The answer can be framed as a Bayesian posterior probability, conditional on observation of the patient's experience following the treatment.

Approaching the concept of cure in this manner faces an immediate difficulty. Accurate assessment of a patient's true underlying state following treatment is not always easy to accomplish. Worse still, the difficulty is quite asymmetric. When the first sign of further disease progression is detected the patient has obviously not been cured. However, continued observations with no evidence of disease progression support increasing hope that the intervention was curative, but mere lack of evidence is rarely dispositive.

It will be instructive to introduce the Bayesian framework in a simpler context, where the patient's true underlying state following a medical intervention is easily ascertained. Insights gained from this analysis can then be expanded to the more complicated task of assessing cure. The success of organ transplants, including whether or not they are initially rejected, will constitute our introductory context to be discussed in section 2 of this book.

1.2 Consequences of the Altered and Selective Focus of PCM

The ultimate goal of PCM is to make separately tailored predictions about individual patients concerning some focal end point. Assessing the (relative) predictive potency of various prognostic factors in some patient population also occurs, but only as a penultimate activity.

This changes the fundamental nature of the questions we ask, the hypotheses we formulate and test, and the way we measure success. Such changes are immediate consequences of PCM's altered and selective focus. Can PCM improve prognostic accuracy? That is the overarching question. If so, by how much and compared to what?

Each patient's probability of experiencing some focal end point will be estimated by a modified form of logistic regression analysis. The time required to reach the end point will be estimated by a modified form of Cox regression. Our principal measures of predictive accuracy will be the percentage rate of correct outcome predictions and timing accuracy enabled by PCM. The relevant hypotheses to formulate and test will be whether or not and the extent to which PCM is successful both in making such predictions accurately and in achieving accuracy improvements compared to similar predictions made by alternative methodologies.

How might one measure the accuracy of a set of probabilistic predictions? We shall do this in three ways.

1. Rank-order the individual probabilistic predictions of experiencing a focal end point generated by logistic regression from largest to smallest. Then test each cut point between adjacent probabilities in the rank order as a possible dichotomous discriminator. Tentatively predict that all patients whose probabilities exceed a given cut point do experience the end point, while all patients with lower probabilities do not. Count the number of correct predictions for that cut point. Repeat the process for each possible cut point. Choose the cut point that offers the highest correct count. Designate this the (not necessarily unique) optimal cut point, and designate its corresponding count the maximum possible number of correct predictions. Divide the maximum count by the number of probabilities in the rank order to compute the percentage rate of correct predictions.

If a receiver operating characteristic (ROC) analysis were performed on the same set of ranked probabilities, an estimated area under the curve (AUC) of 1.00 would correspond to a 100 percent correct prediction rate, and vice versa. ROC/AUC analysis is frequently performed and widely reported in the medical research literature. Our percentage rate of correct predictions is conceptually close to and very highly correlated with an AUC score calculated from the same data set. We shall sometimes present both statistics side by side. However, we prefer the percentage rate of correct predictions because it seems to reflect the overarching goal of achieving predictive accuracy in an intuitively more obvious and straightforward manner.

2. The US Weather Bureau faces a similar task in assessing its probabilistic predictions for accuracy and reliability. It makes daily forecasts covering all kinds of weather. Imagine that the chance of rain for a given day at some location is announced to be a number between 20 and 30 percent. As more and more forecasts are made, the mean of all daily probabilistic predictions announcing the chance of rain to fall between 20 and 30 percent should gradually converge toward the actual incidence of rain at that same location during those same days. Also, the actual incidence should fall within the 20-to-30 percent interval. In like manner, mean probabilistic predictions in all other intervals throughout the entire range of forecasts should gradually converge toward their corresponding actual incidences, and the incidences eventually realized should always fall within their respective intervals.

We shall divide the set of rank-ordered probabilistic predictions of achieving a specified end point into quartiles. The mean of the probabilities in each quartile will be compared with the actual prevalence of correct predictions among the patients in that quartile. These two numbers should be about the same in each quartile. The maximum and mean absolute differences between corresponding mean probabilities and actual prevalence will serve as measures of predictive inaccuracy for PCM. The pattern of prediction errors observed in different quartiles will also be used to assess predictive reliability at different locations along the probability scale.

When there are only a few distinctly different probability values in a data set, partitioning the scale into a small number of subscales (such as quartiles) may be an appropriate procedure. However, when there are many more distinctly different probabilistic predictions, we can investigate their scale characteristics much more thoroughly. The scale partitioning and spacing algorithm (SPSA is part of PCM) will be executed to partition the individual patient probabilistic prediction scale into as many subscales as possible, as long as each subscale encompasses predicted probabilities for at least enough patients to permit reasonably accurate prevalence estimates. Our analysis will succeed in generating mean prediction probabilities that converge toward each corresponding actual prevalence in all subscales. When actual prevalence is regressed against mean prediction probability (simple linear regression), an R-squared value (coefficient of determination) in excess of 95 percent will frequently be achieved, thanks to the improved accuracy of PCM.

3. Whether or not one methodology produces more accurate predictions than another will be tested, statistically, by matched-sample comparisons. Each sample will contain the set of individually tailored probabilistic predictions of experiencing focal end points assigned by a particular

methodology to each patient. Matching occurs patient by patient. Alternative methodologies assign separate probabilities to each patient. A Wilcoxon matched-pairs, signed-ranks test will be adopted to compare two methodologies.

In all such statistical tests, the uniform null hypothesis will be that no difference in predictive accuracy exists between or among alternative methodologies.

Formal hypothesis tests will generally be nondirectional (i.e., two-tailed tests). It is the existence versus nonexistence of any systematic difference in accuracy that is being tested.

The direction and magnitude of differences in predictive accuracy will be measured by the absolute value of probabilistic prediction errors. A prediction error is the difference between whatever probability some methodology assigns to the experience of a focal end point by a patient and its 0/1 actual occurrence. Zero signifies nonoccurrence. One signifies occurrence. The more accurate methodology is the one that generates systematically smaller absolute error differences.

Using probabilistic errors to quantify predictive accuracy can introduce outliers (i.e., extreme values) into the analysis. When a patient actually experiences a rare focal event, the difference between that patient's (typically close to zero) assigned probability and the 1.0 signifying actual occurrence can be much larger than the error differences assigned to the many other patients who do not experience it. Outliers can also arise, although in the reverse manner, with very frequently occurring focal events.

The occurrence of outliers complicates the determination of systematically smaller or larger error differences when means are calculated and compared. It can also undermine the presumption of normally distributed test statistics underlying many parametric procedures (e.g., the analysis of variance and t tests).

Via the magic of the central limit theorem, difficulty with outliers is reduced as sample sizes increase. It will sometimes be necessary, however, to assess the direction and magnitude of differences in predictive accuracy by comparing samples of small-to-intermediate size.

The Wilcoxon matched-pairs, signed-ranks test is less sensitive to outliers than the parametric matched-pairs t test. It is based on mean differences in the ranks of matched-pair differences rather than on mean differences between each pair of probabilities, which might include outliers. Another possible test, the binomial sign test, is not at all sensitive to outliers when performing a matched-pair comparison.

The Wilcoxon matched-pairs, signed-ranks test has a very high relative efficiency (in the neighborhood of 95 percent) in its ability to reject the null hypothesis. Hence, very little needs to be sacrificed to protect effectively against troublesome outliers.

Nonparametric tests will be regularly performed throughout the remainder of this book. Occasionally their slightly more powerful equivalent parametric tests will also be performed and reported, especially when sample sizes are quite adequate.

That the binomial sign test is insensitive to outliers suggests a uniform way to calibrate both the direction and the magnitude of predictive accuracy when comparing different methodologies. Relative predictive accuracy can be encapsulated in an index of error reduction. The index is designed to resemble an ordinary correlation coefficient. It is the signed proportion of net error reductions in any set of matched-pair comparisons calculated as follows.

1. First, select one of two methodologies as more likely to make accurate predictions (e.g., by comparing percentage rates of correct predictions).
2. Then count the number of matched pairs wherein the selected methodology generates the smaller absolute probabilistic prediction error. These are labeled error reductions.
3. Subtract from this the number of matched pairs wherein the selected methodology generates the larger absolute error. These are labeled error increases.
4. Ignore matched pairs with equal absolute errors.
5. Finally, divide the difference between these two counts by their sum (i.e., the number of matched pairs containing nonidentical absolute errors).

The index ranges in value from -1.0, when all comparisons produce (unanticipated) error increases, to +1.0, when all comparisons produce (anticipated) error reductions. Analogous to a correlation coefficient, it has a value of 0.0 when the number of error reductions is exactly offset by an equal number of error increases.

The index of error reduction can be calculated for any set of matched prediction errors. Its sign and magnitude indicate which of any two methodologies generates the more accurate probabilistic predictions. It is normalized to fall between -1.0 and +1.0. The relative predictive accuracy of several different methodologies may be determined at a glance. Alternative methodologies may be ranked according to their relative predictive accuracy.

The distribution of the Wilcoxon test statistic rapidly approaches normality as the number of nontied matched-pair comparisons increases. Whenever the count exceeds twenty-five, this approximation becomes quite satisfactory. Hence, an equivalent standardized Z statistic will generally be computed and referred to the unit normal distribution for statistical significance testing. The Z statistic is the Wilcoxon test statistic divided by its standard deviation. Only for small counts (twenty-five or fewer nontied matched pairs) will an exact probability be computed for Wilcoxon p values.

PCM has been specifically designed to anticipate nontrivial amounts of missing patient data. No patient record is required to possess complete data on all prognostic factors. The SPSA algorithm associates specific probabilistic outcome estimates with every missing observation. This can introduce a substantial number of tied outcome probabilities into the analysis, which, in turn, can also skew or otherwise undermine the presumption of normally distributed test statistics.

The Wilcoxon test eliminates within-pair tied observations. The Kruskal-Wallis test, the Mann-Whitney test, and both the Spearman and Kendall rank correlation tests contain explicit procedures that correct for tied observations. Their parametric equivalents lack such procedures and, typically, assume normal distributions.

These considerations constitute a second reason to systematically substitute nonparametric for parametric statistical tests in assessing PCM.

2.0   THE RESULTS OF 469 KIDNEY TRANSPLANTS

Some years ago 469 patients underwent kidney transplants. The survival of their transplanted kidneys was assessed by Kaplan-Meier analysis. The results were not surprising. In fact, they were typical of that historical time period.

1. Eventual failure occurred in 192 kidneys.
2. The earliest failure occurred in the first month following transplant.
3. The last recorded failure occurred 180 months after transplant.
4. The longest-surviving transplanted kidney was observed to be still functioning properly after two hundred months.
5. Almost half (91 of 192 or 47.4 percent) of the kidneys that eventually failed did so within the first six months, due mostly to rejection of the transplanted tissue.
6. The Kaplan-Meier kidney survival curve displayed a noticeably decreasing (as opposed to increasing or stable) hazard rate over time.
7. That the hazard rate was decreasing was highly significant.
8. If modeled as a Weibull distribution with a declining hazard rate, the survival curve fit the 469-patient sample data quite closely. Its unadjusted coefficient of determination (R-squared) was 0.9490.
9. The Kaplan-Meier cumulative survival plot for these 469 transplanted kidneys is shown as figure 1 on the next page.

Organ transplant technology has improved dramatically since these data were collected. Survival times have improved commensurately. Figure 1 does not reflect these recent improvements, quantitatively, but it likely does reflect contemporary kidney survival in a qualitative (e.g., shape-related) manner.

The success and failure of the 469 kidney transplants will now be investigated in some detail. The purpose is to introduce statistical analysis of medical outcomes in the less familiar Bayesian framework. Cure assessment, to be presented in later sections of this book, will be imbedded in the same Bayesian framework.

Both transplant outcome analysis and cure assessment require lengthy follow-up. From our methodological perspective, therefore, data collected in earlier time periods are not only appropriate they are essential.

To understand better how and why differing transplant outcomes came about, data were also collected for each of the 469 patients on eight prognostic factors:

1. age of patient at the time of transplant;
2. sex of patient;
3. duration in days of hemodialysis prior to transplant;
4. presence or absence of diabetes;
5. number of prior kidney transplants;
6. amount in blood units of blood transfusion;
7. a mismatch score indicating the degree of antibody mismatch (such as differing blood type) with the transplanted kidney; and
8. use or nonuse of an immune suppression drug referred to as ALG.

These eight prognostic factors were submitted as independent variables to a conventional Cox (proportional hazards) regression analysis. The dependent variable was the time in months after transplant until either failure of the kidney graft or some other observation-censoring event occurred.

Age, diabetes, and the use of ALG emerged as the significant and independent predictors of kidney graft survival time.

Figure 1

Kaplan-Meier Survival Analysis of 469 Transplanted Kidneys

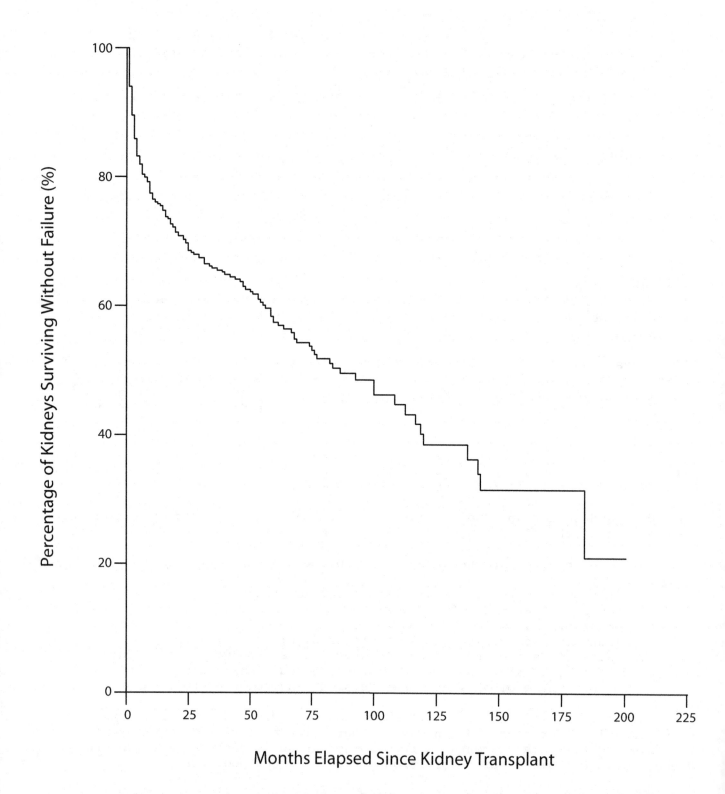

The high incidence of failure during the first six months raised an obvious question. Did these data reflect a single biological phenomenon applying to all patients and operating uniformly over more than fifteen years? Alternatively, was something more complicated going on that differed either between patients or across time periods? This is yet another "does one shoe fit all?" question.

The Kaplan-Meier analysis and the survival curve displayed in figure 1 made the single-phenomenon-operating-uniformly-over-time assumption for all 469 patients. The Cox regression previously reported made the same assumption. Something similar is regularly assumed in the outcome analyses of many organ transplants. A convincingly close fit to the observed data was achieved by further assuming that the single, uniformly operating phenomenon was appropriately characterized by a hazard rate that declined consistently over time.

Alternatively, is there some benefit in viewing the same data as evidence of two separate, though closely related, phenomena operating in two separate, sequential time periods? Would it be useful to interpret figure 1 as depicting the juxtaposition of an early accommodation period lasting less than a year after transplant followed by a subsequent period lasting more than a decade?

Selectively partitioning the 469-patient sample and reanalyzing the same data, separately, is one way to answer this question. If both of the two separate analyses provide a closer fit to the data compared to the single, unpartitioned analysis, then patient partitioning and time separation do enable a distinct improvement. Otherwise, parsimony suggests retaining the simpler assumption.

To check the possibility of distinguishable phenomena operating in sequential time periods successive cut points between five and ten months were tested. Both R-squared fit statistics generated by the two separate analyses had to exceed the R-squared value of 0.9490 achieved by the unseparated analysis in order for a cut point to qualify as enabling an improved interpretation.

Six months turned out to provide the most credible separation. Most credible was interpreted as achieving the highest mean value of the two separate R-squared fit statistics derived from qualifying (i.e., interpretation improving) cut points.

Detailed results of the most credible separation analysis were as follows.

1. A period lasting six months after the transplant was designated the early accommodation period for each patient.
2. All observations made seven or more months after the transplant were designated as falling in the subsequent time period.
3. Patients who managed to survive with a functioning transplanted kidney for more than six months were designated early accommodation successes.
4. Patients who failed to enter the seventh month with a still-functioning kidney were designated early accommodation failures.
5. Separate Kaplan-Meier analyses focusing on transplant survival were then performed on data from the partitioned sample in each of the two successive time periods. The two Kaplan-Meier cumulative survival plots are shown as figures 2 and 3.
6. Surprisingly, exponential distributions (representing a constant hazard rate over time) provided the closest fit to data from both of the patient-partitioned and time-separated subsamples.
7. As anticipated, the hazard rate optimally fitted to kidney failures occurring during the six-month accommodation period (figure 2) far exceeded the hazard rate optimally fitted to failures occurring during the subsequent period (figure 3).

8. Each exponential distribution fit the separated data more closely than when all data were combined into a single time period. Both R-squared fit statistics were higher than 95 percent.
9. Perhaps most dramatic was that evidence of a decreasing hazard rate vanished completely from the survival curves derived from both patient-partitioned and time-separated subsamples. When separated, both underlying hazard rates appeared to be constant over time, although the two rates were decidedly different in magnitude.

There was no difficulty ascertaining which of the 469 patients continued to enjoy properly functioning kidneys for more than six months. The number was 347 (just under 74 percent). These were the early accommodation successes shown in figure 3. The remaining 122 patients (just over 26 percent) suffered early failure and are shown in figure 2.

Comparing figure 1 with figures 2 and 3, the first six monthly data points in figure 1 (obtained from the 122 early failure patients) reappeared in recalculated form as the six data points in figure 2. All remaining monthly data points in figure 1 (obtained from the 347 early success patients) reappeared in recalculated form as the many more data points in figure 3.

No claim is made that all organ transplant data will demonstrate so obvious a separation into a short early accommodation period, followed by a longer subsequent period, as depicted in figures 1, 2, and 3. This particular data set was selected just because it does show an obvious separation. In the absence of such a separation no Bayesian analysis would be appropriate. Recall that the primary purpose of our detailed transplant outcome analysis was to introduce and motivate the Bayesian framework for later use in modeling cure assessment.

Notice also that early success and early failure describe two different kinds of patient experience. They are in large part determined by and, therefore, closely related to survival of the patient's transplanted kidney. They are, however, not quite the same thing. Overall patient status and specific kidney status are distinguishable concepts.

Distinguishing the two concepts made it possible to recharacterize patient survival data as conditional on patient status. Separate conditional survival functions could then be constructed for patients enjoying early accommodation success and patients suffering early accommodation failure.

The fact that all data could be recharacterized as conditional on patient status is what made this an excellent vehicle for introducing the Bayesian framework. That patient status could be distinguished from kidney status made it even more interesting from a patient-centered perspective. Conclusions drawn from a Bayesian analysis of the early accommodation period would then be about the 469 patients, not just about their kidneys.

More familiar conclusions about the long-term survival of transplanted kidneys could then be drawn from traditional Kaplan-Meier and Cox regression analyses, but they would be based on the experience of only the 347 patients who survived the early accommodation period with functioning kidneys. They would also be based exclusively on long-term data drawn from the subsequent period, following the accommodation period. It is to support these long-term conclusions that lengthy follow-up and, therefore, older data are required.

Figure 2

Kaplan-Meier Survival Analysis of 122 Early Accommodation Failure Kidney Transplant Patients

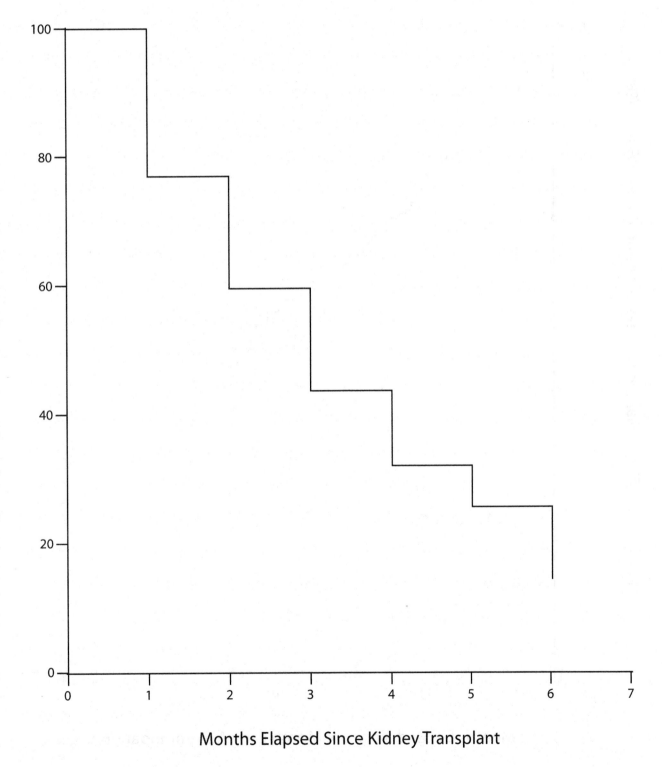

Figure 3

Kaplan-Meier Survival Analysis of 347 Early Accommodation Success Kidney Transplant Patients

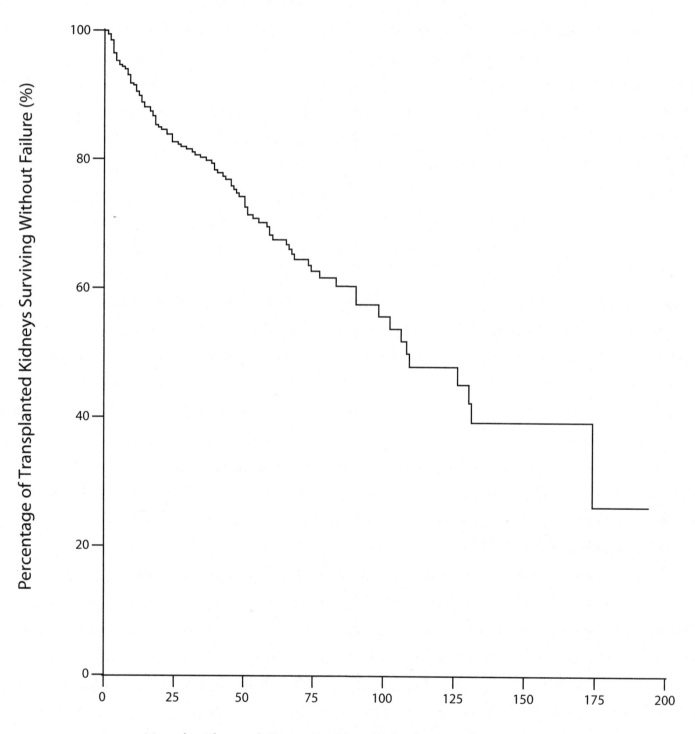

Percentage of Transplanted Kidneys Surviving Without Failure (%)

Months Elapsed Since Six-Month Early Accommodation Success

2.1 A Bayesian Kidney Transplant Model

OUTCOME OBSERVED DURING SIX MONTHS AFTER TRANSPLANT	TRUE PATIENT STATUS AFTER KIDNEY TRANSPLANT		PROBABILITY OF OBSERVED OUTCOME
	EARLY SUCCESS: WILL EXPERIENCE MORE THAN SIX MONTHS OF SUCCESS	EARLY FAILURE: SOME SERIOUS PROBLEM(S) IN FIRST SIX MONTHS	
A SERIOUS PROBLEM OCCURS WITHIN t MONTHS AFTER THE KIDNEY TRANSPLANT THAT PRECLUDES A DECLARATION OF EARLY SUCCESS FOR THE ith PATIENT	$[SP_i]0 = 0$ 0.0 0 {Definition}	$[1 - SP_i] \times [1 - S_i(t)]$ 1.0 $1 - S_i(t)$	$1 - SP_i - S_i(t) + SP_i \times S_i(t)$
THE ith PATIENT SURVIVES FOR MORE THAN t MONTHS AFTER THE KIDNEY TRANSPLANT WITH NO PROBLEM THAT QUALIFIES AS AN EARLY FAILURE	$[SP_i]1 = SP_i$ $RSP_i(t)$ $1 - 0 = 1$	$[1 - SP_i]S_i(t)$ $1 - RSP_i(t)$ $S_i(t)$ {Cox}	$SP_i + S_i(t) - SP_i \times S_i(t)$
INITIAL (PRIOR) PROBABILITY OF THE ith PATIENT'S TRUE STATUS	SP_i {Logit}	$FP_i = 1 - SP_i$	1.0

Explanatory Notes:

1. The larger (upper-left) triangle in each cell contains the joint probability that a patient's transplant experience will fall in that cell (i.e., be classified as both in that row and in that column of the table).
2. Upward-pointing triangles in (the lower portion of) each cell contain the conditional probability that a patient will fall in the indicated row, given that the patient falls in the status-defining column pointed to above.
3. Zero (0) in the upward-pointing triangle of the northwest cell embodies the model's operational definition of what it means for a patient's experience to be classified as an early success. More than six months must elapse after the transplant occurs without encountering any problem sufficiently serious to preclude recording the transplanted kidney as still functioning properly within the patient's body. Furthermore, the patient must then be coping adequately with any complications that did arise during the first six months. Of the 469 patients in the data set to which the Bayesian model was applied 347 were recorded as having properly functioning transplanted kidneys for more than six months. Such patients could not have suffered an

insurmountable early problem. Therefore, they could not have been observed to fall in the first row of the table (i.e., zero conditional probability).

4. The S(t) function in the upward-pointing triangle of the southeast cell is a tailored survival function constructed for each patient, separately, via Cox regression analysis. Cox regression was performed only on the 122 patients out of the 469 total patients classified in the second column of the preceding table. They were the patients known to have emerged from the transplant procedure in some condition that would result in their early failure. Each of them would experience failure in one of the six months constituting the accommodation period. Only which month varied from patient to patient. Hence, each patient's S(t) function can be interpreted as generating a survival probability conditional on that patient's being at clear, but probabilistic risk of early failure for some reason.

5. S(t) indicates that the survival function is defined in terms of the time in months elapsed since the transplant procedure. Values of t are integers ranging from one to six months.

6. The S(t) survival function is indexed with an "i" to indicate that each patient possesses a separately tailored individual survival function. Cox regression first estimates a baseline survival function for the patient population from which the 122 patients at risk of failure sometime during the first six months were obtained. Cox regression then estimates for each such patient an individualized proportionality factor embodying Cox's underlying proportional hazards modeling assumption. The assumed shared baseline survival function is then exponentiated by each patient's individualized proportionality factor to obtain that patient's separately tailored conditional survival function.

7. Leftward-pointing triangles in (the right-hand portion of) each cell contain the conditional probability that a patient will fall in the indicated column, given that the patient falls in the row pointed to at the left. These are probabilities that the transplant experience will be deemed either an early success or an early failure for each patient, conditional upon what the patient experiences during the six-month accommodation period.

8. The 0.0 and 1.0 conditional probabilities in the leftward-pointing triangles of the first row serve to elaborate further in probabilistic terms what it means for a patient experience to be declared an early success versus an early failure. These are very close to definitional probabilities. Their determination follows immediately from the model's operational definition of success and failure, but they are written as 0.0 and 1.0 to indicate that they are determined by observation to be either zero or one, rather than initially stipulated as such by the operational definition. They remain as still conditional values unless or until a patient experiences an insurmountable problem during the accommodation period (i.e., falls into the first row of the table). When that occurs, a 0.0 probability of early success is then assigned to that patient for that and all successive months.

9. Far more interesting are the leftward-pointing triangles in the second row. They contain early success and early failure probabilities revised on the basis of observing each patient during each of the first six months. To revise a probability means to update it (recalculate it, conditionally) on the basis of each successive month that passes without encountering an insurmountable problem (i.e., so long as the patient remains in the second row of the table).

10. RSP stands for revised early success probability. It is designated RSP(t) to indicate that it, too, is a function of time elapsed since the transplant procedure and that it, too, generates a separate output value for each of the six months constituting the six-month accommodation period. It is also indexed with an "i" to indicate that each patient possesses a separately tailored RSP function.

11. The RSP function is constructed for each patient who remains in the second row of the table by a simple application of Bayes' theorem to the other

probabilities in the table. Because of this the probability model is characterized as Bayesian. The RSP function generates the Bayesian posterior early success probability applicable to each such patient. It is a conditional probability because it is based on the observation that the patient has survived for t full months following the kidney transplant without experiencing an insurmountable problem.

12. The calculation formula is $RSP(t) = SP/[SP + (1 - SP) \times S(t)]$, where SP stands for a patient's initial success probability. SP does not change over successive months during the accommodation period. Exactly how each patient's initial SP probability is determined will be explained shortly.

13. Since $S(t)$ is a survival function and because all survival functions begin with a survival probability of 1.0 (when elapsed time t is zero), inserting t = 0 into the formula shows that all $RSP(t)$ functions start at an individual patient's initial SP probability.

14. Because SP and (1 - SP) are positive numbers and because $S(t)$ will be constructed by Cox regression to fall monotonically during each of the successive six months (eventually to zero), $RSP(t)$ will rise monotonically from its initial SP probability to a final end-six-month value of 1.0. This will be true for every patient whose monthly postoperative observations remain consistently in the second row of the table.

15. As soon as any patient's monthly observation drops into the first row, that patient's transplant experience will be deemed an early failure. This does not mean that nothing further can be done to improve the patient's condition. It only means that this particular transplant procedure is interpreted as resulting in an early failure for this particular patient. Subsequent improvements are interpreted by the Bayesian model as belonging to a different procedure.

16. The SP probability contained in the bottom row of the first column is the initial probability that a patient's transplant experience will turn out to be an early success.

17. The FP probability contained in the bottom row of the second column is the initial probability that a patient's transplant experience will turn out to be an early failure. It is simply 1 minus the SP probability.

18. The SP and FP probabilities are labeled initial probabilities because they are assessed prior to or at the beginning of the six-month accommodation period and without the benefit of any patient observations made during that period. Both are indexed with an "i" to indicate individual tailoring.

19. Separate SP (and complementary FP) values are obtained for each patient via logistic regression analysis (Logit). The analysis is performed on all patients (the entire sample of 469 patients in this data set).

20. Complete data on eight prognostic factors for each patient were also available in the data set. There were no missing factor values. These eight prognostic factors served as the independent variables of logistic regression. Whether each patient actually experienced an early success (N = 367) or an early failure (N = 122) served as the dependent variable.

21. Because values of all eight prognostic factors were known prior to the beginning of the six-month accommodation period, values for each patient's initial SP probability could be calculated in advance. For the same reason, these may be treated as Bayesian prior probabilities that each patient's transplant experience would turn out to be an early success or an early failure.

22. No other prognostic factors were included in the 469-patient data set. By necessity, therefore, the same eight factors constituted the independent variables available to the Cox regression analysis. Utilizing the same set of prognostic factors for both regressions is definitely not a requirement of the Bayesian model. In general, the two factor sets may possess only partial or even no overlap.

23. The calculated probabilities in the last column indicate how likely it is that a patient will fall in each of the two rows (i.e., experience which

type of observable outcome) as a function of t. These constitute the patient's Bayesian preposterior probabilities. Putting first t = 0 and then t = 6 into the formulas shows that every patient begins in the second row with probability 1.0 at time t = 0 (when the kidney has just been transplanted), but that the probability of remaining in the second row (i.e., of not experiencing an insurmountable problem) declines monotonically to the level of that patient's initial SP probability at the end of the sixth month.

24. In contrast, the probability that a patient will have switched into the first row (i.e., will have experienced at least one insurmountable problem) within t months begins at 0.0 and rises monotonically to FP = 1 - SP at the end of six months.

25. Time-sequenced values of the Bayesian posterior probability function generated for each of the 469 patients in each of the first six months were quite illuminating. Each patient's initial SP probability anchored the sequence. It became that patient's initial posterior probability (i.e., when t = 0). The mean of these 469 equal-in-value initial SP and initial posterior probabilities was exactly 347/469, the proportion of patients who eventually experienced early success. By uniformly setting posterior probabilities to zero for each patient in the month when an insurmountable problem first occurred (if one occurred) and then replicating that zero in all succeeding months, the mean posterior probability calculated for all 469 patients remained at exactly 347/469 during each of the six months. Apart from computer rounding discrepancies, the mathematics of logistic regression, Cox regression, and Bayes' theorem, acting together, guaranteed this consistent result. It was used to verify that all computations implementing the model had been properly executed.

26. Although their mean value remained constant, the predictive accuracy of successive posterior probabilities increased monotonically each month and eventually achieved 100 percent by the end of month six. We defined predictive error as the absolute value of each patient's difference between calculated monthly posterior probability and the actual one (for early success) or zero (for early failure) experienced at the end of the accommodation period. The mean predictive error calculated for all 469 patients fell steadily from an initial value of 0.3727 to a final end-six-month value of zero.

27. Separate patients were observed to display noticeably different and individually distinctive patterns of time-sequenced posterior probabilities. Obtaining these individually tailored patterns is the grand payoff derived from performing a Bayesian analysis in the manner just outlined.

28. Until experiencing an insurmountable problem all patients' posterior probabilities rose monotonically over time, but with noticeably different patterns of ascent. Differentiated ascent patterns were determined by each patient's separate collection of prognostic factor inputs to either or both logistic regression and Cox regression.

29. Despite these differences, all patients who eventually achieved early success received a 100 percent posterior probability at the end of their sixth month. All patients who experienced one or more insurmountable problems at some time during the accommodation period received a zero end-sixth-month posterior probability.

30. Suppose a patient not included in the sample of 469 (but drawn from the same or from a similar population) is considering a kidney transplant that will be performed in a manner similar to the manner in which the 469 transplants in this data set were performed. A sequence of individually tailored posterior probabilities could then be generated from that prospective patient's prognostic factors, using the estimated statistical parameters derived from the logistic and Cox regressions. That could help both the patient and the patient's physician decide whether or not to have

a kidney transplant. The patient's initial SP probability is likely to be a salient item of information from a decision making perspective. The distinctive pattern of successive posterior probabilities that the patient could anticipate during the six-month accommodation period might also serve as a credible (since individually tailored) "report card" with which to assess positive initial progress. Assuming that early success is achieved, an individually tailored transplant survival function covering the time period starting in the seventh month would "fill out" the projection of likely outcomes. Such a projected pattern of personalized probabilities over time (including both the accommodation and subsequent periods) would be quite informative in choosing whether or not to receive a transplant.

Presenting the Bayesian transplant model in tabular form has several advantages.

First, it provides a comprehensive visual display of how the conditional, joint, and unconditional (marginal) probabilities involved in executing Bayes' theorem relate to one another. All of the relevant probabilities are entered into designated locations of a single table.

Second, it provides a computational template to guide the sequential calculation of all such probabilities. This will be demonstrated.

Third, applying Bayes' theorem to generate Bayesian posterior probabilities constitutes the final step in the computational sequence. The table illustrates how straightforward and obvious Bayes' theorem really is. It lies but a short computational distance from the fundamental definitions of conditional, joint, and unconditional probabilities and the standard calculation rules governing their manipulation.

The table is decidedly "busy." Hopefully, being able to summarize all of these concepts, relationships, and sequential computational steps in a single display compensates for its busyness.

2.2 How Can a Table Be Constructed to Implement Such a Model?

A step-by-step procedure is outlined below and in the next few pages to illustrate the table construction process as it applies to the kidney transplant data set.

STEP 1

The first step is to focus on how success and failure are defined in this illustrative example. Both are defined as patient-centered concepts. Neither is just an organ-centered concept. Receiving a kidney that continues to function properly for more than six months is a necessary precondition to declaring early success. Yes, it is a success from the kidney's perspective. However, it may not be a success from the patient's perspective. Should the patient die from a blood clot or be unable to cope with infection or drugs relating to the transplant during the accommodation period, the Bayesian model would record an early failure. To declare the transplant experience an early success, the transplanted kidney must function properly in the patient's body for more than six months, and the patient must then be coping adequately with any complications that may have arisen during the six-month accommodation period.

Defining success and failure in this manner has definite implications. If the analysis were to focus on kidneys rather than on patients, death from a blood clot that compromised a different organ might not be considered a failure of the kidney. The kidney might be viewed as continuing to function properly, while the fatal blood clot might be regarded as just an observation-censoring event. By causing death it would preclude making further observations of the patient and, therefore, of the otherwise successfully transplanted kidney.

Suppose that there had been less dramatic evidence of distinct time periods in the data set. Distinguishing between the kidney's and the patient's perspective would then have been less compelling for that reason, too. However, the data pointed dramatically in the opposite direction. This provided additional support for separating the two perspectives.

Our preliminary Kaplan-Meier analysis from the kidney's perspective suggested two distinct postoperative time periods. They have been labeled the initial accommodation and subsequent periods, respectively. Almost half (91 of 192 or 47.4 percent) of the total transplant failures in the entire data set occurred within the first six months following the transplant procedure. This was the dramatic evidence suggesting distinct time periods. Trial cutoffs at each successive monthly interval between five and ten months showed six months to be the best way to separate the initial accommodation from the subsequent period.

Without separation a Weibull kidney survival function with a statistically significant (two-tailed p value < 0.00005) decreasing hazard rate over time fit the combined data set very well. The Weibull model demonstrated an unadjusted coefficient of determination (R-squared) of 0.9490.

With separation, evidence of a decreasing hazard rate disappeared from both the accommodation and the subsequent time periods. This equally dramatic observation served to reinforce viewing the data as falling into two separate and distinct time periods.

An exponential survival function (constant hazard rate over time) fit the first six-month accommodation period slightly better than the combined Weibull function without separation. It demonstrated an unadjusted coefficient of determination (R-squared) of 0.9674. An exponential survival function provided a still better fit with the subsequent time period, demonstrating an unadjusted coefficient of determination (R-squared) of 0.9814.

The statistical fit of neither exponential function was significantly improved by substituting a Weibull function that would have permitted a decreasing hazard rate.

Organ transplants are typically viewed as possessing survival functions with decreasing hazard rates. Such was indeed the case with the 469 kidney transplants recorded in this data set. That was without separation into different time periods. With separation, however, the story changed. The apparently decreasing hazard rate associated with the undifferentiated data seems only to have been a statistical artifact resulting from a failure to recognize the two separate and distinct time periods.

It was to correct this apparent oversight that the analysis was separated into an initial accommodation period modeled in a Bayesian framework specifically designed to reflect the patient's perspective, followed by a subsequent period modeled in the traditional manner focusing on the transplanted kidney.

The intent of the Bayesian revision procedure was to provide each of the 469 patients with a continually updated, month-by-month assessment of the likelihood that the entire six-month accommodation period would end successfully. That is what the model defined as early success. No distinction was made between separate causes of failure. What might be treated as a censoring event from the kidney's perspective was treated by the Bayesian model as just another kind of failure, relatively indistinguishable from the patient's point of view. Time-sequenced values of the posterior probability function would not otherwise have displayed the same pleasant properties previously reported.

The subsequent period was then modeled in the traditional manner, from the transplanted kidney's perspective, but starting in month seven for each of the 347 patients who achieved early success. Only data from these 347 patients were included in a Cox regression analysis that estimated both a baseline kidney transplant survival function for the population from which these 347 patients were obtained and the proportional hazard factor used to tailor the baseline survival function via exponentiation to each patient, separately.

STEP 2

The next step is to summarize the rules that define joint, conditional, and unconditional (marginal) probabilities and their proper manipulation. Although completely general conceptually, these rules will be interpreted here in terms of specific table entries and how to calculate them.

1. Every probability is a real number between 0.0 and 1.0, inclusive.
2. The joint probabilities in the large triangles of each cell in the table must add to 1.0.
3. The conditional probabilities in upward-pointing triangles in every column must add to 1.0.
4. The conditional probabilities in leftward-pointing triangles in every row must add to 1.0.
5. Unconditional probabilities of observed patient outcomes are recorded along the right-hand margin of the table. Each unconditional probability is the sum of the joint probabilities along its row of the table.
6. Unconditional probabilities of the patient's true postoperative status are recorded along the bottom margin of the table. Each unconditional probability is the sum of the joint probabilities down its column of the table.
7. The unconditional probabilities up and down the right-hand margin must add to 1.0.
8. The unconditional probabilities along the bottom margin must add to 1.0.
9. Every joint probability in a cell is the product of its upward-pointing conditional probability times its unconditional true patient status probability (marginal column sum). This is how the relationships between joint, conditional, and unconditional probabilities are defined, viewing the table column by column.
10. Every joint probability in a cell is equivalently the product of its leftward-pointing conditional probability times its unconditional observed patient outcome probability (marginal row sum). This is how the relationships between joint, conditional, and unconditional probabilities are defined, viewing the same table row by row.
11. Bayes' theorem is simply a direct implication of the above equivalence. By setting equal the equivalent formulas for calculating each cell's joint probability and manipulating the equation algebraically, the conditional probabilities up and down every column of the table may be calculated in terms of the corresponding reverse conditional probabilities across every row (and vice versa), in concert with the

appropriate unconditional (row and column sum) probabilities. The only restriction is that all unconditional probabilities must be strictly positive numbers. This will avoid dividing by zero in any calculation. It means that no table is permitted to possess either a solid row or a solid column of zero joint probabilities. In practice there would be little temptation to set up a model-reflecting table that violates this rather mild restriction.

STEP 3

The next step is to enter into the table the probabilities that will apply uniformly to all patients during all successive months. These are the probabilities that define the model operationally.

1. A zero is placed in the conditional upward-pointing triangle of the northwest cell. This defines operationally what the model means by a successful patient transplant experience during the six-month accommodation period. If a patient's experience is to be declared an early success, no insurmountable problems can arise during any of the first six months.
2. By rule 9, the large joint probability triangle of the northwest cell must also be filled with a zero.
3. By rule 10, the conditional leftward-pointing triangle of the northwest cell must also be filled with a zero, since all unconditional (row sum) probabilities must be strictly positive numbers.
4. By rule 3, a one must be placed in the conditional upward-pointing triangle of the southwest cell.
5. By rule 4, a one must be placed in the conditional leftward-pointing triangle of the northeast cell.

Conceptually, there is a separate table for each separate patient in each separate month of the accommodation period. Entering a probability into the table therefore means entering it into the table that applies to the particular patient currently being considered in the particular month currently being considered, as both are considered sequentially.

STEP 4

The next step is to enter into the table the probabilities that will apply only to a single patient, but will apply to all six months of the accommodation period.

1. From the logistic regression (Logit) analysis of all 469 patients, each patient's early success probability (SP) is obtained and entered as an unconditional probability into the bottom location of the first column.
2. By rule 8, its complement (FP = 1 - SP) is entered into the bottom location of the second column.
3. These two entries are made for each patient separately.

STEP 5

The final step is to enter into the table the probabilities that will apply separately to each patient and separately to each successive month of the accommodation period.

1. From the Cox regression analysis performed only on the 122 patients who experienced early failure, a sequence of baseline survival probabilities is obtained. The sequence contains a baseline probability for each of the first six months. The sequence decreases monotonically,

as all such time-sequenced survival probabilities must. The sixth-month baseline probability is zero, since the 122 patients were selected as those among the 469-patient data set who experienced at least one insurmountable problem sometime during the first six months.

The same Cox regression analysis estimates a regression coefficient for each of the patient prognostic factors input as its independent variables. These are used to calculate a separate proportionality factor (implied by the proportional hazards modeling assumption underlying Cox regression) for each of the 469 patients. Each patient's prognostic factor values are multiplied by the associated regression coefficients, and the products are added. The sum is then used to exponentiate the base e (base of the natural logarithm system). The result is that patient's proportionality factor.

A tailored survival function is then constructed for each of the 469 patients in each of the first six months. Each baseline probability is exponentiated by that patient's proportionality factor. These tailored $S(t)$ survival probabilities are entered into the conditional upward-pointing triangle in the southeast cell of the table. They are conditional because they are calculated under the assumption that the patient would suffer an early failure in one of the first six months.

2. By rule 3, the complementary $1 - S(t)$ probability is entered as the conditional upward-pointing triangle in the northeast cell of the table.
3. By rule 9, the large joint probability triangles of both the northeast and the southeast cells are filled in with properly multiplied values.
4. By rule 5, both unconditional probabilities in the right-hand margin of the table are added up and filled in.
5. That leaves only the Bayesian posterior RSP probabilities in the leftward-pointing triangles of the southwest and southeast cells still to be calculated and filled in. Rule 10 determines how to make each calculation. Rule 10 also defines as a calculation formula the way Bayes' theorem applies to this illustrative kidney transplant analysis.

2.3 By How Much Did PCM Improve the Accuracy of Predicting Early Success?

A conventional stepwise multivariate logistic regression analysis with backward elimination was executed to predict the early outcomes of all 469 patients who underwent kidney transplants. The early success or failure of each patient's experience during the six-month accommodation period was entered as the dependent variable (end point to be predicted). The eight prognostic factors were entered as independent variables (predictors).

Backward elimination reduced the set of predictors to include as important only age and the use or nonuse of ALG to suppress an immune response. This was not a surprising result. Recall that a conventional multivariate Cox regression was originally executed on the same data drawn from the same 469 patients to predict the overall survival time of their kidney grafts. Diabetes was included, along with age and the use or nonuse of ALG, among the important predictors of that different (although intimately related) end point.

PCM extends the conventional analytical framework. It is not primarily designed to draw conclusions about prognostic factors and the predictive potency of their connections with interesting end points in some patient population. That is the conventional factor-centered focus. PCM assumes that potent predictors have already been identified and selects an admissible collection of them to make as accurate as possible separate end point predictions about individual patients. That is what patient centered as opposed to factor centered means.

PCM's conclusions are always stated as probabilities that an individual patient will experience a stipulated end point of interest. To improve the accuracy of its probabilistic predictions, PCM relies on three procedural devices.

1. Selective Stratification

Refocusing and extending traditional methodology in the PCM manner fundamentally alters what it means for a sample of empirical observations to be representative. It is no longer sufficient just to be population-based. It may even be inappropriate. In the patient-centered context, being population-based may serve the penultimate goal of identifying potent prognostic factors, but not necessarily the ultimate goal. To be representative now means to be specifically applicable to supporting accurate predictions relating to a targeted individual patient. This strongly suggests regularly reconceiving the fundamental concept of a patient population in stratified terms. Equally strongly it suggests determining the appropriate principle of stratification separately on the basis of whichever particular focal question is being asked. Doing both then requires tailoring all supporting analyses accordingly.

In many cancers, for example, there exists a single prognostic factor or a single prognostic index constructed from more than one factor that is widely understood within the medical profession and regularly recorded for most patients. Primary tumor size or thickness is such a single factor. Stage of disease progression is such an index.

PCM selects from among such widely understood and regularly recorded factors and indexes the one that appears to possess the greatest univariate impact. Greatest impact means greatest ability to discriminate reliably among different patients in terms of predicting whether or not and when each one will experience the focal end point.

The selected factor or index is then used to stratify the overall patient population. Separate strata contain distinct subpopulations of patients, where the strata differ significantly in terms of the prevalence of and elapsed time to reach the focal end point.

A sample is drawn from the stratum (subpopulation) regarded as most similar to the targeted patient. Similarity refers to accuracy in predicting the focal end point. A prognostic model is trained on (fitted to data within) the similar-patient sample to produce an explicit prognostic algorithm.

Selective stratification serves to homogenize data relationships within subpopulations. Statistical modeling is then performed separately and independently within homogeneous, but externally heterogeneous, data sets. This tends to improve the fit of prognostic models (e.g., of logistic regression and Cox regression models) to separately drawn data samples. Missing observations are also handled separately across heterogeneous subpopulations. The likely value of a missing observation related to a prognostic factor can then be estimated more accurately.

If no suitable factor or index exists for a given prediction, the patient population is not stratified. When performed, the differentiating consequences of stratification are verified. The differential prevalence of and elapsed time to reach the focal end point across subpopulations are both tested statistically.

A second reason to omit stratification is too small a sample. Due to its increased risk of statistical overfitting, PCM requires sample sizes at least in the hundreds. The smallest sample drawn from a subpopulation (or whole population) needs to be at least that large.

2. SPSA Conversion

The scale partitioning and spacing algorithm (SPSA) is another device to improve prognostic accuracy. Scale partitioning means that the set of possible raw measurement values of a prognostic factor is subdivided into two or more distinct subscales. Scale partitioning is optimized so as to produce the most sensitive and specific prediction of the focal end point. Spacing means ascertaining the apparent "distances" separating partitioned subscales that reveal the "shape" of the univariate relationship linking a prognostic factor to the focal end point. The result is a univariate impact-reflecting index (UIRI). The raw measurement values of most prognostic factors are automatically converted by SPSA into a corresponding UIRI.

A UIRI indicates the direction, the shape, and the clinical potency of whatever univariate relationship the sample data suggest may exist in the similar-patient population stratum, linking each prognostic factor to the focal end point. Direction of impact indicates how more or less of the factor relates to more or less of its impact on the focal end point. Shape of relationship indicates whether the factor's impact is exerted at a constant, accelerating, or decelerating rate at different factor levels. Potency of impact indicates the factor's clinical importance (material influence) relative to the focal end point.

A UIRI is depicted both graphically and algebraically. Its algebraic form is normally incorporated into the prognostic model (explicit algorithm) produced by PCM for a sample of similar patients. Its graphical depiction serves as a visual aid to enhance understanding.

SPSA is a useful tool to the extent that a prognostic factor's impact on some focal end point is genuine, though incompletely understood. A UIRI suggests some form of association or correlation. It may or may not also signal a causal connection linking the prognostic factor to the focal end point in the population stratum containing similar patients. Fortunately, since prediction is the goal of PCM, association or correlation, when genuine, can be useful; but it must be systematic. The underlying biology need not be understood in complete detail.

Genuine means that the apparent linkage relationship is more than a statistical artifact resulting from overfitting a prognostic model to inadequate sample data. Quite large samples are required to distinguish genuine relationships (even if only correlational) from spurious correlations. Only large samples can support split-sample reliability testing, whereby the predictive improvements seemingly achieved in an algorithm-fitting sample can be shown to carry over to a completely distinct validation sample drawn from the same population stratum.

On the other hand, if the detailed biological mechanisms mediating a factor's impact were thoroughly understood, data conversion via SPSA would not be helpful. It would not be performed. Yet detailed knowledge of the underlying pathways and connections linking commonly used prognostic factors to popular focal end points is, today, largely nonexistent. Even the shape (as opposed to just the existence and direction) of many linkage relationships remains poorly understood.

PCM, therefore, converts prognostic factor data into corresponding UIRI scores. This does not improve the univariate predictive accuracy of dichotomous prognostic factors such as whether or not an immunosuppressive drug (e.g., ALG) is used during a transplant procedure. Such factors possess a directional relationship but without any distinctive shape. In contrast, the predictive accuracy of genuinely quantitative prognostic factors such as age and the number of days a patient has previously undergone dialysis is sometimes improved substantially. Quantitative factors can display quite distinctive and predictively useful shapes.

3. Dealing with Missing Observations

A sample may contain missing observations on one or more prognostic factors. If not too many observations were missing and if the goal of the analysis were factor-centered, it would be tempting simply to delete patients with missing observations from the analysis.

Becoming patient-centered, however, precludes such a strategy. The goal is to make a specific prediction, even if imprecise, for all patients.

SPSA includes detailed procedures to estimate likely end point values for missing observations of all prognostic factors. The efficacy of these procedures is considerably enhanced by selective stratification, especially when the total patient population is composed of internally homogeneous, but externally heterogeneous, subpopulations.

In the fortunate situation where a collected sample contains no missing data, SPSA omits such missing-observation estimation procedures.

PCM always begins by looking for a way to partition a heterogeneous patient population into relatively homogeneous subpopulations. That is what it means to execute selective stratification.

Selective stratification is successful to the extent that it succeeds in transforming what begins as a less definitive analysis of a single heterogeneous population into more definitive analyses of two or more relatively homogeneous subpopulations.

In the kidney transplant application, selective stratification of patients was into early accommodation success and early accommodation failure subpopulations. The success of selective stratification was signaled both by the improved statistical fit (R-squared) achieved in each separated subsample compared to the total, unpartitioned sample of 469 patients (a quantitative benefit) and by the dramatic disappearance of a declining hazard rate over time from both subsamples (an unanticipated qualitative insight).

Even more important, this particular form of selective stratification enabled the analysis to be performed in a Bayesian framework. To showcase the Bayesian framework was the principal reason for selecting the kidney transplant data in the first place. PCM's initial attempt to homogenize via selective stratification renders it especially compatible with Bayesian analysis if and when a Bayesian framework is appropriate.

Further substratification might have achieved further homogenization. However, the total sample size of 469 was not quite large enough to subdivide the patient population further into relatively homogeneous substrata.

All eight prognostic factors could be and were converted by SPSA into corresponding UIRIs. There were no missing observations on any of the eight factors for any patient. Consequently, PCM's ability to improve predictive accuracy was restricted to the homogenizing impact of the initial selective stratification and to indicating via SPSA conversion the underlying shape of the impact of the four genuinely quantitative prognostic factors on achieving early success.

SPSA reanalysis of the same 469-patient sample data was executed. A stepwise multivariate logistic regression analysis with backward elimination was again performed. Corresponding UIRI values were substituted for the raw data inputs of all eight prognostic factors. The early success or failure of each patient's experience during the six-month accommodation period remained as the end point.

SPSA achieved a modest, but statistically significant, further improvement in predictive accuracy. Matched pairs of individualized patient probabilities of achieving early success were constructed from the two logistic regression analyses for each of the 469 patients. In terms of the accuracy improvement measures outlined in section 1.2, the results were as follows.

1. SPSA predicted correctly about the same percentage (74 percent) of early successes as the traditional methodology. There was no further subdivision of the patient population into relatively homogeneous substrata, so both logistic regressions shared the same dependent variable.
2. However, SPSA did achieve an AUC correct prediction score 3.6 percentage points higher than the conventional methodology.
3. Looking at matched pairs of probabilistic prediction errors, PCM's index of error reduction (based just on SPSA) was a favorable 0.049.
4. According to the Wilcoxon matched-pairs, signed ranks test, this modest reduction generated an equivalent Z value of 3.11, with a two-tailed p value of 0.0019.

The total sample size of 469 also seemed not quite large enough to perform a split-sample reliability analysis. If evenly split, the training and validation subsamples would have numbered 235 and 234 patients, respectively. Based on our past experience with split-sample testing of PCM's improved accuracy, these would have been marginally adequate, at best. At least several hundred each has generally been our required minimum sample size.

Regrettably, with neither a separate-sample validation nor a split-sample replication, the interpretation of SPSA's efficacy remains constrained. Yes, the null hypothesis of no systematic predictive accuracy improvement could be and was statistically tested. If no significantly improved accuracy had resulted, the story would have ended there. Yet SPSA did provide significantly improved accuracy. Only because of this did its proper attribution then become important. How much of the improvement was due to statistical overfitting?

A separate-sample validation or split-sample replication would have permitted (or failed to permit) ruling out statistical overfitting as the sole source of apparent improvement. Being able to rule out overfitting would have bolstered our confidence in the existence of a systematic underlying basis for SPSA's superior predictive accuracy. It is too bad this could not have been done.

Because they were more accurate, the SPSA-estimated probabilities of each patient's early success (SP) were adopted for inclusion in the Bayesian model. These probabilities ranged from a minimum of 0.5239 to a maximum of 0.9061, with a median of 0.7219 and a mean of 0.7399.

Early failure probabilities (FP = 1 - SP) were somewhat more convenient to analyze. The 469 individually tailored FP probabilities were first ranked and divided into quartiles. The mean probability in each quartile was then compared with the actual prevalence of early failure among patients in that quartile.

These two numbers should converge statistically and become approximately equal as the number of patients in each quartile increases. The maximum absolute difference was 3.33 percentage points. The mean absolute difference was 1.19 percentage points. Furthermore, there was no striking pattern or trend in the succession of quartile probabilities and prevalence.

The SPSA algorithm was executed to partition the scale of individually tailored FP probabilities into as many subscales as possible, as long as each subscale encompassed FP probabilities for at least fifty patients. Four separate subscales were produced. They differed noticeably from the four quartiles.

When successive subscale means were plotted along the horizontal X-axis and each corresponding actual prevalence was plotted along the vertical Y-axis of a graph, all four points fell close to the straight line through the origin that makes a 45-degree angle with each axis. This line assumes that every actual prevalence exactly equals its corresponding subscale mean. Prediction errors are vertical deviations from the line. The uncorrected R-squared value (coefficient of determination) associated with this line, interpreted as a simple linear regression equation constrained to pass through the origin of the graph, was 0.9609 (equivalent to a 0.9803 linear correlation coefficient).

The closeness of statistical fit of the PCM-estimated FP probabilities was most encouraging. Figure 4 provides visual confirmation of their predictive accuracy.

A conventional stepwise multivariate Cox regression analysis with backward elimination was executed to predict how many months were required by the 122 early failure patients to experience an early failure. Failures occurred in either the first, second, third, fourth, fifth, or sixth month following each patient's transplant procedure. Raw data values of the same eight prognostic factors were used as predictors (independent variables).

The use or nonuse of ALG emerged as the only statistically significant predictor of time to failure (i.e., number of months elapsed during the accommodation period until failure occurred). No other factors made an important predictive contribution in the multivariate context.

Repeating the same analysis with UIRIs substituted for unconverted factor inputs generated the same outcome. Because of this and because the sole important predictor was dichotomous, it is legitimate both to interpret the unconverted results in a traditional hypothesis-testing framework and to utilize them simultaneously as if they were PCM-generated.

Figure 4

Scattergram of Predictive Accuracy of Mean Early Accommodation Failure Probability for 469 Kidney Transplant Patients

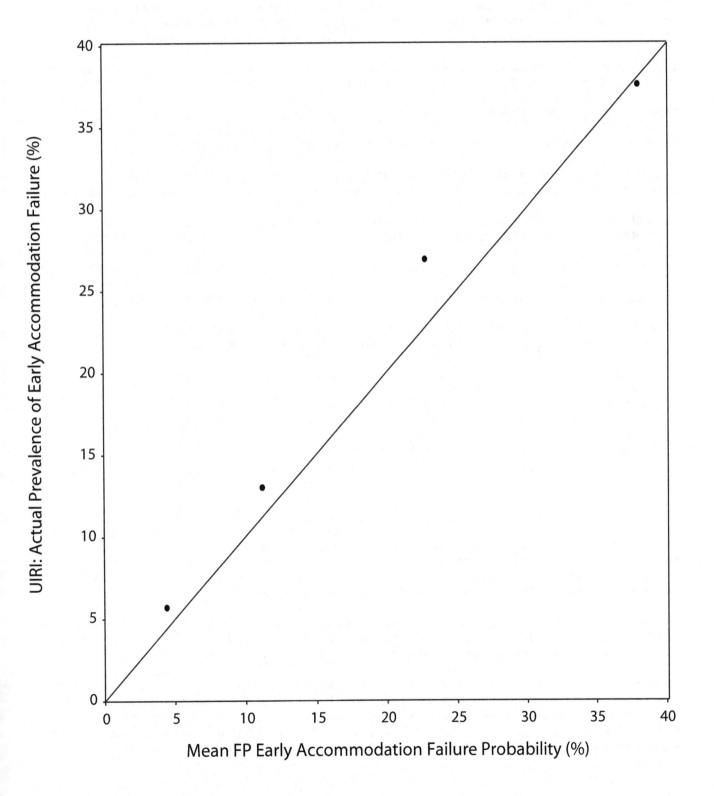

UIRI: Actual Prevalence of Early Accommodation Failure (%)

Mean FP Early Accommodation Failure Probability (%)

Slightly edited computer-generated output for the single important predictor (use of ALG) is shown below and on the next page between the horizontal lines.

RESULTS OF COX REGRESSION ANALYSIS (PROPORTIONAL HAZARDS MODEL)

The dependent variable is the time elapsed in months until the focal event occurs. All 122 PATIENTs experienced the focal event during some month within the six-month accommodation period. The focal event was early failure.

The independent variable IMSPDX is coded 1, if ALG was used to suppress an immune response; or 0, if ALG was not used.

Likelihood ratio chi-square statistic: 3.770, two-tailed p value: 0.0522.
Score chi-square statistic: 4.191, two-tailed p value: 0.0407.
Wald chi-square statistic: 4.119, two-tailed p value: 0.0424.

All three chi-square statistics are based on 1 degree of freedom and 122 observations, encompassing 6 distinct focal event times (measured in months).

INDEPENDENT VARIABLE	REGRESSION COEFFICIENT	STANDARD DEVIATION	CHI-SQUARE (DF = 1)	2-TAIL P VALUE	RELATIVE RISK
IMSPDX	−0.4619	0.2276	4.1192	0.0424	0.6301

COMPARISON OF KAPLAN-MEIER (PRODUCT LIMIT) AND BASELINE SURVIVAL RATES

ELAPSED TIME UNITS	NUMBER OF EVENTS	NUMBER AT RISK	KAPLAN-MEIER SURVIVAL RATE	BASELINE SURVIVAL RATE
0.0000	N/A	122	1.0000	1.0000
1.0000	29	122	0.7623	0.7633
2.0000	29	93	0.5246	0.5235
3.0000	19	64	0.3689	0.3664
4.0000	15	45	0.2459	0.2405
5.0000	14	30	0.1311	0.1235
6.0000	16	16	0.0000	0.0000
TOTAL	122			

If the population of elapsed time intervals until an event occurs is assumed to follow an exponential distribution, implying a constant hazard rate throughout every observation subwindow, the maximum likelihood estimate of the ordinary hazard rate is 0.3297, with a standard error of 0.0299.

The assumption of an exponential distribution with a constant hazard rate produces a VERY GOOD fit with the observed data. The analogue of an unadjusted coefficient of determination (R-squared) would be 0.9486.

An attempt was made to fit a Weibull distribution to the same data. A Weibull distribution permits either an increasing or a decreasing hazard rate over all observation subwindows. This additional flexibility failed to provide a substantially better fit. Consequently, the constant hazard rate assumed by the exponential distribution appears reasonable for this complete observation window.

If the population of elapsed time intervals until an event occurs is assumed to follow an exponential distribution, implying a constant hazard rate throughout every observation subwindow, the maximum likelihood estimate of the BASELINE hazard rate is 0.3319, with a standard error of 0.0301.

The assumption of an exponential distribution with a constant hazard rate produces a VERY GOOD fit with the observed data. The analogue of an unadjusted coefficient of determination (R-squared) would be 0.9479.

An attempt was made to fit a Weibull distribution to the same data. A Weibull distribution permits either an increasing or a decreasing hazard rate over all observation subwindows. This additional flexibility failed to provide a substantially better fit. Consequently, the constant hazard rate assumed by the exponential distribution appears reasonable for this complete observation window.

Notice that successive monthly values of the baseline survival rate estimated by Cox regression track very closely the corresponding monthly Kaplan-Meier product-limit values. This means that estimates of each monthly baseline survival rate are based on the "typical" or "average" patient in the 122-patient sample. They are not based on the "null" patient who did not receive ALG to suppress an immune response. The computer program can be instructed to generate outputs for the "null" patient, instead, but then a different sequence of six monthly baseline survival rates would be printed out. These would not match the corresponding Kaplan-Meier survival rates.

Because of this each patient's individual hazard rate proportionality multiplier (HAZPROP) must be calculated as the exponentiated (base e) product of that patient's deviation from the mean value of IMSPDX for the 122 patients who experienced early failure multiplied by the regression coefficient generated by Cox regression for these 122 patients. The 469 values of HAZPROP are summarized below.

SUMMARY STATISTICS	ATTRIBUTE HAZPROP
n DEFINED	469
MINIMUM	0.9097
MEDIAN	0.9097
MAXIMUM	1.4437
MEAN	0.9985
STD. DEV.	0.1989

All data required to calculate each of the 469 patients' Bayesian posterior early success probabilities RSP(t) are now available. The six revised monthly probabilities are designated POSTPR1, POSTPR2, POSTPR3, POSTPR4, POSTPR5, and POSTPR6. Their values are summarized on the next page.

SUMMARY STATISTICS	ATTRIBUTE POSTPR1	ATTRIBUTE POSTPR2	ATTRIBUTE POSTPR3	ATTRIBUTE POSTPR4	ATTRIBUTE POSTPR5	ATTRIBUTE POSTPR6
n DEFINED	469	469	469	469	469	469
MINIMUM	0.0000	0.0000	0.0000	0.0000	0.0000	0.0000
MEDIAN	0.7679	0.8234	0.8661	0.9044	0.9455	1.0000
MAXIMUM	0.9250	0.9456	0.9639	0.9800	0.9923	1.0000
MEAN	0.7392	0.7395	0.7394	0.7402	0.7404	0.7399
STD. DEV.	0.2007	0.2820	0.3298	0.3666	0.4004	0.4387

Apart from computer rounding discrepancies, the mean values remain constant over the entire six-month accommodation period. That constant mean value is the proportion (347/469 = 0.7399) of patients who experienced early success. It is also the mean SP value of initial early success probabilities (Bayesian prior probabilities) for the total 469-patient sample.

SUMMARY STATISTICS	ATTRIBUTE SP
n DEFINED	469
MINIMUM	0.5239
MEDIAN	0.7219
MAXIMUM	0.9061
MEAN	0.7399
STD. DEV.	0.0802

The maximum computer rounding discrepancy was less than 0.001. This verifies not only that HAZPROP and SP values have been consistently and properly calculated; it also verifies the consistent and proper calculation of RSP(t) posterior probabilities for all 469 patients in all six months of the accommodation period.

Even though Bayesian posterior RSP(t) probabilities remain constant when averaged over all 469 patients, they change quite differently over time for the 347 early success patients compared to the 122 early failure patients.

Posterior probabilities for the 347 early success patients are summarized below.

SUMMARY STATISTICS	ATTRIBUTE POSTPR1	ATTRIBUTE POSTPR2	ATTRIBUTE POSTPR3	ATTRIBUTE POSTPR4	ATTRIBUTE POSTPR5	ATTRIBUTE POSTPR6
n DEFINED	347	347	347	347	347	347
MINIMUM	0.6190	0.7324	0.7911	0.8474	0.9106	1.0000
MEDIAN	0.7685	0.8239	0.8773	0.9242	0.9572	1.0000
MAXIMUM	0.9250	0.9456	0.9639	0.9800	0.9923	1.0000
MEAN	0.7943	0.8479	0.8874	0.9221	0.9572	1.0000
STD. DEV.	0.0678	0.0516	0.0398	0.0295	0.0182	0.0000

Posterior probabilities for the 122 early failure patients are summarized on the next page.

SUMMARY STATISTICS	ATTRIBUTE POSTPR1	ATTRIBUTE POSTPR2	ATTRIBUTE POSTPR3	ATTRIBUTE POSTPR4	ATTRIBUTE POSTPR5	ATTRIBUTE POSTPR6
n DEFINED	122	122	122	122	122	122
MINIMUM	0.0000	0.0000	0.0000	0.0000	0.0000	0.0000
MEDIAN	0.7679	0.7369	0.0000	0.0000	0.0000	0.0000
MAXIMUM	0.9250	0.9456	0.9601	0.9724	0.9742	0.0000
MEAN	0.5824	0.4314	0.3185	0.2227	0.1237	0.0000
STD. DEV.	0.3295	0.4121	0.4172	0.3903	0.3183	0.0000

Posterior probabilities converge to the right final outcome for both early success and early failure patients. This implies that probabilistic errors must be converging to zero for all 469 patients.

Absolute differences between monthly posterior success probabilities and the right final outcome (0, if early failure; 1, if early success) were as follows.

SUMMARY STATISTICS	MONTH 1	MONTH 2	MONTH 3	MONTH 4	MONTH 5	MONTH 6
n DEFINED	469	469	469	469	469	469
MINIMUM	0.0000	0.0000	0.0000	0.0000	0.0000	0.0000
MEDIAN	0.2321	0.1761	0.1223	0.0708	0.0325	0.0000
MAXIMUM	0.9250	0.9456	0.9601	0.9724	0.9742	0.0000
MEAN	0.3037	0.2248	0.1661	0.1156	0.0638	0.0000
STD. DEV.	0.2428	0.2473	0.2337	0.2105	0.1669	0.0000

Comparable absolute error differences for initial SP early success probabilities were as follows.

SUMMARY STATISTICS	ABSOLUTE SP ERROR
n DEFINED	469
MINIMUM	0.0939
MEDIAN	0.2788
MAXIMUM	0.9061
MEAN	0.3727
STD. DEV.	0.2186

2.4 What Do the Tailored Bayesian Posterior Success Probabilities Look Like?

Tabled in appendix A are the initial early success probabilities (SP) and the six succeeding monthly Bayesian posterior RSP(t) probabilities (POSTPR1 through POSTPR6) for all 469 patients. Patient data have been arranged in ascending order by initial SP probability. All probabilities apply to the six-month accommodation period.

Three representative examples of these six-month probability sequences are depicted graphically in figure 5. The three examples show how different patients, each of whom eventually experiences early success, can nonetheless approach that common outcome in noticeably different ways via curves with different shapes. Once again, one shoe does not fit all.

  1. The sequence labeled LOWRISK describes the patient possessing the highest initial SP early success probability who then did experience early success.

2. The sequence labeled MEDRISK describes a patient possessing a "typical" (medium-valued) initial SP probability who also experienced early success.
3. The sequence labeled HIGHRISK describes the patient possessing the lowest initial SP probability who nonetheless did experience early success.

Figure 6 depicts graphically the sequence of estimated kidney transplant survival probabilities that apply to the subsequent time period for these same LOWRISK, MEDRISK, and HIGHRISK patients. Figure 6 is a patient-by-patient extension of figure 5.

How each patient's transplant survival probability is estimated for the subsequent time period will be explained after the presentation of figures 5 and 6.

Figure 5

Illustrative Sequences of Monthly Bayesian Posterior Early Accommodation
Success Probabilities for a Low-Risk, a Medium-Risk, and a High-Risk Patient,
Each of Whom Achieved Early Accommodation Success

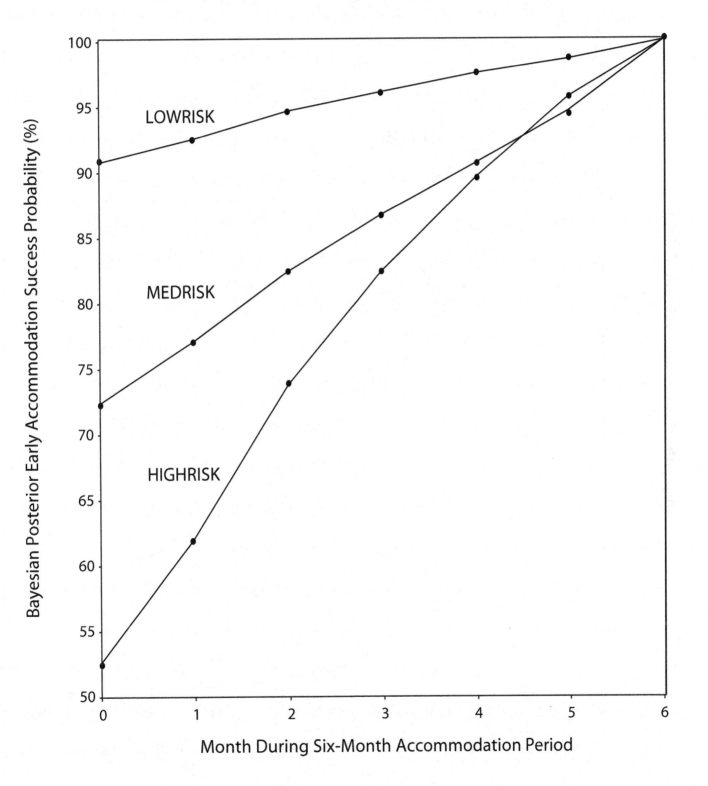

Month During Six-Month Accommodation Period

Figure 6

Transplanted Kidney Survival Probabilities During the Subsequent Period for the Same Low-Risk, Medium-Risk, and High-Risk Patients Who Achieved Early Accommodation Success

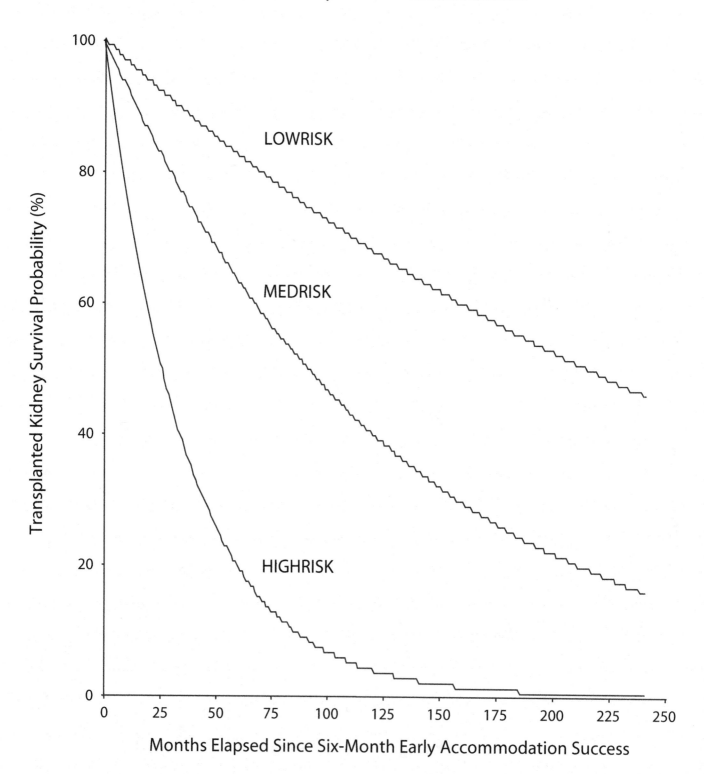

Months Elapsed Since Six-Month Early Accommodation Success

2.5 What Probabilities Apply to the Subsequent Time Period?

A patient who experiences early success survives the six-month accommodation period. The seventh month following the transplant procedure is entered with a properly functioning kidney. Furthermore, the patient is satisfactorily coping with any problems that may have arisen during the accommodation period.

Although currently functioning properly, the transplanted kidney is nevertheless at some risk of future failure. The risk is permanent. Patients generally continue to take immunosuppressive drugs for the rest of their kidney's life to combat this risk.

There remain, of course, competing risks from the patient's perspective. The patient could later die of something completely unrelated to the kidney transplant.

These are exactly the conditions that support the traditional organ-centered survival analysis typically performed in clinical research. A personalized Cox regression executed in the traditional manner but applied only to long-term survivors (i.e., the 347 patients in the data set analyzed here) will generate appropriate probabilistic predictions of kidney survival.

Personalized means that the same Cox regression procedure previously applied to the 122 early failure patients will be replicated for the 347 long-term survivors, with some modifications.

1. Data on whatever prognostic factors prove predictive of long-term kidney survival will be included in the analysis. The factor set may well differ from the factor set appropriate for predicting early success and failure (although that did not occur in this example).
2. Patients will also need to be followed up for decades, not just for a few months. Many transplanted kidneys survive that long.
3. A baseline survival function and individual proportionality factors will then be estimated, just as for the 122 patients suffering early failure, but survival will now refer to long-term kidney survival instead of to a successful six-month patient accommodation experience.
4. An attempt will also be made to improve predictive accuracy through PCM.

A conventional stepwise multivariate Cox regression analysis with backward elimination was executed to predict for how many additional months transplanted kidneys received by the 347 long-term survivors continued to function properly.

Raw data values of the same eight prognostic factors were again used as predictors (independent variables), since no other data were available in this data set.

This time, however, patient age, number of days of prior hemodialysis, and use or nonuse of ALG emerged from the conventional analysis as the statistically significant predictors of time to failure of the transplanted kidney.

Repeating the same analysis with SPSA-generated UIRIs substituted for unconverted factor inputs generated better results. Also, the number of blood units used during transfusion replaced the use or nonuse of ALG as a statistically significant predictor.

When predicting whether or not a transplanted kidney would fail in the subsequent period, PCM produced both a substantial and a statistically

significant improvement in accuracy compared to conventional stepwise
multivariate logistic regression with backward elimination. In terms of the
accuracy improvement measures outlined in section 1.2, the matched-pair
comparisons (with and without the benefit of PCM) were as follows.

1. PCM predicted correctly a slightly higher percentage (74.64) of
   long-term failures than the conventional methodology (72.62 percent
   correct).
2. PCM also achieved an AUC correct prediction score 3.36 percentage
   points higher than the conventional methodology.
3. Looking at matched pairs of probabilistic prediction errors, PCM's
   index of error reduction was a favorable 0.2507.
4. According to the Wilcoxon matched-pairs, signed ranks test this
   reduction generated an equivalent Z value of 4.70, with a two-tailed p
   value less than 0.00005.

The long-term survivor sample of 347 patients also seemed too small to perform
a split-sample reliability analysis. Given that the total sample of 469 was
judged inadequate, the 347-patient subsample was even less adequate. No such
analysis was therefore executed.

As previously acknowledged the 469 patients in this data set experienced
twentieth-century kidney transplant technology. There have been important
advances during the twenty-first century. Survival probabilities have become
decidedly more favorable. Much of the improvement has resulted from better ways
to suppress the receiving body's natural immune response. That renders this
particular data set inappropriate as a vehicle to showcase the efficacy of
contemporary transplant technology.

Nevertheless, to the extent that contemporary transplant technology related to
at least some organs continues to produce outcomes that may conveniently be
viewed as arising from temporally separated biological phenomena, the Bayesian
analysis introduced here remains novel and informative. Especially interesting
would be persistence in the elimination of (or even the substantial diminution
of) a decreasing hazard rate from both sequential time periods.

Comparison of figures 5 and 6 suggests how diverse the transplant experiences
of a low-risk, a medium-risk, and a high-risk patient can be.

1. The LOWRISK patient had a 90.61 percent chance of surviving the
   six-month accommodation period and reaching the seventh month with a
   functioning kidney. Given that early success, the transplanted kidney
   then had a 50 percent chance of continuing to function properly for an
   additional 213.69 months (17.81 years).
2. The MEDRISK patient had a 72.12 percent chance of surviving the
   six-month accommodation period. Given that early success, the
   transplanted kidney then had a 50 percent chance of continuing to
   function properly for an additional 90.30 months (7.52 years).
3. The HIGHRISK patient had a 52.39 percent chance of surviving the
   six-month accommodation period. Given that early success, the
   transplanted kidney then had a 50 percent chance of continuing to
   function properly for an additional 25.49 months (2.12 years).

To the extent that modern kidney and other organ transplant patients continue
to experience such large disparities, graphical presentations, as illustrated
in figures 5 and 6, could also be quite illuminating. The same single shoe
definitely does not seem to fit all transplant patients. These graphs, along
with personalized supporting data as tabled in appendix A, could help both
patients and their physicians make better informed treatment selection choices.

2.6 A Brief Summary of Some Useful Statistical Concepts and Procedures

The analysis of 469 kidney transplants served as an introduction to and an illustration of a particular Bayesian framework for the statistical analysis of medical data. The next section will apply the same Bayesian framework to the concept of cure.

Both PCM and this Bayesian framework are being offered as extensions to statistical concepts and procedures routinely applied in medicine today. Neither is being offered as a substitute or replacement. Both involve modifications and enhancements.

Neither is it claimed that this particular way of applying Bayes' theorem to analyzing medical records is unique. Other forms of Bayesian analysis have been successfully applied to medicine, to business, and in numerous other contexts for many years. This particular application of Bayes' theorem, however, is not a routine component of contemporary clinical research.

Appendixes B through F summarize several of the standard statistical concepts and procedures already discussed (e.g., Kaplan-Meier, logistic regression, and Cox regression analysis). Additional concepts and procedures that will become useful in the assessment of cure are also presented. These appendixes are provided strictly for review. They do not purport to offer either original or complete expositions of the relevant material.

Interested readers may find it helpful to browse through these appendixes before proceeding to the next section. They may also be helpful in clarifying what has already been presented in this section.

3.0   THE CONCEPT OF CURE

A cure is a fundamental change in state. In the context of a progressive and potentially fatal disease such as cancer, a patient may be characterized as cured if:

1. the patient gets the disease in the first place, thus becoming transformed into a state of being at substantial risk (designated SR) of various forms of disease progression, including the possibility of dying because of it; and
2. the patient is subsequently retransformed, this time from being at risk into a cured state; where
3. cured means now at very low or no risk (minimal risk, designated MR) of experiencing further progression of that particular bout with that particular disease; and where
4. the curative retransformation may result from either a medical intervention; a nonmedical intervention; or no intervention at all (it may occur spontaneously).

The important idea is that a patient must undergo a change in state in order to become cured. The Bayesian model introduced in section 2 requires an underlying state change. Detecting if, when, and for whom a particular medical intervention succeeds in producing such a favorable state change is the central task of the remainder of this book.

Typically a cured patient must have undergone some initial change in state to become sick in the first place. This is not always true. For example, it is not true in the case of a hereditary disease or a congenital defect that is operative at birth. When true, however, the initial change in state is generally regarded as an unfavorable event. It is common to speak of the "risk" of getting a disease (i.e., of experiencing that unfavorable change of state).

The subsequent change in state (becoming cured) is generally regarded as a favorable event. The "risk" lies in just the opposite direction. It denotes the possibility of not being cured and of suffering continuing disease progression.

Because these two changes in state are asymmetrically related to the concept of risk it is important to distinguish clearly between the two types of risk:

1. the initial risk of getting a progressive disease; and
2. having gotten it, the subsequent risk of not being cured and of experiencing, instead, further disease progression.

This book focuses on the second type of risk, on the risk of disease progression and on the efficacy of a medical intervention in eliminating that risk. High-risk and low-risk factors refer to prognostic indicators of the likelihood, the nature, and the timing of disease progression rather than to whether or when a patient gets a disease in the first place.

3.1   What Constitutes a Focal Event in the Cure Context?

Curing a progressive disease requires that its progress be halted. That is a minimum requirement. Consequently, it is appropriate to pay particular attention to any evidence of disease progression contained in patient records. Data on disease progression also provide a good basis for making a prognosis of the outcomes most important both to a doctor and to a patient.

Of particular relevance to the prognosis of important patient outcomes is the time required for any such disease to make a transition from its current stage to any one of its subsequent stages. The following analytical framework has been designed to describe both whether or not and the time elapsed until a patient diagnosed with a progressive disease experiences some characteristic event that provides clear evidence of further disease progression. This will serve as our framework for cure assessment.

1. Many progressive diseases are characterized by a sequence of developmental stages. Various forms of cancer (although not all cancer patients) typically progress through successive stages, such as I, II, III, and IV of melanoma and breast cancer.

2. Successive stages of the disease are indicated by certain observable events. Examples include its original diagnosis, its recurrence, its becoming systemic, and death as a direct result of it. Many of these observable events are among the most salient of patient outcomes.

3. Once a patient is diagnosed with a progressive disease that patient is regarded as at substantial risk (SR) of experiencing further disease progression. That further disease progression has actually occurred is inferred when the patient experiences one or more in the sequence of observable events that indicate its sequential stages.

4. Unless something occurs to alter a patient's risk state from substantial (SR) to being at very low or no such risk (MR), that patient is presumed to remain in the SR state.

5. Any observable event experienced by a patient at some particular stage of disease progression that provides clear evidence of still further progression is designated a focal event. Focal simply means worth focusing attention upon because it signals continuing progression.

6. Further progression does not require advancement to the next stage of disease development. Any evidence of continuing progression, even if restricted to a given stage of development, constitutes a focal event.

7. A patient in the SR state is presumed to possess a nontrivial probability of experiencing one or more focal events. Thus, an untreated stage IV melanoma or breast cancer patient may eventually die of the disease. Disease-specific death would constitute a regrettably possible focal event for any patient in stage IV.

8. In sharp contrast a patient in the MR state has an essentially zero probability of experiencing one or more focal events. The likelihood that a female patient will go through any stage of prostate cancer (much less die of it) may be treated as zero.

9. The occurrence of a focal event is either observed or not observed. Sometimes a focal event occurs but remains unobserved. The primary tumor in melanoma sometimes remains undetected until it metastasizes to a local lymph node. Occasionally the primary tumor is never identified. This can cause both diagnostic and prognostic problems, as discussed in appendix B.

10. Of great interest also is the time required for a focal event to occur, when it occurs. This refers to the time elapsed between some reference event (e.g., original diagnosis or a specific treatment) and observation of the focal event (e.g., relapse, recurrence, or disease-specific death).

Our cure assessment methodology is elaborated in appendixes B through F at the end of this book. Both the occurrence versus nonoccurrence of a focal event and the time elapsed until its occurrence are given a probabilistic interpretation. Both are imbedded within the framework of several probabilistic models commonly employed in medicine. At least scanning these appendixes is recommended for all readers at this time, if only to pick up the terminology adopted throughout the remainder of the book.

4.0 A FIRST ILLUSTRATIVE ANALYSIS

Medical records of more than twenty-two hundred cancer patients were collected between 1945 and 1996 from the region of Turku, Finland. All of these patients were diagnosed with some form of breast cancer. The earliest diagnosis occurred in January 1945. The latest diagnosis occurred in January 1992. After deleting duplicated and otherwise unusable records, clean (but sometimes incomplete) data for 2,192 patients of relatively homogeneous genetic stock remained.

Less than 2 percent of the patients in this cleaned data set were lost to regularly scheduled follow-up at any time for any reason excluding their death. The last follow-up date was June 1996. Consequently, the entire data set spanned 51.4 years. Both its relatively homogeneous genetic composition and its thorough and lengthy follow-up period rendered the Turku data set ideal for assessing the curative impact of a medical intervention.

4.1 Selecting the Target Intervention

Medical interventions recorded in the Turku data set included five types of surgery, radiation therapy, and four types of adjuvant therapy. Virtually all patients underwent some type of surgical procedure. Almost 85 percent received either a radical mastectomy (Halsted procedure) or a modified radical mastectomy. Approximately 60 percent of the patients received radiation therapy. No type of adjuvant therapy was recorded for any patients diagnosed before 1966, and fewer than 20 percent of the patients diagnosed thereafter received adjuvant therapy in any form.

Based on these data set characteristics, either radical or modified radical mastectomy (both of which included lymph node dissection, accompanied by radiation therapy, but without any form of adjuvant therapy) emerged as the medical intervention whose curative impact could most conveniently be assessed. Selecting this as the target intervention resulted in the largest possible subsample of patients who received identical medical treatment.

The target intervention was judged to be potentially curative. It seemed plausible to expect an appreciable proportion (although by no means all) of the patients so treated to be cured. The target intervention was the standard of care for invasive breast cancer during much of that historical time period. More to the point, a previous analysis of the same patients in the same Turku data set (entry 4, "ANNOTATED REFERENCES"), although not focusing exclusively on the target intervention, clearly indicated a substantial rate of cure.

It seemed likely that no significant differences would arise between radical mastectomy and modified radical mastectomy in terms of either the nature or timing of subsequent focal events. This, of course, needed to be verified in the Turku data. If verified, it would allow treating these two types of mastectomy as equivalent in effect in terms of disease progression. Both types of patients could then be combined to form a single intervention sample.

Preliminary inspection of the data showed an abrupt reversal in the mid-1980s in the relative mix of radical mastectomies versus modified radical mastectomies performed. On patients diagnosed prior to 1985, approximately three radical mastectomies were performed for every one modified radical mastectomy. This ratio remained reasonably stable from 1945 through 1984. For patients diagnosed thereafter, this ratio changed to approximately nine modified radical mastectomies for every one radical mastectomy.

Such an abrupt reversal would normally require detailed investigation, most especially of its consequences. An equally dramatic change occurred elsewhere in the Turku data set with potentially misleading results.

Recall that no type of adjuvant therapy was recorded for any patients diagnosed before 1966. Tamoxifen was the principal form of adjuvant therapy introduced after 1966. Initially, it seems, tamoxifen was prescribed in a very selective manner, mostly to the "sickest" patients in relatively advanced stages of disease progression. These patients had the poorest prognoses.

A raw comparison of outcomes between patients who initially received tamoxifen and those who did not suggested that tamoxifen hastened both the recurrence of breast cancer and disease-specific death. This seemingly harmful impact was both strong and statistically significant. Only after the same comparison was restricted to matched pairs of patients diagnosed in the same stage of disease progression was the true impact of the drug revealed. Tamoxifen was then shown to have a strong and significant beneficial impact.

Fortunately, a similar modification was not required to facilitate cure assessment. It was only necessary to show that, regardless of what inspired the historical reversal in surgical practice, the two procedures were equivalent in terms of their respective impacts on disease progression in whatever subset of patients was finally selected for analysis. Then the two subsamples of patients might legitimately be merged into a single sample.

A sufficiently lengthy follow-up period is always required to assess the curative impact of any medical intervention. At least seven years would seem minimally adequate in the present context. This observation suggests an easy way to resolve the issue. Restricting the analysis to patients diagnosed before 1985 not only ensured the required follow-up period; it simultaneously avoided mixing prereversal and postreversal patients in the same sample. It will be shown in section 4.4 that there are no discernible differences in terms of impact on disease progression between radical mastectomy and modified radical mastectomy patients diagnosed prior to 1985. Therefore, the two subsamples can and will be combined to form a single intervention sample.

4.2 Additional Steps to Homogenize the Analysis

A small proportion of the 2,192 Turku patients (about 7 percent) experienced breast cancer bilaterally. In most cases (about 83 percent) there was a distinct interval of time (at least one month) separating the initial diagnosis of breast cancer and the subsequent detection of cancer in the other breast. The median time interval between these two events was about five years. For one patient the time interval exceeded thirty years.

Including bilateral patients in the analysis could cause confusion. It was not universally clear whether instances of bilaterality should be treated as separately and independently developing cancers or as evidence of disease progression (i.e., as a focal event relative to the original diagnosis of cancer in the other breast). To eliminate any such confusion, all bilateral patients were deleted from the intervention sample.

Approximately 87 percent of the Turku patients were women diagnosed with either ductal or lobular breast cancer. The remaining 13 percent were diagnosed with a variety of "special" breast problems. "Special" problems were not clearly identified in the data set. Therefore, the intervention sample was also restricted to female ductal and lobular breast cancer patients.

4.3 The First Intervention Sample

A subsample of 550 patients was selected from the Turku data set according to the preceding criteria. All 550 patients shared the following characteristics:

1. women diagnosed with invasive breast cancer (either ductal or lobular) between 1945 and the end of 1984 in Turku, Finland;
2. no bilaterality (as of the time last observed);
3. received a mastectomy (either radical or modified radical);
4. along with radiation therapy; but
5. not followed by any form of adjuvant therapy; and
6. patient status when last observed known and properly recorded.

Variable characteristics of these 550 patients are summarized in appendix G.

4.4 Verifying No Differences Between Radical and Modified Radical Mastectomy

Once the intervention sample had been selected, it was important to verify the legitimacy of having combined radical and modified radical mastectomy patients. There must be no evidence that these somewhat different surgical procedures had a differential impact on disease progression. Comparisons of the two patient subsamples should show no systematic differences in relevant patient outcomes.

A cross tabulation of surgical procedures and patient outcomes is shown below, along with conditional relative frequencies (proportions) for each procedure.

PATIENT STATUS WHEN LAST OBSERVED	MODIFIED RADICAL MASTECTOMY	RADICAL MASTECTOMY	TOTAL
DIED OF BREAST CANCER	66	212	278
DIED OF OTHER CANCER	6	21	27
DIED OF OTHER CAUSE	36	98	134
STILL ALIVE	17	94	111
TOTAL	125	425	550

PATIENT STATUS WHEN LAST OBSERVED	MODIFIED RADICAL MASTECTOMY	RADICAL MASTECTOMY
DIED OF BREAST CANCER	0.5280	0.4988
DIED OF OTHER CANCER	0.0480	0.0494
DIED OF OTHER CAUSE	0.2880	0.2306
STILL ALIVE	0.1360	0.2212
TOTAL	1.0000	1.0000

A chi-square statistical test was performed on the above table. The computed value of the chi-square statistic was 4.95 with three degrees of freedom. The associated two-tailed p value was 0.1758, indicating no significant difference.

Four additional tests were performed. Each test produced a pair of Kaplan-Meier curves with respect to a separate focal event. The first Kaplan-Meier curve in each pair was based on modified radical mastectomy patients. The second curve was based on radical mastectomy patients. The significance of the difference between the two curves in each pair was then assessed via the log-rank test.

Computed chi-square values and associated p values derived from the log-rank tests are shown below for each of the four separate focal events. In all four cases, the null hypothesis tested was that survival outcomes were identical in the modified radical mastectomy and the radical mastectomy populations from which the two patient subsamples were drawn.

1. When the focal event was the first relapse or recurrence of breast cancer following the intervention, the log-rank test generated a chi-square value of 0.91 with one degree of freedom and an associated two-tailed p value of 0.3396, again indicating no significant difference.
2. When the focal event was death due to breast cancer, the log-rank test generated a chi-square value of 0.46 with one degree of freedom and an associated two-tailed p value of 0.4970, again indicating no significant difference.
3. When the focal event was either the first relapse or recurrence of breast cancer or death due to breast cancer, whichever occurred first following the intervention (if either occurred), the log-rank test generated a chi-square value of 0.43 with one degree of freedom and an associated two-tailed p value of 0.5134, again indicating no significant difference.
4. When the focal event was death from any cause (including breast cancer), the log-rank test generated a chi-square value of 1.96 with one degree of freedom and an associated two-tailed p value of 0.1620, again indicating no significant difference.

Because all four tests generated insignificant results, the corresponding graphical representations (i.e., the four pairs of Kaplan-Meier curves) are not shown.

The message seems clear. There were no discernible differences between the radical and the modified radical mastectomy in terms of their impact on disease progression. It seems entirely reasonable to combine the two subsamples.

Due to the abrupt reversal in surgical practice that occurred with patients diagnosed beginning in 1985 and in order to obtain a lengthy follow-up period, the intervention sample was restricted to patients diagnosed no later than 1984. Some of the other (homogenizing) restrictions applied to selecting the intervention sample pushed the latest date of diagnosis back even further to 1980. As a result, the subsequent follow-up period was extended to 16.16 years (February 1980 to April 1996).

4.5 Executing an Initial Kaplan-Meier Survival Analysis

The next step was to define a focal event specifically tailored to facilitate cure assessment and to execute an initial Kaplan-Meier survival analysis in terms of it.

Any patient who experienced either a relapse or recurrence of breast cancer or death due to breast cancer following mastectomy and radiation was clearly not cured by that intervention. Each of these events constituted an unambiguous indication of further disease progression. Each provided indisputable proof that the patient remained at substantial risk (SR) despite the intervention.

The focal event was therefore defined as whichever of these events occurred first (if any occurred). Its elapsed time since the patient was originally diagnosed became the focal event time. If none of these events had (yet) occurred when the patient was last seen, the time elapsed between diagnosis and last follow-up alive (or other death) was treated as a censored observation.

The KAPM (Kaplan-Meier) procedure was invoked to produce a Kaplan-Meier survival analysis. Annotated outputs of the procedure are shown below and on the next several pages between the horizontal lines. A graphical representation of exactly the same output appears later in figure 7 as the corresponding Kaplan-Meier survival curve.

Keep in mind, however, that any MR patients who were cured by the intervention would show up among the censored observations. Because the Kaplan-Meier analysis assumes that all patients remain at risk (SR), there is no way at this point in the analysis to discriminate between:

1. a censored observation signifying that an SR patient has not yet experienced the focal event, but would if observed for a sufficiently long time in the absence of competing-risk censoring events; and
2. a censored observation signifying that an MR patient has been cured by the intervention and, therefore, is no longer at substantial risk of experiencing the focal event, no matter how long observed.

DESCRIPTIVE SUMMARY OF ELAPSED TIME INTERVALS

The set of strictly positive elapsed observation time intervals relating to 550 PATIENTs constitutes the effective sample for the descriptive summary. There are 401 distinct elapsed time intervals in this set. The complete observation window (i.e., the longest elapsed time interval observed) is 43.0837 elapsed time unit(s). The time unit is one full year.

The MINIMUM number of elapsed time units observed is 0.0821.
The MEDIAN number of elapsed time units observed is 6.5819.
The MAXIMUM number of elapsed time units observed is 43.0837.
The MEAN number of elapsed time units observed is 10.0460,
with a STANDARD DEVIATION of 9.1527.

KAPLAN-MEIER ANALYSIS (SURVIVAL RATE ESTIMATED VIA THE PRODUCT-LIMIT METHOD)

The same set of strictly positive elapsed observation time intervals relating to 550 PATIENTs constitutes the effective sample for the Kaplan-Meier analysis. It focuses on the particular subset of 197 distinct intervals that terminate with the occurrence of at least one focal event. In addition, the analysis considers all truncated-observation intervals that terminate before a focal event has occurred (censored observations), if any exist. A total of 293 focal events occur during the observation subwindow that encompasses all events. This observation subwindow spans 24.2524 elapsed time unit(s).

ELAPSED TIME UNITS	NUMBER OF EVENTS	NUMBER AT RISK	HAZARD RATE	CUMULATIVE HAZARD RATE	KAPLAN–MEIER SURVIVAL RATE	STANDARD ERROR
0.0000	N/A	550	N/A	N/A	1.0000	N/A
0.0821	1	550	0.0018	0.0018	0.9982	0.0018
0.0849	2	549	0.0036	0.0055	0.9945	0.0031
0.1615	1	547	0.0018	0.0073	0.9927	0.0036
0.1670	2	546	0.0037	0.0110	0.9891	0.0044
0.1698	1	544	0.0018	0.0128	0.9873	0.0048
0.2491	1	543	0.0018	0.0146	0.9855	0.0051
0.2519	3	542	0.0055	0.0202	0.9800	0.0060
0.3285	1	539	0.0019	0.0220	0.9782	0.0062
0.3313	3	538	0.0056	0.0276	0.9727	0.0069
0.3340	3	535	0.0056	0.0332	0.9673	0.0076
0.4107	1	532	0.0019	0.0351	0.9655	0.0078
0.4134	4	531	0.0075	0.0426	0.9582	0.0085
0.4189	3	527	0.0057	0.0483	0.9527	0.0090
0.4956	1	524	0.0019	0.0502	0.9509	0.0092
0.5010	1	523	0.0019	0.0521	0.9491	0.0094
0.5804	3	521	0.0058	0.0579	0.9436	0.0098
0.5832	1	518	0.0019	0.0598	0.9418	0.0100
0.5859	1	517	0.0019	0.0618	0.9400	0.0101
0.5887	1	515	0.0019	0.0637	0.9382	0.0103
0.6626	2	514	0.0039	0.0676	0.9345	0.0106
0.6653	3	512	0.0059	0.0734	0.9290	0.0110
0.6680	2	509	0.0039	0.0774	0.9254	0.0112
0.6708	1	507	0.0020	0.0793	0.9236	0.0113
0.7529	1	506	0.0020	0.0813	0.9217	0.0115
0.7557	1	505	0.0020	0.0833	0.9199	0.0116
0.8296	1	504	0.0020	0.0853	0.9181	0.0117
0.8323	4	503	0.0080	0.0932	0.9108	0.0122
0.8351	2	499	0.0040	0.0972	0.9071	0.0124
0.8378	3	497	0.0060	0.1033	0.9017	0.0127
0.9145	2	494	0.0040	0.1073	0.8980	0.0129
0.9172	4	492	0.0081	0.1155	0.8907	0.0133
0.9199	2	488	0.0041	0.1196	0.8871	0.0135
0.9993	1	486	0.0021	0.1216	0.8852	0.0136
1.0815	1	484	0.0021	0.1237	0.8834	0.0137
1.0842	3	483	0.0062	0.1299	0.8779	0.0140
1.1609	2	480	0.0042	0.1341	0.8743	0.0142
1.1663	3	478	0.0063	0.1403	0.8688	0.0144
1.1691	2	475	0.0042	0.1446	0.8651	0.0146
1.2457	1	473	0.0021	0.1467	0.8633	0.0147
1.2485	1	472	0.0021	0.1488	0.8614	0.0148
1.2512	4	471	0.0085	0.1573	0.8541	0.0151
1.2540	2	467	0.0043	0.1616	0.8505	0.0152
1.3306	1	465	0.0022	0.1637	0.8486	0.0153
1.3334	3	464	0.0065	0.1702	0.8432	0.0155
1.3361	2	461	0.0043	0.1745	0.8395	0.0157
1.4100	1	459	0.0022	0.1767	0.8377	0.0158
1.4128	2	458	0.0044	0.1811	0.8340	0.0159
1.4182	2	456	0.0044	0.1854	0.8304	0.0160
1.4210	2	454	0.0044	0.1899	0.8267	0.0162
1.4976	1	452	0.0022	0.1921	0.8249	0.0162
1.5004	1	451	0.0022	0.1943	0.8230	0.0163
1.5031	1	450	0.0022	0.1965	0.8212	0.0164
1.5058	1	449	0.0022	0.1987	0.8194	0.0164
1.5798	2	448	0.0045	0.2032	0.8157	0.0166

ELAPSED TIME UNITS	NUMBER OF EVENTS	NUMBER AT RISK	HAZARD RATE	CUMULATIVE HAZARD RATE	KAPLAN-MEIER SURVIVAL RATE	STANDARD ERROR
1.5825	2	446	0.0045	0.2077	0.8121	0.0167
1.5852	2	444	0.0045	0.2122	0.8084	0.0168
1.6619	1	442	0.0023	0.2144	0.8066	0.0169
1.6674	2	441	0.0045	0.2190	0.8029	0.0170
1.6701	3	439	0.0068	0.2258	0.7974	0.0172
1.7468	1	436	0.0023	0.2281	0.7956	0.0172
1.7495	3	435	0.0069	0.2350	0.7901	0.0174
1.8317	1	432	0.0023	0.2373	0.7883	0.0175
1.8344	2	431	0.0046	0.2420	0.7846	0.0176
1.8371	1	429	0.0023	0.2443	0.7828	0.0176
1.9138	1	428	0.0023	0.2466	0.7810	0.0177
1.9165	1	427	0.0023	0.2490	0.7791	0.0177
1.9220	1	425	0.0024	0.2513	0.7773	0.0178
1.9247	1	424	0.0024	0.2537	0.7755	0.0178
1.9987	1	423	0.0024	0.2560	0.7736	0.0179
2.0014	3	422	0.0071	0.2632	0.7681	0.0180
2.0835	1	417	0.0024	0.2656	0.7663	0.0181
2.1629	1	415	0.0024	0.2680	0.7645	0.0181
2.1684	2	414	0.0048	0.2728	0.7608	0.0182
2.2451	1	412	0.0024	0.2752	0.7589	0.0183
2.2478	2	411	0.0049	0.2801	0.7552	0.0184
2.2506	2	408	0.0049	0.2850	0.7515	0.0185
2.2533	1	406	0.0025	0.2874	0.7497	0.0185
2.3300	1	405	0.0025	0.2899	0.7478	0.0186
2.3327	1	404	0.0025	0.2924	0.7460	0.0186
2.4176	1	403	0.0025	0.2949	0.7441	0.0187
2.4203	3	402	0.0075	0.3023	0.7386	0.0188
2.4970	1	399	0.0025	0.3048	0.7367	0.0188
2.4997	1	398	0.0025	0.3074	0.7349	0.0189
2.5024	1	397	0.0025	0.3099	0.7330	0.0189
2.5818	1	396	0.0025	0.3124	0.7312	0.0190
2.5873	2	395	0.0051	0.3175	0.7275	0.0191
2.6667	3	393	0.0076	0.3251	0.7219	0.0192
2.6722	1	390	0.0026	0.3277	0.7201	0.0192
2.7489	2	389	0.0051	0.3328	0.7164	0.0193
2.8337	3	387	0.0078	0.3406	0.7108	0.0194
2.8392	1	383	0.0026	0.3432	0.7089	0.0194
2.9131	1	382	0.0026	0.3458	0.7071	0.0195
2.9159	1	381	0.0026	0.3484	0.7052	0.0195
2.9186	2	379	0.0053	0.3537	0.7015	0.0196
3.0007	4	377	0.0106	0.3643	0.6941	0.0197
3.0829	1	373	0.0027	0.3670	0.6922	0.0198
3.1678	2	371	0.0054	0.3724	0.6885	0.0198
3.2444	1	369	0.0027	0.3751	0.6866	0.0199
3.2526	1	368	0.0027	0.3778	0.6847	0.0199
3.3293	1	366	0.0027	0.3805	0.6829	0.0199
3.3348	2	365	0.0055	0.3860	0.6791	0.0200
3.4142	2	362	0.0055	0.3915	0.6754	0.0201
3.4169	1	360	0.0028	0.3943	0.6735	0.0201
3.4196	1	359	0.0028	0.3971	0.6716	0.0201
3.4963	2	358	0.0056	0.4027	0.6679	0.0202
3.5867	1	356	0.0028	0.4055	0.6660	0.0202
3.6715	1	354	0.0028	0.4083	0.6641	0.0203
3.7482	3	353	0.0085	0.4168	0.6585	0.0203
3.7564	1	350	0.0029	0.4197	0.6566	0.0204
3.8303	1	349	0.0029	0.4225	0.6547	0.0204

ELAPSED TIME UNITS	NUMBER OF EVENTS	NUMBER AT RISK	HAZARD RATE	CUMULATIVE HAZARD RATE	KAPLAN-MEIER SURVIVAL RATE	STANDARD ERROR
3.8331	1	348	0.0029	0.4254	0.6528	0.0204
3.8385	1	346	0.0029	0.4283	0.6509	0.0205
3.9152	3	345	0.0087	0.4370	0.6453	0.0205
3.9179	1	341	0.0029	0.4399	0.6434	0.0206
3.9234	1	340	0.0029	0.4429	0.6415	0.0206
4.0001	3	339	0.0088	0.4517	0.6358	0.0207
4.0822	1	336	0.0030	0.4547	0.6339	0.0207
4.1671	1	335	0.0030	0.4577	0.6320	0.0207
4.2465	1	334	0.0030	0.4607	0.6301	0.0207
4.2492	1	333	0.0030	0.4637	0.6283	0.0208
4.2520	2	332	0.0060	0.4697	0.6245	0.0208
4.3341	2	330	0.0061	0.4758	0.6207	0.0209
4.3368	1	328	0.0030	0.4788	0.6188	0.0209
4.4135	1	327	0.0031	0.4819	0.6169	0.0209
4.5011	1	324	0.0031	0.4850	0.6150	0.0209
4.5039	1	323	0.0031	0.4881	0.6131	0.0209
4.5805	2	320	0.0063	0.4943	0.6093	0.0210
4.6654	1	317	0.0032	0.4975	0.6073	0.0210
4.7475	1	316	0.0032	0.5006	0.6054	0.0210
4.7503	1	315	0.0032	0.5038	0.6035	0.0211
4.8324	2	314	0.0064	0.5102	0.5996	0.0211
4.8351	1	311	0.0032	0.5134	0.5977	0.0211
5.0022	1	309	0.0032	0.5166	0.5958	0.0211
5.0843	1	308	0.0032	0.5199	0.5939	0.0212
5.0870	1	306	0.0033	0.5231	0.5919	0.0212
5.2513	2	304	0.0066	0.5297	0.5880	0.0212
5.4211	1	301	0.0033	0.5330	0.5861	0.0212
5.5032	1	299	0.0033	0.5364	0.5841	0.0213
5.6647	1	297	0.0034	0.5397	0.5821	0.0213
5.6702	1	296	0.0034	0.5431	0.5802	0.0213
5.8345	1	294	0.0034	0.5465	0.5782	0.0213
5.9139	2	292	0.0068	0.5534	0.5742	0.0213
5.9166	1	290	0.0034	0.5568	0.5723	0.0214
5.9988	2	289	0.0069	0.5637	0.5683	0.0214
6.0015	1	286	0.0035	0.5672	0.5663	0.0214
6.0782	1	285	0.0035	0.5707	0.5643	0.0214
6.0809	1	284	0.0035	0.5743	0.5623	0.0214
6.1630	2	283	0.0071	0.5813	0.5584	0.0215
6.2534	1	280	0.0036	0.5849	0.5564	0.0215
6.4943	1	279	0.0036	0.5885	0.5544	0.0215
6.4998	1	278	0.0036	0.5921	0.5524	0.0215
6.5025	1	277	0.0036	0.5957	0.5504	0.0215
6.5053	1	276	0.0036	0.5993	0.5484	0.0216
6.5819	1	275	0.0036	0.6030	0.5464	0.0216
6.6641	1	274	0.0036	0.6066	0.5444	0.0216
6.8338	1	273	0.0037	0.6103	0.5424	0.0216
7.0008	2	271	0.0074	0.6177	0.5384	0.0216
7.1678	2	267	0.0075	0.6251	0.5344	0.0216
7.2445	1	265	0.0038	0.6289	0.5324	0.0217
7.3321	1	264	0.0038	0.6327	0.5303	0.0217
7.4143	3	263	0.0114	0.6441	0.5243	0.0217
7.4197	1	259	0.0039	0.6480	0.5223	0.0217
7.5867	1	258	0.0039	0.6518	0.5202	0.0217
7.6661	1	256	0.0039	0.6558	0.5182	0.0217
7.6716	1	255	0.0039	0.6597	0.5162	0.0217
7.7483	1	254	0.0039	0.6636	0.5141	0.0217

ELAPSED TIME UNITS	NUMBER OF EVENTS	NUMBER AT RISK	HAZARD RATE	CUMULATIVE HAZARD RATE	KAPLAN-MEIER SURVIVAL RATE	STANDARD ERROR
7.7510	1	253	0.0040	0.6676	0.5121	0.0218
7.8332	2	252	0.0079	0.6755	0.5080	0.0218
8.0850	1	249	0.0040	0.6795	0.5060	0.0218
8.1699	1	248	0.0040	0.6835	0.5040	0.0218
8.4191	2	246	0.0081	0.6917	0.4999	0.0218
8.4985	1	244	0.0041	0.6958	0.4978	0.0218
8.7504	1	240	0.0042	0.6999	0.4957	0.0218
8.8325	1	239	0.0042	0.7041	0.4937	0.0218
8.9174	1	237	0.0042	0.7083	0.4916	0.0218
9.7469	1	230	0.0043	0.7127	0.4895	0.0218
10.1658	1	225	0.0044	0.7171	0.4873	0.0219
10.2507	1	224	0.0045	0.7216	0.4851	0.0219
10.2535	1	223	0.0045	0.7261	0.4829	0.0219
10.3356	1	221	0.0045	0.7306	0.4807	0.0219
10.7518	1	218	0.0046	0.7352	0.4785	0.0219
11.3349	1	210	0.0048	0.7400	0.4763	0.0219
11.7484	1	206	0.0049	0.7448	0.4739	0.0219
11.8332	1	203	0.0049	0.7497	0.4716	0.0219
12.1700	1	201	0.0050	0.7547	0.4693	0.0220
12.3370	1	198	0.0051	0.7598	0.4669	0.0220
12.7477	1	196	0.0051	0.7649	0.4645	0.0220
12.8298	1	194	0.0052	0.7700	0.4621	0.0220
12.9147	1	193	0.0052	0.7752	0.4597	0.0220
13.5828	1	189	0.0053	0.7805	0.4573	0.0220
14.9161	1	178	0.0056	0.7861	0.4547	0.0221
17.3364	1	138	0.0072	0.7934	0.4514	0.0221
17.6622	1	133	0.0075	0.8009	0.4480	0.0222
17.6705	1	131	0.0076	0.8085	0.4446	0.0223
18.6643	1	115	0.0087	0.8172	0.4407	0.0225
20.4193	1	88	0.0114	0.8286	0.4357	0.0228
24.2524	1	38	0.0263	0.8549	0.4243	0.0249

TOTAL   293

ELAPSED TIME UNITS identifies the length of each distinct time interval that is terminated by one or more focal events. All focal events that occur within such an interval occur at the end of that interval, at the exact moment when the interval expires. All times are elapsed times from some initiating event, such as date of birth, date of onset of some illness, date of diagnosis, date of some therapeutic intervention, and so on. Typical time units are days, weeks, months, and years.

NUMBER OF EVENTS is a count of the number of focal events that occur at the end of an elapsed time interval, thus terminating that interval. Typical focal events are death due to a specific cause, death due to any cause, relapse, and recurrence. The focal event count does not include instances where the observation process becomes truncated for one reason or another (i.e., where observations become censored).

NUMBER AT RISK is a count of the number of entities (e.g., patients) observed that have not yet experienced the focal event just prior to the end of the time interval, but that are at risk of experiencing it before that interval ends.

HAZARD RATE is the proportion of those entities at risk just prior to the end of the time interval that do experience the focal event when the interval ends. It is simply the NUMBER OF EVENTS divided by the NUMBER AT RISK.

CUMULATIVE HAZARD RATE is the cumulative sum of the HAZARD RATEs over successive time intervals. It is useful in fitting, statistically, various hazard functions (such as the exponential and Weibull functions) to observed data.

KAPLAN-MEIER SURVIVAL RATE indicates the proportion of those entities (e.g., patients) that have survived up to and through the end of an interval without experiencing the focal event. If the focal event occurs, it occurs after the end of that interval. It is computed by first subtracting each HAZARD RATE up to and including the current HAZARD RATE from 1.0 and then multiplying together all these differences. The resulting product is called the Kaplan-Meier product-limit survival rate.

STANDARD ERROR is the standard deviation of the distribution of a KAPLAN-MEIER SURVIVAL RATE estimate around its true population value. Each estimated survival rate is based on sample data and, therefore, is likely to be somewhat in error. When the sample size is large enough (hundreds of observations), the distribution of these errors of estimation approximates a normal distribution. As the sample size grows very large, this normal approximation improves asymptotically.

Estimates of the above KAPLAN-MEIER SURVIVAL RATE(s) and the associated STANDARD ERROR(s) are based on the assumption that both the sample of elapsed focal event time intervals and the sample of truncated-observation (censored) time intervals are randomly and independently drawn from their respective populations and that these two samples are drawn independently of each other.

If the population of elapsed time intervals until an event occurs is assumed to follow an exponential distribution, implying a constant hazard rate throughout every observation subwindow, the maximum likelihood estimate of that hazard rate is 0.0530, with a standard error of 0.003098.

The assumption of an exponential distribution with a constant hazard rate produces a MARGINALLY ACCEPTABLE fit with the observed data. The analogue of an unadjusted coefficient of determination (R-squared) would be 0.4082.

If the population of elapsed time intervals until an event occurs is assumed to follow a Weibull distribution, which permits either an increasing or a decreasing hazard rate over all observation subwindows, the maximum likelihood estimate of the intensity parameter (analogous to the constant hazard rate parameter characterizing an exponential distribution) is 0.0430, with a standard error of 0.004354. In addition, there appears to be a DECREASING trend in the hazard rate over time. The maximum likelihood estimate of the trend parameter is 0.6142, with a standard error of 0.031207.

The assumption of a Weibull distribution with a DECREASING hazard rate produces a better fit with the data, at least in this complete observation window (two-tailed p value less than 0.00005). The improved value of the analogue of an unadjusted coefficient of determination (R-squared) is 0.8864, indicating a GOOD fit.

Figure 7

Kaplan-Meier Survival Analysis of 550 Patients from Turku, Finland, Initially Diagnosed With Invasive Breast Cancer and Subsequently Treated With Both Mastectomy and Radiation

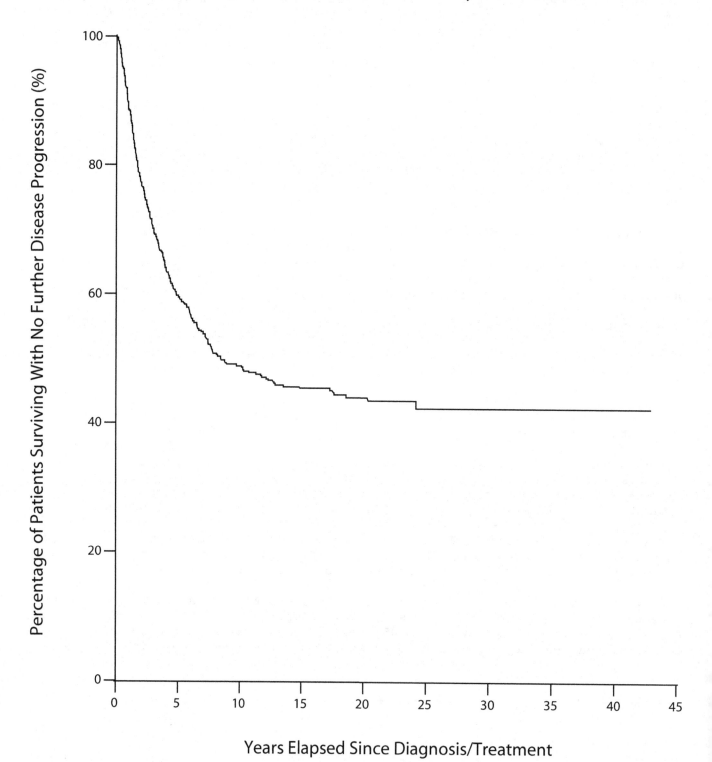

4.6 A Preliminary Interpretation of the Kaplan-Meier Survival Analysis

Looking at figure 7, the single most striking observation is that the curve seems to be falling toward a limiting survival probability (horizontal asymptote). However, that limiting probability is somewhat below 0.42 rather than anywhere near zero. The last focal event occurred after 24.2524 years, yielding an estimated survival probability of 0.4243. After that the curve appears to flatten out (i.e., become virtually horizontal).

The bottom entry in the Kaplan-Meier survival table indicates that thirty-seven other patients were followed up for more than twenty-four years to a maximum of about forty-three years. None of them had yet experienced the focal event when last seen. Because the data suggested the existence of a limiting survival probability (horizontal asymptote), because this probability fell well above zero (somewhat below 0.42), and because enough patients (thirty-seven) were followed up for a long enough time without evidence of further disease progression, it seems quite plausible to suppose that an appreciable proportion of the 550 patients in the intervention sample were actually cured.

Exactly what proportion is not yet clear. The estimate of 0.42 based only on the flattening of the Kaplan-Meier survival curve provides an upper bound. One or more of the 109 survivors among alive censored patients could conceivably still have experienced the focal event, even after a decade or two.

A detailed analysis of the eventual outcomes of the 550 patients in the total intervention sample yielded the following results.

Suffered relapse/recurrence and died of breast cancer	112	
Suffered relapse/recurrence but died of something else	13	
Suffered relapse/recurrence but still alive when last seen	2	
Suffered no relapse/recurrence but died of breast cancer	166	
Total number of patients who experienced the focal event		293
Experienced no relapse/recurrence and died of something else	148	
Experienced no relapse/recurrence and still alive when last seen	109	
Total number of censored patients (no focal event when last seen)		257
Total number of patients in the intervention sample		550
Long-term survivors among censored patients	37	
Other than long-term survivors among censored patients	220	
	257	
Long-term survivors among dead censored patients	15	
Other than long-term survivors among dead censored patients	133	
	148	
Long-term survivors among alive censored patients	22	
Other than long-term survivors among alive censored patients	87	
	109	

These results lend further support to the notion that the intervention did cure an appreciable proportion of the 550 patients. Due to the lengthy follow-up, the eventual outcome of 441 patients (over 80 percent of the 550) became clear. Four hundred thirty-nine had already died (with or without having experienced the focal event), and two had already suffered either a relapse or a recurrence but were still alive when last seen. It was only the 550 - 441 = 109 patients who had suffered neither a relapse nor a recurrence and who were still alive when last seen whose eventual fate remained unclear.

As previously discussed, some way now had to be found to partition the total intervention sample into:

1. a cured MR subsample of patients for whom the intervention was successful in altering their state from substantial risk to little or no risk of experiencing further disease progression; and
2. an SR subsample of patients for whom the intervention was not curative and who, therefore, remained at substantial risk of experiencing further disease progression despite the intervention.

Because the concept of cure had been defined as a change in state, partitioning the total intervention sample in this manner would permit applying the traditional Kaplan-Meier paradigm in a more focused way. The underlying statistical model would be reformulated in Bayesian terms. The Bayesian framework enabled by reformulation would then restrict applying both Kaplan-Meier and Cox regression analyses only to SR patients (i.e., only to the SR subsample).

The Bayesian framework would provide three additional benefits.

1. It would produce an estimate of the curative impact of mastectomy and radiation on the population of patients from which the sample was drawn (i.e., an estimate of the population proportion cured by that medical intervention).
2. It would produce an initial estimate of the (prior) probability that each individual patient was, in fact, cured by mastectomy and radiation. Each initial cure probability would be tailored on the basis of whatever of prognostic significance was known about that patient and recorded in the data set. This would be accomplished by a multiple logistic regression analysis executed on the entire sample of 550 patients.
3. By combining the results of multiple Cox regression (applied selectively to only the SR subsample) with multiple logistic regression (applied to all patients in the sample) according to Bayes' theorem, the framework would also produce a time-phased estimate of each patient's (posterior) cure probability.

It is the production of a Bayesian posterior cure probability that answers in individually tailored and time-phased probabilistic terms the question so often posed by so many patients:

> "For how long must I wait with no evidence of further disease progression before concluding that my treatment was successful; that I beat the cancer; and that I have actually been cured?"

Before exploiting the Bayesian framework to partition the intervention sample into MR and SR subsamples, however, we must first establish that at least some of the 550 Turku patients were very likely cured.

4.7   The RISKTEST Simulator

The luxury of long-term follow-up in the Turku data set offered an additional benefit. Because the complete history and final outcome of almost 80 percent of the patients in the intervention sample were known as of April 1996, the process of acquiring them, diagnosing them, treating them, and following them up may be simulated in some detail. The RISKTEST simulator described in appendix H accomplishes this task.

RISKTEST was designed to mimic as closely as possible the entire sequence of events occurring between 1945 and 1996.

1. The patient acquisition period spanned 34.84 years between April 1945, when the first of the 550 patients was diagnosed and treated, and February 1980, when the last patient was diagnosed and treated.
2. The follow-up period began in February 1980 and ended in April 1996, spanning 16.16 years.
3. The focal event was actually experienced by 293 of the 550 patients.
4. An analysis of the 111 patients still alive in April 1996 showed the following rather distinct pattern of follow-up.

   A. Thirty-three (29.7 percent) were last seen at a uniform rate of approximately two each month over the previous sixteen months.
   B. Sixty-one (55.0 percent) were last seen during December 1994.
   C. Ten (9.0 percent) were last seen during December 1992.
   D. Seven (6.3 percent) were apparently lost to regular follow-up (an overall loss to follow-up of 7/550 = 1.3 percent).

5. This pattern was coded within a specially constructed subroutine of the RISKTEST simulator. The subroutine was executed whenever RISKTEST was invoked with a -1 entry to designate its follow-up cycle.
6. Simulation of the focal event was based on the results of the Kaplan-Meier analysis of all 550 patients presented in section 4.5. The parameters of the best-fitting Weibull distribution with a significantly decreasing hazard rate over time (R-squared = 0.8864) served as inputs to RISKTEST. The Weibull intensity parameter for the focal event was 0.0430. The corresponding Weibull trend parameter was 0.6142.
7. A second Kaplan-Meier analysis was performed on the same 550-patient data to obtain separate simulation parameters for death due to other cancers and death due to other causes. Several statistical tests were first performed to ensure that there were no significant differences between patients who experienced these two separate events.

   A. A chi-square test comparing the T staging distributions of twenty-seven patients who died of some other cancer with 134 patients who died of some other (noncancer) cause showed no significant difference (two-tailed p value = 0.9774).
   B. A chi-square test comparing their N staging distributions also showed no significant difference (two-tailed p value = 0.6873).
   C. A Fisher exact test comparing their M staging distributions also showed no significant difference (two-tailed p value = 0.8323).
   D. A t test of the difference between their mean tumor sizes also showed no significant difference (two-tailed p value = 0.4590). This result was reinforced by a Mann-Whitney test (two-tailed p value = 0.6586) and by a median test (two-tailed p value = 0.9857).

E. A chi-square test comparing their tumor grade distributions also showed no significant difference (two-tailed p value = 0.8156).

F. A chi-square test comparing their degree of necrosis distributions also showed no significant difference (two-tailed p value = 0.2238).

G. A t test of the difference between their mean times (in years) elapsed between diagnosis and death (all causes) also showed no significant difference (two-tailed p value = .7363). This result was reinforced by a Mann-Whitney test (two-tailed p value = 0.8777) and by a median test (two-tailed p value = 1.0000).

H. A chi-square test comparing their mitotic rate distributions showed a suggestive, but not a significant, difference (two-tailed p value = 0.0824). Patients who died of another cancer tended to have somewhat higher mitotic rates than patients who died of a cause other than cancer.

8. Since no significant differences emerged in any of these tests, the two events were treated as a single composite event, death from other than breast cancer, experienced by 27 + 134 = 161 of the 550 patients.

9. In the second Kaplan-Meier analysis, death from other than breast cancer was treated as the focal event, while death due to breast cancer was treated as just another censoring event. The best fit to the data was achieved by a Weibull distribution with a significantly increasing hazard rate over time (R-squared = 0.9957). The Weibull intensity parameter for death from other than breast cancer was 0.0370. The corresponding Weibull trend parameter was 1.6950.

The RISKTEST simulator may be used to investigate the Turku intervention sample for evidence that mastectomy and radiation succeeded in curing at least some patients. RISKTEST will enable execution of a simulation-based hypothesis test.

The null hypothesis will be that no patients were cured. This means that all 550 patients are presumed to have remained at substantial risk (in the SR category) despite their mastectomy and radiation.

The alternate hypothesis will be that at least some patients were cured. It is directional relative to the actual number of patients who experienced the focal event. The higher the number of patients presumed to have been cured, the lower will be the number simulated as experiencing the focal event.

The test statistic will be the simulated number of patients experiencing the focal event. The distribution of this test statistic expected under the null hypothesis will be generated by the RISKTEST simulator, fitted to the Turku data as described above via maximum likelihood estimation.

RISKTEST will execute a simulation run of one hundred thousand trials. With that many trials, a symmetric, unimodal, quite normal-looking distribution of simulated focal event counts will be generated.

Exactly where within the one-hundred-thousand-trial simulated distribution the observed number of 293 Turku patients actually experiencing the focal event falls will constitute the test of the hypothesis. Evidence favoring the null hypothesis will be closeness of the observed count of 293 to the middle of the simulated distribution. Due to the unimodality and symmetry imposed by the central limit theorem, the mode and mean of the simulated distribution will coincide (approximately) to form its midpoint (median).

Downward displacement of 293 below the combined mode, median, and mean will constitute evidence favoring the alternate hypothesis.

The exact percentile location in the simulated distribution where 293 falls will serve as a one-tailed p value. Thus, if 293 falls at or below the fifth percentile, the null hypothesis (that all 550 patients remained at risk and that none were cured) may be rejected at the conventional 5 percent significance level. Otherwise, the null hypothesis cannot be rejected.

Because the null and alternate hypotheses are strictly directional in this context, it makes little sense to calculate a bidirectional two-tailed p value. What does it mean to contemplate more than all the patients remaining at risk of further disease progression after their mastectomy and radiation?

A run of one hundred thousand simulation trials was made by the RISKTEST simulator with the following inputs.

NUMBER OF PATIENTS ACQUIRED: 550
NUMBER OF MR PATIENTS AT VERY LOW/NO RISK: 0
OBSERVED NUMBER OF PATIENTS ACTUALLY EXPERIENCING THE FOCAL EVENT: 293
NUMBER OF YEARS CONSTITUTING PATIENT ACQUISITION PERIOD: 34.8371
NUMBER OF YEARS CONSTITUTING PATIENT FOLLOW-UP PERIOD: 16.1646
NUMBER OF YEARS CONSTITUTING PATIENT FOLLOW-UP CYCLE: -1
WEIBULL INTENSITY PARAMETER FOR FOCAL EVENT: 0.0430
WEIBULL TREND PARAMETER FOR FOCAL EVENT: 0.6142
WEIBULL INTENSITY PARAMETER FOR DEATH NOT DUE TO BREAST CANCER: 0.0370
WEIBULL TREND PARAMETER FOR DEATH NOT DUE TO BREAST CANCER: 1.6950

Results are presented below and on the next two pages. Lightly edited computer output appears between the horizontal lines.

The simulated number of patients experiencing the focal event was less than the observed number (293) in 3,492 trials.
The simulated number of patients experiencing the focal event was equal to the observed number (293) in 714 trials.
The simulated number of patients experiencing the focal event was more than the observed number (293) in 95,794 trials.

If interpreted as a statistical test of the goodness of fit of the hypothesized (i.e., no cure) simulation model with the target number of patients actually observed to have experienced the focal event (293), the fit is not very close, with a directional (one-tailed) p value of (3,492 + 714) / 100,000 = 0.04206.

Below are tabled the detailed results of the one hundred thousand simulation trials. The second column counts the number of such trials (out of one hundred thousand) in which the number of patients who experience the focal event is as indicated in the first column. The third and fourth columns show these counts as equivalent relative and cumulative relative frequencies, respectively.

NUMBER OF PATIENTS WHO EXPERIENCE THE FOCAL EVENT	ABSOLUTE FREQUENCIES (COUNTS)	RELATIVE FREQUENCIES (PROPORTIONS)	CUMULATIVE RELATIVE FREQUENCIES
263	1	0.00001	0.00001
265	1	0.00001	0.00002
266	1	0.00001	0.00003
268	1	0.00001	0.00004

NUMBER OF PATIENTS WHO EXPERIENCE THE FOCAL EVENT	ABSOLUTE FREQUENCIES (COUNTS)	RELATIVE FREQUENCIES (PROPORTIONS)	CUMULATIVE RELATIVE FREQUENCIES
269	5	0.00005	0.00009
270	3	0.00003	0.00012
271	3	0.00003	0.00015
272	4	0.00004	0.00019
273	5	0.00005	0.00024
274	11	0.00011	0.00035
275	12	0.00012	0.00047
276	18	0.00018	0.00065
277	28	0.00028	0.00093
278	23	0.00023	0.00116
279	54	0.00054	0.00170
280	52	0.00052	0.00222
281	74	0.00074	0.00296
282	78	0.00078	0.00374
283	108	0.00108	0.00482
284	141	0.00141	0.00623
285	148	0.00148	0.00771
286	190	0.00190	0.00961
287	223	0.00223	0.01184
288	294	0.00294	0.01478
289	392	0.00392	0.01870
290	460	0.00460	0.02330
291	493	0.00493	0.02823
292	669	0.00669	0.03492
293	714	0.00714	0.04206
294	795	0.00795	0.05001
295	975	0.00975	0.05976
296	1048	0.01048	0.07024
297	1166	0.01166	0.08190
298	1399	0.01399	0.09589
299	1579	0.01579	0.11168
300	1734	0.01734	0.12902
301	1871	0.01871	0.14773
302	2078	0.02078	0.16851
303	2267	0.02267	0.19118
304	2432	0.02432	0.21550
305	2463	0.02463	0.24013
306	2682	0.02682	0.26695
307	2964	0.02964	0.29659
308	3053	0.03053	0.32712
309	3117	0.03117	0.35829
310	3297	0.03297	0.39126
311	3370	0.03370	0.42496
312	3471	0.03471	0.45967
313	3371	0.03371	0.49338
314	3489	0.03489	0.52827
315	3469	0.03469	0.56296
316	3369	0.03369	0.59665
317	3311	0.03311	0.62976
318	3321	0.03321	0.66297
319	3084	0.03084	0.69381
320	2915	0.02915	0.72296
321	2764	0.02764	0.75060
322	2697	0.02697	0.77757
323	2487	0.02487	0.80244

NUMBER OF PATIENTS WHO EXPERIENCE THE FOCAL EVENT	ABSOLUTE FREQUENCIES (COUNTS)	RELATIVE FREQUENCIES (PROPORTIONS)	CUMULATIVE RELATIVE FREQUENCIES
324	2360	0.02360	0.82604
325	2167	0.02167	0.84771
326	1982	0.01982	0.86753
327	1754	0.01754	0.88507
328	1627	0.01627	0.90134
329	1497	0.01497	0.91631
330	1249	0.01249	0.92880
331	1114	0.01114	0.93994
332	919	0.00919	0.94913
333	856	0.00856	0.95769
334	707	0.00707	0.96476
335	635	0.00635	0.97111
336	532	0.00532	0.97643
337	467	0.00467	0.98110
338	365	0.00365	0.98475
339	333	0.00333	0.98808
340	249	0.00249	0.99057
341	188	0.00188	0.99245
342	162	0.00162	0.99407
343	131	0.00131	0.99538
344	95	0.00095	0.99633
345	77	0.00077	0.99710
346	57	0.00057	0.99767
347	68	0.00068	0.99835
348	37	0.00037	0.99872
349	31	0.00031	0.99903
350	28	0.00028	0.99931
351	15	0.00015	0.99946
352	14	0.00014	0.99960
353	13	0.00013	0.99973
354	10	0.00010	0.99983
355	8	0.00008	0.99991
356	2	0.00002	0.99993
358	2	0.00002	0.99995
359	1	0.00001	0.99996
360	1	0.00001	0.99997
361	1	0.00001	0.99998
362	1	0.00001	0.99999
363	1	0.00001	1.00000
TOTAL	100000	1.00000	

The 293 patients actually observed to have experienced the focal event were fewer than the most frequently occurring simulated number of 314. The median number of simulated patients experiencing the focal event was also 314. That the mode and median of the simulated distribution would coincide was essentially guaranteed by virtue of the central limit theorem operating on such a very large number of Monte Carlo simulation trials. For the same reason, the simulated distribution appeared symmetric, unimodal, and quite normal-looking.

It would be difficult, although not impossible, to interpret these results as supporting the presumption that none of the 550 Turku patients was cured by mastectomy and radiation. Someone strongly committed to the notion that invasive breast cancer cannot be permanently cured might take solace in the observation that the null hypothesis could only be rejected on a directional (one-tailed), but not on a "less biased" (two-tailed), basis.

Rather than debate the convincingness of these simulated results, taken in isolation, it would seem far more productive to reexecute RISKTEST with different inputs embodying the presumption that at least some of the 550 Turku patients were cured by their mastectomy and radiation. Comparing the results of the two separate simulation runs fitted, respectively, to the competing presumptions of possible versus impossible cure should prove much more illuminating. To accomplish this, we need an estimate of how many and which patients were probably cured.

4.8 A Systematic Search for Evidence of Cure

The initial Kaplan-Meier survival outputs tabled in section 4.5 and depicted graphically in figure 7 produced the results summarized below.

1. The focal event (further disease progression) was experienced by 293 of the 550 patients in the Turku intervention sample. These were clearly SR patients.
2. The remaining 550 - 293 = 257 patients had not experienced the focal event when they were last observed. These were the censored patients. Any MR patients would have been included among them.
3. The detailed analysis in section 4.6 showed that 148 of these 257 patients were censored because they died of something other than their breast cancer. The remaining 257 - 148 = 109 patients were censored because, when patient follow-up terminated in April 1996, they had been last seen still alive without evidence of disease progression.
4. The longest focal event time was 24.25 years after initial diagnosis.
5. Of the 257 censored patients, thirty-seven were characterized as long-term survivors. Each of them was followed up without evidence of disease progression for longer than the longest focal event time. Fifteen of the thirty-seven eventually died of something other than their breast cancer, and twenty-two were last seen still alive. These thirty-seven long-term survivors are the most likely candidates for classification as MR patients cured by their mastectomy and radiation.
6. The 257 - 37 = 220 censored patients who were not long-term survivors are more difficult to classify. One hundred thirty-three died of something other than their breast cancer, and eighty-seven were last seen still alive without evidence of disease progression. Some of the 220 censored patients were probably cured by their treatment (MR), while others probably remained at substantial risk (SR).

Based on these results the 550 patients may be divided into the following three risk categories. This is a tentative classification. It follows from the observations just summarized.

PATIENT'S LEVEL OF RISK	ABSOLUTE FREQUENCIES (COUNTS)	RELATIVE FREQUENCIES (PROPORTIONS)	CUMULATIVE RELATIVE FREQUENCIES
CERTAIN RISK (SR)	293	0.5327	0.5327
QUESTIONABLE RISK	220	0.4000	0.9327
MINIMAL RISK (MR)	37	0.0673	1.0000
TOTAL	550	1.0000	

Including only the thirty-seven long-term survivors would imply that the proportion of patients cured by the intervention was 0.0673. This seems much too low. Figure 7 suggests visually a proportion somewhat below 0.42. If there is reasonable evidence that some of the 220 QUESTIONABLE RISK patients were also cured, they need to be reclassified (moved down into the MR category).

However, not all QUESTIONABLE RISK patients are reasonable candidates for reclassification. For example, a patient whose cancer has already become metastatic and systemic seems quite unlikely to be cured by mastectomy and radiation alone or by any other kind of strictly locoregional therapy.

This suggests looking at the state of disease progression of each of the 220 QUESTIONABLE RISK patients at the time of diagnosis and treatment. Based on their T, N, and M staging, some of them may be considered inappropriately reclassifiable.

PATIENT'S LEVEL OF RISK	T LEVEL OF STAGING				
	T=0 OR 1	T=2	T=3	T=4	TOTAL
CERTAIN RISK (SR)	37	141	70	42	290
QUESTIONABLE RISK	93	108	6	7	214
MINIMAL RISK (MR)	10	21	4	2	37
TOTAL	140	270	80	51	541

PATIENT'S LEVEL OF RISK	N LEVEL OF STAGING			
	N=0	N=1	N=2	TOTAL
CERTAIN RISK (SR)	74	175	41	290
QUESTIONABLE RISK	164	51	2	217
MINIMAL RISK (MR)	26	11	0	37
TOTAL	264	237	43	544

PATIENT'S LEVEL OF RISK	M LEVEL OF STAGING		
	M=0	M=1	TOTAL
CERTAIN RISK (SR)	271	22	293
QUESTIONABLE RISK	219	1	220
MINIMAL RISK (MR)	37	0	37
TOTAL	527	23	550

The picture painted by these three tables is already quite encouraging. There is a clear tendency in each table for higher levels of patient risk to be associated with later stages of disease progression. This tendency is extremely significant in all three tables.

Based on chi-square tests for the statistical independence of each table's row and column attributes, two-tailed p values associated with the T and N staging tables were both less than 0.00005. The two-tailed p value associated with the M staging table was 0.0002.

The total patient counts in the T and N staging tables added to slightly less than 550 because T and N staging data were missing for a small number of patients. Also, only one patient was recorded as T0. That patient was therefore combined with the 139 T1 patients. Appendix G summarizes these data as originally tabulated.

Medical judgment suggests that two kinds of restrictions might reasonably be placed on permissible risk category reclassifications.

1. Some QUESTIONABLE RISK patients may have been diagnosed in such an advanced stage of disease progression prior to the intervention as to rob the intervention of any plausible curative potential.

   Such is the case with the single M1 QUESTIONABLE RISK patient in the M staging table. That patient was therefore judged to be an inappropriate candidate for reclassification into the MR category.

2. Some MR patients, even though they survived for a very long time without evidence of further disease progression, may have been initially diagnosed in such an advanced stage as to render a cure unlikely. If so, they should be moved into and permanently retained in the QUESTIONABLE RISK category.

   The two T4 patients in the MR category (two of the thirty-seven long-term survivors) could have been viewed this way. However, one of them was N1 and M0, while the other was N0 and M0. Consequently, they were not so restricted.

   No other examples like this were compelling in any of the three staging tables.

Both the continuing search for a pattern of cure described in sections 4.9 and 4.10 and subsequent execution of the minimal risk partitioning algorithm (MRPA) to be introduced in section 5 will be explicitly constrained to ensure that no QUESTIONABLE RISK patients diagnosed in the M1 stage are inadvertently reclassified into the MR category.

No restrictions limiting reclassification of MR patients into the QUESTIONABLE RISK category will be imposed.

4.9 Executing the CURE Option of the KAPM Procedure

The KAPM procedure executed to produce the initial Kaplan-Meier survival analysis possesses a CURE option. When enabled, the CURE option makes a systematic search of whatever patient survival data it receives for a time-phased pattern of cure. The KAPM procedure with the CURE option enabled was applied to the Turku intervention sample. An edited version of the report it generated is presented in the next five pages.

SEARCH FOR A PATTERN OF CURE (VERY LOW/NO RISK) AMONG CENSORED OBSERVATIONS

Patient survival data suggest a pattern of cure if the following conditions are satisfied.

First, the focal event targeted by the Kaplan-Meier analysis must be inherently avoidable. It must be possible never to experience it. Thus, death (all causes) would definitely not qualify as permanently avoidable. Progression of a curable disease (including eventual death because of it) would qualify.

The focal event chosen for the intervention sample (any evidence of further disease progression) does qualify, assuming the possibility of cure.

Second, if the purpose of the Kaplan-Meier analysis is to search for evidence of a curative impact of some particular medical intervention, it must be plausible to expect an appreciable proportion of the patient population from which sample data were obtained to have been cured by virtue of that intervention. Furthermore, the plausibility of its curative impact must have been established prior to obtaining and without reference to actual sample observations.

Radical and modified radical mastectomy with radiation was preestablished as satisfying this condition for this population of patients (entry 4, "ANNOTATED REFERENCES").

Failure to satisfy the prior plausibility criterion might be appropriate if a particular set of observations was collected for the express purpose of challenging conventional wisdom.

Third, the survival data submitted to the Kaplan-Meier analysis must be tested by the RISKTEST simulator. RISKTEST results must render it at least plausible to reject the null hypothesis of no patients cured (in this case that all patients remained in the SR category, despite their mastectomy and radiation).

A one-hundred-thousand-trial run of the RISKTEST simulator permitted rejection of the null hypothesis with a one-tailed p value of 0.04206.

Fourth, the nature of the progressive disease and the choice of a focal event must be such that patient survival curves are reasonably described by a Weibull distribution, including as a special case the exponential distribution. Use of the Weibull distribution permits hazard rates either to rise consistently or to fall consistently or to remain uniformly constant over time.

This is a flexibility and convenience criterion, not a hard-and-fast logical requirement. It is, however, an essential precondition if survival data are submitted to the KAPM procedure with the CURE option enabled.

The R-squared value of 0.8864 reported at the end of section 4.5 satisfies this condition.

Fifth, the sequence of Kaplan-Meier survival rates obtained from the sample data via the product-limit method must approach a horizontal asymptote at some decidedly positive survival probability. The same sequence must also fit a Weibull distribution with a decreasing trend in hazard rate distinctly better (in terms of comparable R-squared values) than it fits an exponential distribution (each distribution fitted to the same sample data submitted for analysis).

The table displayed in section 4.5 and the corresponding survival curve shown in figure 7 satisfy this condition.

Sixth, analysis of the residuals (fitted Weibull survival probabilities subtracted from corresponding Kaplan-Meier survival rates) must show a statistically significant pattern wherein positive residuals are concentrated among the earlier observations (i.e., survival times of relatively short duration), while negative residuals are concentrated among the later observations (i.e., survival times of relatively long duration).

This pattern is directionally consistent with, but by no means guarantees, the convergence over time of the sequence of Kaplan-Meier survival rates to a horizontal asymptote at a decidedly positive probability.

With patient follow-up of sufficiently long duration, the existence of an apparent horizontal asymptote provides a reasonable estimate of the proportion in the parent population cured by the intervention.

The cross table of residuals analyzed below satisfies this condition.

Seventh, and most compelling, if the preceding six conditions are satisfied, it is worth repeating the Kaplan-Meier analysis a number of times, each successive time with the remaining censored observations of longest duration selectively culled. If the total sample contains a substantial subset of cured patients, such a sequence of analyses should gradually eliminate them.

1. Over the sequence of analyses, the initial advantage of the fitted Weibull model over the fitted exponential model (difference in R-squared values) should decline.
2. It should then stabilize at some level, possibly at zero.
3. The sharpness of decrease of the fitted Weibull hazard rate over time should also decline initially and then stabilize at some level, possibly at zero (where the Weibull trend parameter = 1.0).
4. Whichever model (Weibull or exponential) eventually fits the set of Kaplan-Meier survival probability estimates better should have its R-squared statistic increase steadily to a maximum value at a contextually plausible cure rate and then stabilize or decline.

Results bearing on this condition are displayed on the next two pages, following the cross-table analysis immediately below.

CROSS TABLE OF RESIDUALS	EARLY RESIDUAL (KAPM - FITTED)	LATE RESIDUAL (KAPM - FITTED)	TOTAL
POSITIVE RESIDUAL	45	6	51
NEGATIVE RESIDUAL	53	93	146
TOTAL	98	99	197

These data display an extremely significant "lean" in the direction of relatively higher cell counts along the table's major diagonal (top-left and bottom-right cells), compared to its off-diagonal (top-right and bottom-left cells).

A Fisher exact statistical test was performed on this table.

The one-tailed p value (directional alternative to the null hypothesis) is less than 0.00005. The two-tailed p value is also less than 0.00005.

Since positive residuals are relatively heavily concentrated among the earlier observations while negative residuals are heavily concentrated among the later observations, it is quite reasonable to interpret the decreasing hazard rate as at least somewhat spurious. The hazard rate specifically applicable to the subset of patients genuinely at risk may decrease over time. It may also increase or remain constant. However, the above pattern of residuals suggests that the actual trend in hazard rate has been distorted by contaminating the sample with an appreciable proportion of cured patients. The exaggerated decreasing trend in hazard rate may be nothing more than a statistical artifact of the maximum likelihood algorithm's attempt to force fit as closely as possible a Weibull function that must fall asymptotically to zero to a sequence of focal event and censored times whose Kaplan-Meier survival probability appears to approach a horizontal asymptote somewhat below 0.42. Contaminating the sample with cured patients appears to have introduced a specification error into the analysis. The Weibull model may not be appropriate for the commingled sample, even though it may be entirely appropriate for the genuine at-risk (SR) subsample if analyzed by itself.

CENSORED TIME BOUND	NUMBER AND PROPORTION SO CURED	WEIBULL INTENSITY PARAMETER	WEIBULL TREND PARAMETER	R-SQUARED VALUE OF WEIBULL	R-SQUARED VALUE OF EXPONENTIAL	R-SQUARED DIFFERENCE IN VALUE
INFINITE	0(.000)	0.0430	0.6142	0.8864	0.4082	0.4781
24.2524	37(.067)	0.0584	0.6662	0.9091	0.6098	0.2994
20.4193	86(.156)	0.0838	0.7330	0.9420	0.7741	0.1679
18.6643	112(.204)	0.1021	0.7793	0.9582	0.8518	0.1064
17.6705	127(.231)	0.1147	0.8110	0.9671	0.8925	0.0745
17.6622	128(.233)	0.1156	0.8132	0.9676	0.8952	0.0724
17.3364	132(.240)	0.1192	0.8224	0.9699	0.9048	0.0650
14.9161	171(.311)	0.1623	0.9369	0.9869	0.9755	0.0114
13.5828	181(.329)	0.1757	0.9740	0.9899	0.9864	0.0035
12.9147	184(.335)	0.1797	0.9849	0.9907	0.9888	0.0019
12.7477	185(.336)	0.1811	0.9883	0.9909	0.9895	0.0014
12.3370	186(.338)	0.1824	0.9917	0.9911	0.9901	0.0010
12.1700	188(.342)	0.1851	0.9982	0.9915	0.9913	0.0002
11.8332	189(.344)	0.1864	1.0000	0.9918	0.9918	0.0000
11.7484	191(.347)	0.1892	1.0000	0.9928	0.9928	0.0000
11.3349	194(.353)	0.1935	1.0000	0.9941	0.9941	0.0000
10.7518	201(.365)	0.2040	1.0000	0.9962	0.9962	0.0000
10.3356	203(.369)	0.2070	1.0000	0.9967	0.9967	0.0000
10.2535	204(.371)	0.2085	1.0000	0.9968	0.9968	0.0000
9.7469	208(.378)	0.2145	1.0000	0.9973	0.9973	0.0000
8.9174	214(.389)	0.2237	1.0000	0.9976	0.9976	0.0000
8.8325	215(.391)	0.2252	1.0000	0.9976	0.9976	0.0000
8.4985	218(.396)	0.2297	1.0000	0.9975	0.9975	0.0000
8.1699	219(.398)	0.2313	1.0000	0.9974	0.9974	0.0000
7.8332	220(.400)	0.2327	1.0000	0.9974	0.9974	0.0000
7.5867	221(.402)	0.2341	1.0000	0.9973	0.9973	0.0000
7.4143	222(.404)	0.2355	1.0000	0.9973	0.9973	0.0000
7.0008	224(.407)	0.2382	1.0000	0.9972	0.9972	0.0000
6.8338	225(.409)	0.2396	1.0000	0.9972	0.9972	0.0000
6.1630	226(.411)	0.2408	1.0000	0.9971	0.9971	0.0000
5.9988	227(.413)	0.2420	1.0000	0.9971	0.9971	0.0000
5.8345	228(.415)	0.2432	1.0000	0.9971	0.9971	0.0000
5.6702	229(.416)	0.2444	1.0000	0.9971	0.9971	0.0000
5.5032	230(.418)	0.2455	1.0000	0.9971	0.9971	0.0000
5.4211	231(.420)	0.2466	1.0000	0.9970	0.9970	0.0000
5.2513	232(.422)	0.2477	1.0000	0.9970	0.9970	0.0000

CENSORED TIME BOUND	NUMBER AND PROPORTION SO CURED	WEIBULL INTENSITY PARAMETER	WEIBULL TREND PARAMETER	R-SQUARED VALUE OF WEIBULL	R-SQUARED VALUE OF EXPONENTIAL	R-SQUARED DIFFERENCE IN VALUE
5.0870	233(.424)	0.2488	1.0000	0.9970	0.9970	0.0000
5.0843	234(.425)	0.2499	1.0000	0.9970	0.9970	0.0000
4.8351	235(.427)	0.2510	1.0000	0.9969	0.9969	0.0000
4.8324	236(.429)	0.2520	1.0000	0.9969	0.9969	0.0000
4.5805	237(.431)	0.2530	1.0000	0.9969	0.9969	0.0000
4.5039	239(.435)	0.2550	1.0000	0.9968	0.9968	0.0000
4.4135	241(.438)	0.2570	1.0000	0.9967	0.9967	0.0000
3.9152	242(.440)	0.2579	1.0000	0.9967	0.9967	0.0000
3.8331	243(.442)	0.2587	1.0000	0.9967	0.9967	0.0000
3.5867	244(.444)	0.2596	1.0000	0.9966	0.9966	0.0000
3.3348	245(.445)	0.2604	1.0000	0.9966	0.9966	0.0000
3.2526	246(.447)	0.2611	1.0000	0.9966	0.9966	0.0000
3.0829	247(.449)	0.2618	1.0000	0.9966	0.9966	0.0000
2.9159	248(.451)	0.2625	1.0000	0.9966	0.9966	0.0000
2.8337	249(.453)	0.2632	1.0000	0.9965	0.9965	0.0000
2.2478	250(.455)	0.2637	1.0000	0.9965	0.9965	0.0000
2.0835	251(.456)	0.2642	1.0000	0.9965	0.9965	0.0000
2.0014	253(.460)	0.2652	1.0000	0.9965	0.9965	0.0000
1.9165	254(.462)	0.2657	1.0000	0.9965	0.9965	0.0000
0.9993	255(.464)	0.2659	1.0000	0.9965	0.9965	0.0000
0.5859	256(.465)	0.2660	1.0000	0.9965	0.9965	0.0000
0.5010	257(.467)	0.2662	1.0000	0.9966	0.9966	0.0000

Explanatory Notes:

1. The top row in the table presumes that no patients in the intervention sample were cured. It recapitulates the results of fitting, first, a Weibull survival function and then an exponential survival function via maximum likelihood to the focal and censored event times, as if all 550 patients remained at risk despite their mastectomy and radiation.
2. Subsequent rows presume that at least some and successively more censored patients were cured, starting with the thirty-seven long-term survivors who lived without evidence of disease progression longer than the longest focal event time (24.25 years) and ending with all 257 censored patients.
3. Of these 257 censored patients, the shortest-term survivor lived without evidence of disease progression for only 0.5010 years (bottom row).
4. The ever-expanding subset of patients presumed cured was culled from each successive Kaplan-Meier analysis. The results of successive analyses appear in successive rows of the table.
5. The CENSORED TIME BOUND is the culling criterion. Those censored patients who survived for at least the CENSORED TIME BOUND (in years) with no evidence of further disease progression were deleted from each successive row of the table.
6. The sequence of CENSORED TIME BOUNDs replicated (in reverse order) the sequence of focal event times occurring in the intervention sample.
7. The NUMBER AND PROPORTION SO CURED records the ever-increasing number of patients culled from each successive Kaplan-Meier analysis.
8. The WEIBULL INTENSITY PARAMETER and the WEIBULL TREND PARAMETER are the two parameters fitted via maximum likelihood to the remaining subset of nonculled patients presumed to be at risk in each successive analysis. See appendix C for a description of the Weibull function and its two parameters (LAMBDA, indicating intensity, and DELTA, indicating trend).
9. The R-SQUARED VALUE OF WEIBULL is the unadjusted coefficient of determination associated with the best-fitting (likelihood maximizing) Weibull function. In calculating R-squared, the Kaplan-Meier survival

probability estimates produced via the product-limit method are taken to be the "correct" survival probabilities that the best-fitting Weibull function is attempting to reproduce.

10. The R-SQUARED VALUE OF EXPONENTIAL is the unadjusted coefficient of determination associated with the best-fitting exponential function (Weibull function whose trend parameter is exactly 1.0). In calculating R-squared, the Kaplan-Meier survival probability estimates produced via the product-limit method are taken to be the "correct" survival probabilities that the best-fitting exponential function is attempting to reproduce.

11. The R-SQUARED DIFFERENCE IN VALUE measures the relative improvement in goodness of fit achieved by the best-fitting Weibull function over the best-fitting exponential function. A Weibull survival function must always fit a given data set at least as well as the more restrictive exponential survival function in terms of maximum likelihood. Therefore, an R-squared difference of zero indicates virtually no relative improvement (i.e., that the best-fitting Weibull function is essentially exponential).

This table reflects a striking pattern of cure.

1. All six of the preconditions stated as necessary before producing such a table were fully satisfied.

2. The compelling pattern of cure specified in the seventh condition was fully realized.

3. The relative improvement in goodness of fit achieved by the best-fitting Weibull function over the best-fitting exponential function, measured by the R-SQUARED DIFFERENCE IN VALUE, declined steadily from an initial value of 0.4781 to a final value of zero.

4. Zero improvement occurred when the longest-surviving 189 of the 257 censored patients were treated as cured and, therefore, removed from the KAPM analysis. The best-fitting Weibull function then became exponential (a Weibull function with trend parameter = 1.0) at a value of R-squared = 0.9918. All 189 patients survived without evidence of further disease progression for at least 11.8332 years. This suggests a minimum proportion cured in the neighborhood of 189/550 = 0.344.

5. The exponential function remained best-fitting until all 257 censored patients were finally removed from the KAPM analysis. This lends further support to the notion that the initial superiority of the Weibull over the exponential function was spurious. It signified nothing more than a model specification error. A large number of cured MR patients, transformed to a state of minimal risk by virtue of their mastectomy and radiation, contaminated the remaining sample of SR patients still at risk despite their treatment.

6. The R-squared goodness-of-fit statistic associated with the best-fitting function increased steadily from an initial value of 0.8864, when none of the 550 patients was treated as cured, to a maximum value of 0.9976, when 214/550 = 38.9 percent were treated as cured. All of these 214 censored patients survived without evidence of further disease progression for at least 8.9174 years.

7. The maximum value of R-squared occurred at a cured proportion (0.389) somewhat below the last proportion (0.4243) on the initial Kaplan-Meier curve shown in figure 7, just where the curve appeared to be approaching a horizontal asymptote.

8. Thereafter, R-squared declined gradually, but only very slightly, to 0.9966, when all 257 CENSORED patients (257/550 = 46.7 percent) were treated as cured.

9. The closeness of successive R-squared values between a 0.344 proportion cured (R-squared = 0.9918) and a 0.467 proportion cured (R-squared = 0.9966) suggests the need for some kind of fine-tuning mechanism to obtain a more precise estimate of the actual proportion cured.

4.10 Fine-Tuning the Initial Estimate of the Actual Proportion Cured

An obvious place to initiate the fine-tuning process is at the CENSORED TIME BOUND that achieved the maximum R-squared value. That occurred at 8.9174 years. There 214 (38.9 percent) of the 550 patients were provisionally regarded as cured (MR). These were the 214 censored patients who survived for at least 8.9174 years after initial diagnosis and treatment without evidence of further disease progression.

Executing the RISKTEST simulator at several smaller and several larger CENSORED TIME BOUNDs will help to produce an appropriate initial estimate of the proportion of the 550 Turku patients who were actually cured by their mastectomy and radiation. It will also serve to identify just who those patients probably were.

Notice that each null hypothesis now being tested by RISKTEST will be unique. Each successive simulation run will be initiated by a sequence of inputs specifying some particular number of patients (out of 550) presumed to have been cured. The particular patients are the censored ones who survived at or beyond each successive CENSORED TIME BOUND.

Changing the nature of the null hypothesis has several important implications.

1. Each corresponding alternate hypothesis is now bidirectional. It makes sense to consider either a smaller or a larger number of cured (MR) patients compared to each successive null-hypothesized number. This suggests focusing on two-tailed rather than on one-tailed p values generated by RISKTEST.
2. Each successive CENSORED TIME BOUND provisionally partitions the 550 patients into different MR and SR subsets. Each separate provisional partitioning requires that separate estimates now be made via maximum likelihood of the appropriate parameters of both the focal event and composite censoring event distributions to serve as inputs to successive runs of the RISKTEST simulator.
3. The best-fitting simulation run will be the one whose corresponding set of inputs to RISKTEST center most closely around 293 the simulated distribution of focal events experienced by the particular patients partitioned into the SR subset by that particular CENSORED TIME BOUND.

Nine simulations runs were executed. Each simulation run consisted of ten thousand trials (RISKTEST's default number). Simulation results are shown below and on the next three pages.

Run Number 1

PROVISIONAL NUMBER OF CURED (MR) PATIENTS: 189 (189/550 = 0.3436)
CENSORED TIME BOUND: 11.8332 years
VALUE OF R-SQUARED: 0.9918
RISKTEST INPUTS: 550 189 293 34.8371 16.1646 -1 0.1864 1 0.0642 1.8115

RISKTEST OUTPUTS:

The simulated number of patients experiencing the focal event was less than the observed number (293) in 1,043 trials.
The simulated number of patients experiencing the focal event was equal to the observed number (293) in 239 trials.
The simulated number of patients experiencing the focal event was more than the observed number (293) in 8,718 trials.

If interpreted as a statistical test of the goodness of fit of the simulation model with the observed number of patients experiencing the focal event, these results are consistent with a bidirectional (two-tailed) p value of 0.2564.

Run Number 2

PROVISIONAL NUMBER OF CURED (MR) PATIENTS: 201 (201/550 = 0.3655)
CENSORED TIME BOUND: 10.7518 years
VALUE OF R-SQUARED: 0.9962
RISKTEST INPUTS: 550 201 293 34.8371 16.1646 -1 0.2040 1 0.0593 1.6691

RISKTEST OUTPUTS:

The simulated number of patients experiencing the focal event was less than the observed number (293) in 1,560 trials.
The simulated number of patients experiencing the focal event was equal to the observed number (293) in 376 trials.
The simulated number of patients experiencing the focal event was more than the observed number (293) in 8,064 trials.

If interpreted as a statistical test of the goodness of fit of the simulation model with the observed number of patients experiencing the focal event, these results are consistent with a bidirectional (two-tailed) p value of 0.3872.

Run Number 3

PROVISIONAL NUMBER OF CURED (MR) PATIENTS: 208 (208/550 = 0.3782)
CENSORED TIME BOUND: 9.7469 years
VALUE OF R-SQUARED: 0.9973
RISKTEST INPUTS: 550 208 293 34.8371 16.1646 -1 0.2145 1 0.0554 1.5837

RISKTEST OUTPUTS:

The simulated number of patients experiencing the focal event was less than the observed number (293) in 2,060 trials.
The simulated number of patients experiencing the focal event was equal to the observed number (293) in 517 trials.
The simulated number of patients experiencing the focal event was more than the observed number (293) in 7,423 trials.

If interpreted as a statistical test of the goodness of fit of the simulation model with the observed number of patients experiencing the focal event, these results are consistent with a bidirectional (two-tailed) p value of 0.5154.

Run Number 4 (highest value of R-squared)

PROVISIONAL NUMBER OF CURED (MR) PATIENTS: 214 (214/550 = 0.3891)
CENSORED TIME BOUND: 8.9174 years
VALUE OF R-SQUARED: 0.9976
RISKTEST INPUTS: 550 214 293 34.8371 16.1646 -1 0.2237 1 0.0514 1.5093

RISKTEST OUTPUTS:

The simulated number of patients experiencing the focal event was less than the observed number (293) in 2,686 trials.
The simulated number of patients experiencing the focal event was equal to the observed number (293) in 573 trials.
The simulated number of patients experiencing the focal event was more than the observed number (293) in 6,741 trials.

If interpreted as a statistical test of the goodness of fit of the simulation model with the observed number of patients experiencing the focal event, these results are consistent with a bidirectional (two-tailed) p value of 0.6518.

Run Number 5

PROVISIONAL NUMBER OF CURED (MR) PATIENTS: 220 (220/550 = 0.4000)
CENSORED TIME BOUND: 7.8332 years
VALUE OF R-SQUARED: 0.9974
RISKTEST INPUTS: 550 220 293 34.8371 16.1646 -1 0.2327 1 0.0467 1.4347

RISKTEST OUTPUTS:

The simulated number of patients experiencing the focal event was less than the observed number (293) in 3,606 trials.
The simulated number of patients experiencing the focal event was equal to the observed number (293) in 689 trials.
The simulated number of patients experiencing the focal event was more than the observed number (293) in 5,705 trials.

If interpreted as a statistical test of the goodness of fit of the simulation model with the observed number of patients experiencing the focal event, these results are consistent with a bidirectional (two-tailed) p value of 0.8590.

Run Number 6 (best-fitting run)

PROVISIONAL NUMBER OF CURED (MR) PATIENTS: 224 (224/550 = 0.4073)
CENSORED TIME BOUND: 7.0008 years
VALUE OF R-SQUARED: 0.9972
RISKTEST INPUTS: 550 224 293 34.8371 16.1646 -1 0.2382 1 0.0433 1.3901

RISKTEST OUTPUTS:

The simulated number of patients experiencing the focal event was less than the observed number (293) in 4,320 trials.
The simulated number of patients experiencing the focal event was equal to the observed number (293) in 687 trials.
The simulated number of patients experiencing the focal event was more than the observed number (293) in 4,993 trials.

If interpreted as a statistical test of the goodness of fit of the simulation model with the observed number of patients experiencing the focal event, these results are consistent with a bidirectional (two-tailed) p value of 1.0000.

Run Number 7

PROVISIONAL NUMBER OF CURED (MR) PATIENTS: 225 (225/550 = 0.4091)
CENSORED TIME BOUND: 6.8338 years
VALUE OF R-SQUARED: 0.9972
RISKTEST INPUTS: 550 225 293 34.8371 16.1646 -1 0.2396 1 0.0282 1

RISKTEST OUTPUTS:

The simulated number of patients experiencing the focal event was less than the observed number (293) in 6,565 trials.
The simulated number of patients experiencing the focal event was equal to the observed number (293) in 646 trials.
The simulated number of patients experiencing the focal event was more than the observed number (293) in 2,789 trials.

If interpreted as a statistical test of the goodness of fit of the simulation model with the observed number of patients experiencing the focal event, these results are consistent with a bidirectional (two-tailed) p value of 0.6870.

Run Number 8

PROVISIONAL NUMBER OF CURED (MR) PATIENTS: 235 (235/550 = 0.4273)
CENSORED TIME BOUND: 4.8351 years
VALUE OF R-SQUARED: 0.9969
RISKTEST INPUTS: 550 235 293 34.8371 16.1646 -1 0.2510 1 0.0337 1.3006

RISKTEST OUTPUTS:

The simulated number of patients experiencing the focal event was less than the observed number (293) in 6,689 trials.
The simulated number of patients experiencing the focal event was equal to the observed number (293) in 725 trials.
The simulated number of patients experiencing the focal event was more than the observed number (293) in 2,586 trials.

If interpreted as a statistical test of the goodness of fit of the simulation model with the observed number of patients experiencing the focal event, these results are consistent with a bidirectional (two-tailed) p value of 0.6622.

Run Number 9

PROVISIONAL NUMBER OF CURED (MR) PATIENTS: 245 (245/550 = 0.4455)
CENSORED TIME BOUND: 3.3348 years
VALUE OF R-SQUARED: 0.9966
RISKTEST INPUTS: 550 245 293 34.8371 16.1646 -1 0.2604 1 0.0260 1.2824

RISKTEST OUTPUTS:

The simulated number of patients experiencing the focal event was less than the observed number (293) in 8,935 trials.
The simulated number of patients experiencing the focal event was equal to the observed number (293) in 428 trials.
The simulated number of patients experiencing the focal event was more than the observed number (293) in 637 trials.

If interpreted as a statistical test of the goodness of fit of the simulation model with the target number of patients experiencing the focal event. these results are consistent with a bidirectional (two-tailed) p value of 0.2130.

On the next page are tabled the results of one hundred thousand simulation trials. Again, the second column counts the number of such trials (out of one hundred thousand) in which the number of patients who experience the focal event is as indicated in the first column.

With one exception, inputs to the best-fitting RISKTEST run (Run Number 6) were replicated precisely to produce this table. The exception was a small reduction in the intensity parameter for the focal event from 0.2382 to 0.2350 (to be explained in section 4.11).

NUMBER OF PATIENTS WHO EXPERIENCE THE FOCAL EVENT	ABSOLUTE FREQUENCIES (COUNTS)	RELATIVE FREQUENCIES (PROPORTIONS)	CUMULATIVE RELATIVE FREQUENCIES
266	1	0.00001	0.00001
268	2	0.00002	0.00003
270	4	0.00004	0.00007
271	2	0.00002	0.00009
272	12	0.00012	0.00021
273	35	0.00035	0.00056
274	48	0.00048	0.00104
275	59	0.00059	0.00163
276	103	0.00103	0.00266
277	148	0.00148	0.00414
278	244	0.00244	0.00658
279	367	0.00367	0.01025
280	492	0.00492	0.01517
281	772	0.00772	0.02289
282	1057	0.01057	0.03346
283	1511	0.01511	0.04857
284	2019	0.02019	0.06876
285	2638	0.02638	0.09514
286	3368	0.03368	0.12882
287	4008	0.04008	0.16890
288	4867	0.04867	0.21757
289	5535	0.05535	0.27292
290	6199	0.06199	0.33491
291	6822	0.06822	0.40313
292	7087	0.07087	0.47400
293	7253	0.07253	0.54653
294	7171	0.07171	0.61824
295	6886	0.06886	0.68710
296	6357	0.06357	0.75067
297	5549	0.05549	0.80616
298	4826	0.04826	0.85442
299	3951	0.03951	0.89393
300	3135	0.03135	0.92528
301	2420	0.02420	0.94948
302	1768	0.01768	0.96716
303	1269	0.01269	0.97985
304	794	0.00794	0.98779
305	547	0.00547	0.99326
306	297	0.00297	0.99623
307	183	0.00183	0.99806
308	105	0.00105	0.99911
309	50	0.00050	0.99961
310	25	0.00025	0.99986
311	8	0.00008	0.99994
312	3	0.00003	0.99997
313	3	0.00003	1.00000
TOTAL	100000	1.00000	

4.11 Convincing Confirmation of the Existence of Cure

The distribution of simulated focal event counts tabled on the previous page is virtually normal. Its modal value is perfectly centered at 293, the target focal event count actually observed in the 550-patient Turku intervention sample. Only a very slight fine-tuning adjustment to the focal event intensity parameter (from 0.2382 to 0.2350) was required to achieve this perfectly centered result. The adjustment moved the center of the simulated distribution down by a single focal event (from 294 to 293).

What rendered it so convincing as confirmation of the existence of cure was that the parameter estimates embodied in the inputs to the best-fitting RISKTEST simulation run were obtained directly from the collected Turku sample data, in conjunction with a trial-and-error sequence of specific assumptions about how many and just which patients were actually cured by their mastectomy and radiation.

Consequently, the initial partitioning into MR and SR subsamples will be as follows:

1. number of MR patients cured by mastectomy and radiation = 224;
2. MR proportion of patients cured = 224/550 = 0.4073;
3. where all MR patients survived without evidence of further disease progression for at least 7.0008 years after their mastectomy and radiation;
4. where the survival function for 326 SR patients who remained at substantial risk despite their mastectomy and radiation was exponential; and
5. where the hazard rate for these 326 SR patients was constant (not decreasing) at 0.2350 focal events per year.

Notice that what originally appeared to be a Weibull survival curve with a decreasing hazard rate over time for the unpartitioned sample of 550 patients turned out to be an exponential survival curve with a constant hazard rate for just the 326 presumed SR patients. The 224 presumed MR patients were not at risk of further disease progression. Their survival curves were forever horizontal at 100 percent survival probability. Purging them from the sample produced the same change in shape of hazard function (although for a different reason) that was demonstrated with kidney transplants in section 2.

Recall that no QUESTIONABLE RISK M1 patients were considered curable by mastectomy and radiation alone. None were supposed to be reclassified into the MR category. The RISKTEST analysis did not violate this restriction. Of the twenty-three patients diagnosed in the M1 stage, all but one was included among the 293 patients who experienced further disease progression. The single exception subsequently died about four and one-half years later of a cause unrelated to cancer. She was not considered a candidate for cure because the best-fitting RISKTEST simulation run excluded all patients (including her) who survived disease-free for less than 7.0008 years from being presumed transformed into the MR state.

Nevertheless, the M1 restriction will remain in effect. Subsequent execution of the MRPA algorithm (to be introduced in section 5) will be explicitly constrained to ensure that no QUESTIONABLE RISK patients diagnosed in the M1 stage are inadvertently reclassified into the MR category.

5.0 THE MINIMAL RISK PARTITIONING ALGORITHM (MRPA)

The initial partitioning of the 550 patients in the intervention sample can be refined still further. Refinement will be accomplished via selective reclassification of patients on the basis of various things we know about them that are recorded in the Turku data set, in concert with each patient's directly observed posttreatment experience.

The 293 patients who experienced the focal event cannot be reclassified. Their experience provides indisputable proof that they belong in the CERTAIN RISK (hence, SR) category. They were and always will remain so classified.

Reclassification can only take place between the QUESTIONABLE RISK and the MINIMAL RISK (MR) categories, and it can only happen to censored patients. Selective reclassification will be performed by the minimal risk partitioning algorithm (MRPA). MRPA is introduced and described in this section.

MRPA operates within a Bayesian framework. Which patients become selectively reclassified will be based on each patient's individually tailored Bayesian posterior cure probability. Her cure probability may be interpreted as the likelihood that a particular Turku patient was actually transformed from the SR state of substantial risk into the MR state of minimal risk of further disease progression following her mastectomy and radiation.

5.1 A Bayesian Cure Model

A Bayesian cure model has been constructed. It is analogous to the kidney transplant model outlined in section 2.1 and operationalized in section 2.2. To operationalize such a model means to apply both the framework and the logic of mathematical probabilities to observational data obtained from patient records.

As with the kidney transplant model, the cure model combines outputs of logistic regression and Cox regression analyses via Bayes' theorem to produce individually tailored posterior cure probabilities. Logistic regression again provides the corresponding prior probabilities, this time that each patient was cured following her mastectomy and radiation. Cox regression again enables the revision (recalculation) of prior probabilities on the basis of follow-up patient observations of the focal event. Individually revised (posterior) cure probabilities are then used by MRPA to reclassify censored patients.

Logistic regression analysis (Logit) can only provide plausible estimates of individually tailored prior cure probabilities when the intervention sample is appropriately prepartitioned into MR and SR subsamples. That is why such great care was taken in section 4.10 to fine-tune the initial partitioning and the estimated proportion cured. The RISKTEST simulator implemented fine-tuning.

Unlike the kidney transplant model, however, the cure model is iterative. MRPA repeats the entire Bayesian analysis as long as consistency with observational data can be improved. Each successive MRPA iteration repartitions the total sample of patients into MR and SR subsamples that are progressively more consistent with the complete collection of patient observations.

The cure model is presented on the next three pages. It is interpreted in terms of the 550 Turku patients diagnosed with invasive breast cancer. Their medical intervention was mastectomy and radiation. The focal event was any form of disease progression observed following their mastectomy and radiation.

OUTCOME OBSERVED AFTER MASTECTOMY AND RADIATION	TRUE PATIENT STATE AFTER MASTECTOMY/RADIATION		PROBABILITY OF OBSERVED OUTCOME
	CURED: TRANSFORMED TO MINIMAL RISK OF DISEASE PROGRESSION	NOT CURED: STILL AT SUBSTANTIAL RISK OF DISEASE PROGRESSION	
THE ith PATIENT'S FIRST EVENT THAT CLEARLY INDICATES SOME DISEASE PROGRESSION OCCURS WITHIN t YEARS AFTER TREATMENT	$[CP_i]0 = 0$ 0.0 "0" {Definition}	$[1 - CP_i] \times [1 - S_i(t)]$ 1.0 $1 - S_i(t)$	$1 - CP_i - S_i(t) + CP_i \times S_i(t)$
THE ith PATIENT SURVIVES FOR MORE THAN t YEARS AFTER TREATMENT WITH NO EVIDENCE OF DISEASE PROGRESSION	$[CP_i]1 = CP_i$ $RCP_i(t)$ $1 - 0 = 1$	$[1 - CP_i]S_i(t)$ $1 - RCP_i(t)$ $S_i(t)$ {Cox}	$CP_i + S_i(t) - CP_i \times S_i(t)$
INITIAL (PRIOR) PROBABILITY OF THE ith PATIENT'S TRUE STATE	CP_i {Logit}	$1 - CP_i$	1.0

Explanatory Notes:

1. The larger triangle in each cell contains the joint probability that a patient will fall in that cell (i.e., both in that row and in that column).
2. Upward-pointing triangles in each cell contain the conditional probability that a patient will fall in the indicated row, given that the patient falls in the state-defining column pointed to above.
3. Zero (0) in the upward-pointing triangle of the northwest cell embodies the model's operational definition of what it means to have been cured by mastectomy and radiation. The zero is a virtual zero, possibly, but not necessarily an actual zero. It is assumed to be at most a very small positive number that may be treated as if it were zero.
4. The $S(t)$ function in the upward-pointing triangle of the southeast cell is a tailored survival function obtained for each patient, separately, via Cox (proportional hazards) regression analysis performed only on the SR subsample of patients deemed by the minimal risk partitioning algorithm (MRPA) to have remained at substantial risk of further disease progression despite their mastectomy and radiation. Elapsed time t is measured in years.
5. Leftward-pointing triangles in each cell contain the conditional probability that a patient will fall in the indicated column, given that the patient falls in the row pointed to at the left. These are revised probabilities

that the patient was, in fact, cured by mastectomy and radiation. A tailored revised cure probability function, RCP(t), is constructed for each patient, separately, by MRPA. Each RCP(t) function is defined on t, the elapsed time following treatment during which a patient is observed with no evidence of further disease progression. Each RCP(t) function evaluated at time t for a particular patient generates the Bayesian posterior cure probability applicable to that patient at that point in elapsed time.

6. The formula used by MRPA to calculate a censored patient's RCP(t) function is RCP(t) = CP/[CP + (1 - CP) x S(t)]. Putting first t = 0, then an infinite value of t, into the formula shows that all RCP(t) functions start at the censored patient's initial CP probability and then rise monotonically (sometimes via an "S-shaped" curve) to an asymptotic probability of 1.0.

7. The CP probability contained in the bottom row of the first column is the initial (posttreatment) probability that a patient was, in fact, cured by mastectomy and radiation. This probability does not change over time. A separate CP value is obtained for each patient via logistic regression analysis (Logit) performed on all 550 patients in the sample. Each such CP value acts as the Bayesian prior cure probability for a particular patient.

8. The calculated probabilities in the last column indicate how likely it is that a patient will fall in each of the two rows (i.e., experience each of the two observable outcomes) as a function of t. These constitute the patient's Bayesian preposterior probabilities. Putting first t = 0, and then an infinite value of t, into the calculations shows that every patient begins in the second row with probability 1.0 at time t = 0 (when mastectomy and radiation are received), but that the probability of remaining in the second row (i.e., of not experiencing any event evidencing further disease progression) declines to an asymptotic level of that patient's initial CP probability. In contrast, the probability that a patient will have switched into the first row (i.e., will have experienced at least one event evidencing further disease progression) within t years after receiving mastectomy and radiation begins at 0 and rises to an asymptotic level of 1 - CP, the complement of that patient's initial CP probability.

9. Although not explicitly shown anywhere in the table, it is interesting to contemplate how a patient's individual hazard rate would be revised over time as more and more time elapses after mastectomy and radiation with no evidence of disease progression. Each patient's hazard rate is either 0 if cured (patient falls in the first column), or obtainable from the tailored hazard function corresponding to that patient's tailored survival function if not cured (patient falls in the second column). Unless or until a patient experiences an event evidencing further disease progression, it remains uncertain whether or not that patient was, in fact, cured. The patient's RCP(t) function indicates the patient's revised cure probability as time elapses with no evidence of disease progression. Therefore, the patient's expected hazard rate would be the relevant statistic to track during this period of uncertainty. The expected hazard rate will normally decline over time with no evidence of disease progression. For sure it will decline monotonically if the patient's individual hazard rate either declines or remains constant over time. However, if the patient's individual hazard rate increases over time and that patient is at high enough risk to have a distinctly "S-shaped" RCP(t) curve, then that patient's expected hazard rate may rise to a maximum initially and then fall asymptotically to zero as time elapses with no further disease progression.

10. Once MRPA has partitioned a sample of patients into separate MR and SR subsamples, a separate initial CP probability may be calculated, and a separate S(t) survival function may be constructed for each patient via logistic regression and Cox regression, respectively. However, neither of these analyses may be performed without first partitioning the sample, at least tentatively. MRPA includes modified versions of both logistic and Cox regression analysis as internal subroutines to accomplish these tasks.

11. After an initial CP probability and a tailored S(t) survival function have been obtained for a given patient, the remaining probabilities shown in the table may be calculated by MRPA according to the standard formulas. This is how a revised RCP(t) function is produced for each separate patient.

12. MRPA is an iterative algorithm. It begins with an initial partitioning that seems plausible on the basis of a refined Kaplan-Meier analysis of patient outcome data. As if the initial partitioning were correct, revised RCP(t) functions are constructed for each censored patient in the sample. Each censored RCP(t) function is then evaluated at the time when that patient was last observed not (yet) to have experienced the focal event. Censored patients are rank-ordered in descending sequence according to their evaluated RCP(t) probabilities. The rank order is scanned to identify the point of vertical separation that, when cross tabulated with the initial partitioning, minimizes the number of inconsistent cross classifications.

13. A cross classification is inconsistent if either an MR patient in the initial partitioning has a RCP(t) value that falls below the point of vertical separation or an SR patient in the initial partitioning has a RCP(t) value that falls above the point of vertical separation. This misclassification-minimizing point defines a revised trial partitioning. All patients who have experienced the focal event are combined with the censored patients whose RCP(t) values fall below the revised trial partitioning point in the rank order. These are defined as belonging to the revised SR subsample. The remaining censored patients whose RCP(t) values fall higher in the rank order are defined as belonging to the revised MR subsample. The process is repeated with the revised trial partitioning playing the role of the initial partitioning. Successive iterations are executed as long as the minimum number of misclassifications can be successively reduced from iteration to iteration. A slight modification (to be explained later) is sometimes required to avoid iterative cycling.

14. MRPA is said to achieve partial convergence if the minimum number of misclassifications found on its last iteration is still positive. It achieves complete convergence if misclassifications can be completely eliminated. MRPA fails if not even a plausible initial partitioning can be found to begin the iterative process. When applied to the 550-patient Turku sample, MRPA achieved complete convergence in three iterations.

5.2 Logistic Regression Analysis (Logit): Obtaining Individually Tailored Prior Cure Probabilities from the Fine-Tuned Initial Partitioning of Patients into MR and SR Subsamples

A number of individual patient characteristics recorded in the Turku data set appeared plausible as prognostic factors that might predict, probabilistically, each patient's membership in the MR and SR subsamples. Annotated values of these candidate factors are summarized in appendix G. The factors included:

1. age of patient at diagnosis and treatment (in years);
2. size of tumor in millimeters of longest dimension;
3. type of tumor (ductal or lobular);
4. grade of tumor (grade 1, grade 2, or grade 3);
5. mitotic rate of tumor per hpf (rare, two or three, or more than three);
6. location of tumor (medial, central, lateral, or diffuse);
7. T stage (T0, T1, T2, T3, or T4);
8. N stage (N0, N1, or N2);
9. M stage (M0 or M1);
10. degree of necrosis (none, spotty, moderate, or severe);
11. ulceration (present or absent, present in only nine patients); and
12. inflammation (present or absent, present in only four patients).

Estrogen receptor (ER) response positivity and progesterone receptor (PR) response positivity were also recorded in the 2,192-patient data set. Unfortunately, ER response observations were missing for all but eleven of the 550 patients in the intervention sample, while PR response observations were missing for all 550 patients. These two factors and ulceration and inflammation were therefore eliminated as candidate predictors due to insufficient data.

Age at diagnosis and M stage were also eliminated, but for logical reasons. Patients treated at an advanced age were unable to survive as long as younger patients simply because of their age. The initial partitioning was defined in terms of both length of survival without evidence of further disease progression and M stage. Including either factor would thus have exploited the logical connections and reflected improperly purely definitional relationships.

Indexes were constructed for four of the remaining factors. Only a single patient was diagnosed in stage T0. Also, only a few patients lacked T stage or N stage data. Consequently, stage T0 was grouped with stage T1, and mean sample values were assigned to patients with missing T or N stage observations. Mean sample values were also substituted for missing observations of tumor size (in millimeters) and degree of risk associated with tumor location on the breast.

A separate univariate analysis was performed on each of the eight remaining factors as the single predictor (independent variable) of logistic regression. The initial partitioning into 224 MR and 326 SR patients served as each dependent variable, which was uniformly coded 0 for MR and 1 for SR.

Coding MR as 0 and SR as 1 ensured that a positive regression coefficient assigned to any prognostic factor would indicate that higher factor values were associated with increasing risk of further disease progression. A negative coefficient would indicate that higher factor values were linked with higher likelihood that a patient was cured following her mastectomy and radiation.

Results of the eight univariate logistic regression analyses are tabled below. Each analysis was based on the factor or factor index scores for the 550 intervention patients. All eight univariate relationships emerged as positive.

PROGNOSTIC FACTOR	REGRESSION COEFFICIENT	STANDARD DEVIATION	CHI-SQUARE (DF = 1)	TWO-TAILED P VALUE	ODDS RATIO
SIZ	0.0536	0.0094	32.5610	0.0000	1.0551
TYP	0.3852	0.2403	2.5693	0.1090	1.4700
GRA	0.5455	0.1261	18.7300	0.0000	1.7255
MIT	0.4788	0.1212	15.6004	0.0001	1.6141
LOC	0.0868	0.1160	0.5597	0.4544	1.0907
TUM	1.2176	0.1417	73.8660	0.0000	3.3792
NOD	2.0164	0.1933	108.7982	0.0000	7.5113
NEC	0.5578	0.1221	20.8759	0.0000	1.7468

Explanatory Notes:

1. TYP was tumor type, coded 0 for lobular and 1 for ductal.
2. MIT was mitotic count, coded 1 for rare, 2 for two or three mitoses per hpf, and 3 for more than three mitoses per hpf.
3. LOC was tumor location, coded 1 for medial, 2 for central, 3 for lateral, and 4 for diffuse, and with substituted mean values.
4. TUM was T stage, and NOD was N stage, both with substituted mean values.
5. NEC was degree of necrosis, coded 0 for none, 1 for spotty, 2 for moderate, and 3 for severe.
6. Notice that all except TYP and LOC yielded highly significant associations.

Conventional stepwise multivariate logistic regression with backward
elimination of the eight prognostic factors produced the following results.
Slightly edited computer output is enclosed between the horizontal lines for
the three factors that survived backward elimination.

Likelihood ratio chi-square statistic: 194.537, two-tailed p value: 0.0000
(based on 3 degrees of freedom and 550 complete observations).

INDEPENDENT VARIABLE	REGRESSION COEFFICIENT	STANDARD DEVIATION	CHI-SQUARE (DF = 1)	2-TAIL P VALUE	ODDS RATIO
intercept	-2.3019	0.3084	55.7261	0.0000	0.1001
TUM	0.8483	0.1536	30.5166	0.0000	2.3356
NOD	1.7549	0.2057	72.7899	0.0000	5.7828
NEC	0.3361	0.1439	5.4543	0.0195	1.3994

Pearson chi-square fit statistic (based on 46 degrees of freedom): 40.805,
p value: 0.6891.

Deviance chi-square fit statistic (based on 46 degrees of freedom): 34.391,
p value: 0.8960.

Classification improvement index (proportional reduction in the number of wrong
classifications enabled by using values of the independent variables): 0.3884.

The above logistic regression coefficients were used to calculate PRMSR0, the
initial probability that each of the 550 intervention patients remained in the
SR state despite her mastectomy and radiation.

DEFINE PRMSR0:
EXP(-2.3019+0.8483*TUM+1.7549*NOD+0.3361*NEC)/
[1+EXP(-2.3019+0.8483*TUM+1.7549*NOD+0.3361*NEC)]

SUMMARY STATISTICS	ATTRIBUTE PRMSR0	ATTRIBUTE MRSR0DX
n DEFINED	550	550
MINIMUM	0.1894	0
MEDIAN	0.5748	1
MAXIMUM	0.9963	1
MEAN	0.5927	0.5927
STD. DEV.	0.2751	0.4913

Values of PRMSR0 ranged from a minimum of 18.94 to a maximum of 99.63 percent,
with a mean of 59.27 percent. The M in the PRMSR0 attribute name indicates
substitution of mean values for missing factor observations wherever
appropriate. The 0 indicates MRPA's initial (as opposed to subsequent
iteration) partitioning. The mean value of PRMSR0 was the complement of the
proportion of patients initially presumed cured (MR = 224/550 = 0.4073).

MRSR0DX (coded 0 for MR and 1 for SR) is a dummy variable encapsulating the
initial partitioning. The mean value of MRSR0DX was the proportion of patients
initially presumed to have remained in the SR state (SR = 326/550 = 0.5927).
Logistic regression ensured identical mean values for PRMSR0 and MRSR0DX.

5.3 By How Much Did PCM Improve the Consistency of the Initial Prior Cure
     Probabilities with the Initial Partitioning of Patients into MR and SR
     Subsamples?

The intervention sample size of 550 was too small to subdivide the patient
population into relatively homogeneous strata. However, all eight prognostic
factors were converted by SPSA into corresponding UIRIs. Minimum subscale sizes
were uniformly set at twenty-five or fifty patient observations. Missing
observations of tumor size, tumor location, T stage, and N stage were replaced
in the usual PCM manner as outlined in section 2.3. Consequently, PCM's ability
to improve the consistency of partitioning probabilities relied on indicating
via SPSA conversion the underlying shape of each factor's discriminating impact
(excluding tumor type, because it was dichotomous), in combination with its
selective replacement of missing observations.

A PCM reanalysis of the same 550-patient intervention sample data was executed.
A stepwise multivariate logistic regression analysis with backward elimination
was performed. Corresponding UIRI values were substituted for all eight
prognostic factors as independent variables. The initial partitioning of the
550 patients into MR and SR subsamples remained as the dependent variable.

UIRIs replacing the same three prognostic factors survived PCM's backward
elimination. The manner in which SPSA converted each factor into its
corresponding UIRI is shown below (see appendix G for their raw data coding).

TUMUIRI's optimal scale partitioning and numeric rescaling were as follows.

42/140 IF T<2 ELSE
160/270 IF T=2 ELSE
124/140 IF T>=3 OR T=UNDEFN (UNDEFN means undefined or missing observation)

NODUIRI's optimal scale partitioning and numeric rescaling were as follows.

95/270 IF N=0 OR N=UNDEFN ELSE (UNDEFN means undefined or missing observation)
189/237 IF N=1 ELSE
42/43 IF N=2

NECUIRI's optimal scale partitioning and numeric rescaling were as follows.

205/383 IF NECROSIS=0 ELSE
59/89 IF NECROSIS=1 ELSE
37/51 IF NECROSIS=2 ELSE
25/27 IF NECROSIS=3

Slightly edited computer output describing the PCM reanalysis is enclosed
between the horizontal lines on the following page. It is shown only to provide
a comparison with the corresponding computer output presented in section 5.2.

SPSA succeeded in either matching or enhancing the goodness of statistical fit
and the classification improvement measures. By converting all three factors to
corresponding UIRIs SPSA also rendered the three odds ratios directly
comparable (i.e., no problem with differing factor measurement scales). SPSA
normally accomplishes all of these things. However, the calculation of UIRIs
made explicit use of predicted end point values. Classical hypothesis testing
and the conventional interpretation of p values was thereby rendered
inapplicable. The underlying reasoning became circular. The reported results
should only be interpreted as descriptive, but not as inferential statistics.

Likelihood ratio chi-square statistic: 199.123, two-tailed p value: 0.0000
(based on 3 degrees of freedom and 550 complete observations).

INDEPENDENT VARIABLE	REGRESSION COEFFICIENT	STANDARD DEVIATION	CHI-SQUARE (DF = 1)	2-TAIL P VALUE	ODDS RATIO
intercept	-5.7379	0.8140	49.6917	0.0000	0.0032
TUMUIRI	3.5749	0.5781	38.2405	0.0000	35.6918
NODUIRI	4.1242	0.4704	76.8782	0.0000	61.8180
NECUIRI	3.0028	1.2792	5.5099	0.0189	20.1409

GOODNESS OF STATISTICAL FIT OF LOGISTIC REGRESSION MODEL

Pearson chi-square fit statistic (based on 27 degrees of freedom): 17.292,
p value: 0.9237.

Deviance chi-square fit statistic (based on 27 degrees of freedom): 20.909,
p value: 0.7906.

Classification improvement index (proportional reduction in the number of wrong
classifications enabled by using values of the independent variables): 0.4018.

Coefficients obtained from the above stepwise multivariate logistic regression
PCM reanalysis with backward elimination were used to calculate PRUSR0. PRUSR0
provides an alternative estimate of the initial probability that each of the
550 intervention patients remained in the SR state despite her mastectomy and
radiation. The operational definition of PRUSR0 is shown below.

DEFINE PRUSR0:
EXP(-5.7379+3.5749*TUMUIRI+4.1242*NODUIRI+3.0028*NECUIRI)/
[1+EXP(-5.7379+3.5749*TUMUIRI+4.1242*NODUIRI+3.0028*NECUIRI)]

SUMMARY STATISTICS	ATTRIBUTE PRUSR0	ATTRIBUTE MRSR0DX
n DEFINED	550	550
MINIMUM	0.1670	0
MEDIAN	0.6193	1
MAXIMUM	0.9858	1
MEAN	0.5927	0.5927
STD. DEV.	0.2798	0.4913

Values of PRUSR0 ranged from a minimum of 16.70 to a maximum of 98.58 percent,
with a mean of 59.27 percent. The U in the PRUSR0 attribute name indicates
substitution of corresponding UIRI's for prognostic factors in the PCM
reanalysis. The 0 again indicates MRPA's initial partitioning.

MRSR0DX (coded as 0 for MR and 1 for SR) is a dummy variable encapsulating the
initial partitioning. Its mean value was the SR proportion of patients presumed
to be still at risk, despite their mastectomy and radiation (326/550 = 0.5927).
Logistic regression again ensured identical mean values for PRUSR0 and MRSR0DX.

Despite omitting the usual first step of subdividing the patient population into relatively homogeneous strata, PCM still achieved a modest, but statistically significant, consistency improvement. Matched pairs of individualized patient probabilities of remaining in the SR state (PRMSR0 and PRUSR0) were analyzed for each of the 550 patients. In terms of the accuracy improvement measures outlined in section 1.2 the results were as follows.

1. Conventional methodology (PRMSR0) produced 133 misclassifications. The remaining 550 - 133 = 417 out of 550 = 75.82 percent were correct.
2. PCM-generated discriminations (PRUSR0) produced 130 misclassifications. The remaining 550 - 130 = 420 out of 550 = 76.36 percent were correct.
3. PCM achieved an AUC correct discrimination score of a very modest 0.4 percentage points higher than conventional methodology (0.8273 versus 0.8233).
4. Nevertheless, looking at matched pairs of probabilistic discrimination errors, PCM's index of error reduction was a favorable 0.1491.
5. According to the Wilcoxon matched-pairs, signed ranks test, this reduction generated an equivalent Z value of 3.56, with a two-tailed p value of 0.0004.

5.4 Converting PCM-Generated UIRIs into Dummy Variables to Drive MRPA

A detailed inspection of misclassifications suggested a way to facilitate MRPA's progress from iteration to iteration and enable its eventual convergence to a solution.

1. MRPA is an iterative algorithm.
2. Posterior probabilities that a patient either was transformed by her mastectomy and radiation into the MR state or remained in the SR state drive successive iterations.
3. Posterior probabilities are revised versions of the prior probabilities that distinguish patients in the MR state from patients in the SR state at the time of their mastectomy and radiation.
4. Logistic regression produces individually tailored prior probabilities on the basis of discriminating factors included in medical records collected for each patient.
5. Cox regression produces the updating information based on prognostic factors also included in patient records indicating how long it will take following the intervention for each patient still in the SR state to display evidence of further disease progression.
6. Bayes' theorem guides the revision by combining appropriately the results of successive logistic and Cox regression analyses.
7. Successive regressions are uniformly designed to reflect the currently presumed partitioning of patients between the MR and SR states.
8. Therefore, in order for MRPA to converge successfully to an effective final partitioning (appropriate cure assessment), it is critical that both prior and posterior probabilities provide an unambiguous reclassification signal.
9. That signal is the misclassification-minimizing posterior cure probability. Patients with equal or higher probabilities are retained within or moved into the MR subsample on the next iteration. Patients with lower probabilities are retained within or moved into the SR subsample.
10. Both the PRMRS0 and PRUSR0 probabilities (complements of the respective prior cure probabilities) produced by multivariate logistic regression with backward elimination made ambiguous contributions to the calculation of the reclassification signal.

11. Ambiguity resulted from nonunique misclassification-minimizing probabilities. PRMRS0 possessed four distinct possibilities, while PRUSR0 possessed two distinct possibilities.
12. One way to eliminate this ambiguity is to convert PCM-generated UIRIs used as independent variable inputs to both logistic and Cox regression into corresponding 0/1 dummy variables. Selective editing of the converted dummy variables can then discriminate more sharply between MR and SR patients in a refined version of the same regression analysis.

The three UIRIs identified in section 5.3 as having survived backward elimination were converted into corresponding 0/1 dummy variables as follows.

```
DEFINE TUMLDV2: 1 IF T=2 ELSE 0
DEFINE TUMLDV34: 1 IF T>=3 OR T=UNDEFN ELSE 0

DEFINE NODLDV1: 1 IF N=1 ELSE 0
DEFINE NODLDV2: 1 IF N=2 ELSE 0

DEFINE NECLDV1: 1 IF NECROSIS=1 ELSE 0
DEFINE NECLDV2: 1 IF NECROSIS=2 ELSE 0
DEFINE NECLDV3: 1 IF NECROSIS=3 ELSE 0
```

L in each dummy variable name indicates that it has been constructed to be an independent variable input to logistic (versus Cox) regression. DV in each name identifies it as a UIRI converted to a corresponding 0/1 dummy variable.

With respect to T stage (TUM):

1. T0 and T1 patients were assigned zeros on both TUMLDV2 and TUMLDV34;
2. T2 patients were assigned a value of one on TUMLDV2 and zero on TUMLDV34; and
3. T3 and T4 patients and patients with missing T stage observations were assigned a value of one on TUMLDV34 and zero on TUMLDV2.

With respect to N stage (NOD):

1. N0 patients and patients with missing N stage observations were assigned zeros on both NODLDV1 and NODLDV2;
2. N1 patients were assigned a value of one on NODLDV1 and zero on NODLDV2; and
3. N2 patients were assigned a value of one on NODLDV2 and zero on NODLDV1.

With respect to necrosis (NEC):

1. patients with no necrosis were assigned zeros on NECLDV1, NECLDV2, and NECLDV3;
2. patients with spotty necrosis were assigned a value of one on NECLDV1 and zeros on NECLDV2 and NECLDV3;
3. patients with mild necrosis were assigned a value of one on NECLDV2 and zeros on NECLDV1 and NECLDV3; and
4. patients with severe necrosis were assigned a value of one on NECLDV3 and zeros on NECLDV1 and NECLDV2.
5. There were no missing observations of necrosis.

A multivariate logistic regression analysis was executed with the seven dummy variables as its discriminating factor inputs and with the initial partitioning of patients into MR and SR subsamples as its end point. Slightly edited computer output is displayed on the next page between the horizontal lines.

Likelihood ratio chi-square statistic: 202.269, two-tailed p value: 0.0000 (based on 7 degrees of freedom and 550 complete observations).

INDEPENDENT VARIABLE	REGRESSION COEFFICIENT	STANDARD DEVIATION	CHI-SQUARE (DF = 1)	2-TAIL P VALUE	ODDS RATIO
intercept	-1.5263	0.2218	47.3528	0.0000	0.2173
TUMLDV2	0.9659	0.2463	15.3773	0.0001	2.6272
TUMLDV34	2.1234	0.3567	35.4442	0.0000	8.3593
NODLDV1	1.7776	0.2189	65.9159	0.0000	5.9156
NODLDV2	3.5596	1.0383	11.7526	0.0006	35.1496
NECLDV1	0.0579	0.3035	0.0363	0.8488	1.0596
NECLDV2	0.6799	0.3941	2.9762	0.0845	1.9737
NECLDV3	1.5024	0.8016	3.5125	0.0609	4.4924

GOODNESS OF STATISTICAL FIT OF LOGISTIC REGRESSION MODEL

Pearson chi-square fit statistic (based on 23 degrees of freedom): 16.224, p value: 0.8455.

Deviance chi-square fit statistic (based on 23 degrees of freedom): 17.762, p value: 0.7703.

Classification improvement index (proportional reduction in the number of wrong classifications enabled by using values of the independent variables): 0.4018.

The purpose of dummy variable editing is to render unique the value of the misclassification-minimizing probability that will be produced from the output of the above logistic regression. A greater likelihood of uniqueness can be accomplished in two ways.

1. Each set of dummy variables associated, respectively, with each separate discriminating factor is first inspected. The dummy variables comprising each set must be in ascending sequence with respect to their estimated REGRESSION COEFFICIENTs. Because the dummy variables were converted from corresponding UIRIs, each set of corresponding REGRESSION COEFFICIENTs would automatically be in ascending sequence under univariate analysis. However, when combined in multivariate analysis, factor intercorrelations can generate rank-order inversions.

   Detected inversions must be eliminated by combining pairs of adjacent dummy variables into a single replacement dummy variable that combines corresponding patients into a single category. The replacement dummy variable is then substituted for the inverted pair.

   In this context the first dummy variable is considered adjacent to the "shadow" dummy variable representing patients with assigned zeros on all explicit variables. Simply eliminating the first dummy variable has the effect of combining it with the "shadow" dummy variable and grouping together all associated patients.

2. After eliminating inversions clear separation of discriminatory impact is sought within each properly sequenced set of dummy variables. P values may be construed as indicators of separation impact. P values

falling below some cutoff level (e.g., 0.05) may then be taken as indicating sufficiently clear separation.

Insufficient separation can be eliminated in the same manner that detected inversions were eliminated. Grouping together adjacent subscales comprising the complete factor scale can be accomplished by defining replacement dummy variables to substitute for adjacent pairs of insufficiently separated variables or by eliminating the first dummy variable.

There were no inversions in the computer output displayed on the previous page. However, separate values of necrosis produced insufficient separation. Grouping together patients with no or spotty necrosis (low necrosis) and patients with mild or severe necrosis (high necrosis) produced adequate separation.

A single replacement dummy variable was defined and substituted for NECLDV1, NECLDV2, and NECLDV3.

DEFINE NECLDV23: 1 IF NECROSIS>=2 ELSE 0

A revised dummy variable logistic regression was performed. Slightly edited computer output is displayed below between the horizontal lines.

Likelihood ratio chi-square statistic: 201.257, two-tailed p value: 0.0000 (based on 5 degrees of freedom and 550 complete observations).

INDEPENDENT VARIABLE	REGRESSION COEFFICIENT	STANDARD DEVIATION	CHI-SQUARE (DF = 1)	2-TAIL P VALUE	ODDS RATIO
intercept	-1.5331	0.2205	48.3379	0.0000	0.2159
TUMLDV2	0.9802	0.2448	16.0254	0.0001	2.6649
TUMLDV34	2.1720	0.3518	38.1154	0.0000	8.7761
NODLDV1	1.7810	0.2188	66.2445	0.0000	5.9355
NODLDV2	3.5780	1.0372	11.9011	0.0006	35.8031
NECLDV23	0.8468	0.3500	5.8550	0.0155	2.3322

GOODNESS OF STATISTICAL FIT OF LOGISTIC REGRESSION MODEL

Pearson chi-square fit statistic (based on 11 degrees of freedom): 11.447, p value: 0.4066.

Deviance chi-square fit statistic (based on 11 degrees of freedom): 12.767, p value: 0.3088.

Classification improvement index (proportional reduction in the number of wrong classifications enabled by using values of the independent variables): 0.4018.

The edited dummy variables satisfied all uniqueness-improving criteria. The revised REGRESSION COEFFICIENTS were used to define PRDVSR0. Values of PRDVSR0 served as individually tailored probabilities that each of the 550 intervention patients would fall into the SR subsample of the initial partitioning.

DEFINE PRDVSR0:
EXP(-1.5331+.9802*TUMLDV2+2.1720*TUMLDV34+1.7810*NODLDV1+
3.5780*NODLDV2+.8468*NECLDV23)/
[1+EXP(-1.5331+.9802*TUMLDV2+2.1720*TUMLDV34+1.7810*NODLDV1+
3.5780*NODLDV2+.8468*NECLDV23)]

Better still, dummy variable editing proved successful, albeit at a small cost.
Inspection of misclassifications resulting from PRDVSR0 probabilities disclosed
a unique minimizing probability. Compared to PRUSR0, however, a single
additional misclassification resulted. The count rose from 130 to 131.

Looking at matched pairs of probabilistic discrimination errors, PRDVSR0's
index of error reduction compared to PRMSR0 was a favorable 0.1855. According
to the Wilcoxon matched-pairs, signed ranks test, this reduction generated an
equivalent Z value of 3.16, with a two-tailed p value of 0.0016. PRDVSR0
achieved an AUC correct discrimination score of 0.8266.

Prior cure probabilities for the initial partitioning (PRECPR0) were then
defined as the complement of the calculated PRDVSR0 probabilities.

DEFINE PRECPR0: 1-PRDVSR0

SUMMARY STATISTICS	ATTRIBUTE PRECPR0
n DEFINED	550
MINIMUM	0.0063
MEDIAN	0.4270
MAXIMUM	0.8225
MEAN	0.4073
STD. DEV.	0.2796

Values of PRECPR0 ranged from a minimum of 0.63 to a maximum of 82.25 percent,
with a mean of 40.73 percent. The PRE in the PRECPR0 attribute name indicates a
prior distribution of probabilities produced from logistic regression in such a
manner as to be suitable for subsequent Bayesian revision via corresponding
survival probabilities generated from Cox regression. CPR stands for cure
probability. The 0 indicates MRPA's initial partitioning.

Notice that logistic regression again ensured identical values for the mean of
PRECPR0 (40.73 percent) and the percentage of intervention patients estimated
to have fallen into the MR subsample of the initial partitioning (224/550).

A cross tabulation of prior cure probabilities with the initial partitioning
was quite encouraging. The table below displays absolute frequencies (counts).
The table on the next page displays corresponding relative frequencies
(proportions).

VALUE OF PRECPR0	MR	SR	TOTAL
CURE JUDGED IMPOSSIBLE (M1 PATIENT)	0	23	23
0% < PRIOR CURE PROBABILITY =< 25%	31	195	226
25% < PRIOR CURE PROBABILITY =< 50%	39	45	84
50% < PRIOR CURE PROBABILITY =< 75%	78	45	123
75% < PRIOR CURE PROBABILITY =< 100%	76	18	94
TOTAL	224	326	550

VALUE OF PRECPR0	MR	SR	TOTAL
CURE JUDGED IMPOSSIBLE (M1 PATIENT)	0.0000	1.0000	1.0000
0% < PRIOR CURE PROBABILITY =< 25%	0.1372	0.8628	1.0000
25% < PRIOR CURE PROBABILITY =< 50%	0.4643	0.5357	1.0000
50% < PRIOR CURE PROBABILITY =< 75%	0.6341	0.3659	1.0000
75% < PRIOR CURE PROBABILITY =< 100%	0.8085	0.1915	1.0000

5.5 Cox Regression Analysis (Cox): Survival Given the Initial Partitioning

Ten univariate Cox regression analyses were performed. All analyses were based on the same patient attributes included in the Turku data set. The same factor indexes constructed by grouping values and by substituting mean values were used again. This time, however, each factor was reinterpreted as a candidate predictor (independent variable) to produce a univariate patient survival function. The end point (dependent variable) of each Cox regression was the time in years elapsed from diagnosis and treatment to the first evidence (if any) of further disease progression (Cox regression's focal event time).

Each patient's age at diagnosis and M stage were reinstated as candidate predictive factors. The dependent variable in Cox regression was no longer defined in terms of a minimum time elapsed since treatment without evidence of disease progression. Neither was it related by stipulation to being diagnosed M0 versus M1. M1 diagnosis would likely reduce the time until experiencing the focal event, thereby rendering it plausible as a prognostic factor of survival.

Each analysis was restricted to the 326 SR patients initially presumed to have remained at substantial risk of further disease progression despite their mastectomy and radiation. The remaining 224 MR patients were presumed to be at little or no such risk and, therefore, were excluded from consideration.

Results of the ten univariate Cox regression analyses were as follows.

PROGNOSTIC FACTOR	REGRESSION COEFFICIENT	STANDARD DEVIATION	CHI-SQUARE (DF = 1)	TWO-TAILED P VALUE	RELATIVE RISK
AGE	-0.0007	0.0054	0.0155	0.9009	0.9993
SIZ	0.0172	0.0046	13.7309	0.0002	1.0173
TYP	0.2752	0.1808	2.3158	0.1281	1.3167
GRA	0.6122	0.0926	43.7491	0.0000	1.8445
MIT	0.4837	0.0792	37.2704	0.0000	1.6221
LOC	-0.0007	0.0840	0.0001	0.9934	0.9993
TUM	0.1803	0.0636	8.0334	0.0046	1.1976
NOD	0.7120	0.1000	50.6907	0.0000	2.0381
MET	1.1904	0.2261	27.7217	0.0000	3.2884
NEC	0.3086	0.0608	25.7240	0.0000	1.3615

Explanatory Notes:

1. TYP was tumor type, coded 0 for lobular and 1 for ductal.
2. MIT was mitotic count, coded 1 for rare, 2 for two or three mitoses per hpf, and 3 for more than three mitoses per hpf.
3. LOC was tumor location, coded 1 for medial, 2 for central, 3 for lateral, and 4 for diffuse, and with substituted mean values.
4. TUM was T stage, and NOD was N stage, both with substituted mean values.
5. MET was M stage, coded 0 for M0 and 1 for M1.

6. NEC was degree of necrosis, coded 0 for none, 1 for spotty, 2 for moderate, and 3 for severe.
7. Notice that all factors except AGE, TYP, and LOC were highly significant univariate predictors pointing in the proper direction (i.e., with positive regression coefficients).
8. In section 5.2 neither tumor type (TYP) nor tumor location (LOC) was shown to discriminate significantly on a univariate basis between being transformed into the MR state versus remaining in the SR state despite mastectomy and radiation. Age at diagnosis (AGE) was not then subjected to univariate logistic regression because it was related definitionally to the criteria by which the MR and SR subsamples were initially identified.

From a conventional stepwise multivariate Cox regression of these ten factor indexes with backward elimination, tumor grade (GRA), N stage (NOD), M stage (MET), and necrosis (NEC) emerged as the significant independent predictors of time elapsed until experiencing the focal event. Slightly edited computer output showing these results is enclosed below between the horizontal lines.

Likelihood ratio chi-square statistic: 99.817, two-tailed p value: 0.0000.
Score chi-square statistic: 112.693, two-tailed p value: 0.0000.
Wald chi-square statistic: 106.850, two-tailed p value: 0.0000.

All three chi-square statistics are based on 4 degrees of freedom and 326 observations, encompassing 197 distinct focal event times.

INDEPENDENT VARIABLE	REGRESSION COEFFICIENT	STANDARD DEVIATION	CHI-SQUARE (DF = 1)	2-TAIL P VALUE	RELATIVE RISK
GRA	0.4385	0.1008	18.9376	0.0000	1.5503
NOD	0.5616	0.1023	30.1470	0.0000	1.7535
MET	0.8918	0.2305	14.9724	0.0001	2.4396
NEC	0.1524	0.0693	4.8422	0.0278	1.1646

The SR subsample size of 326 was too small to subdivide the patient population into relatively homogeneous strata. However, all ten predictive factors were converted by SPSA into corresponding UIRIs. This time the end point used by SPSA to generate UIRIs was whether or not each of the 326 SR patients had experienced any kind of disease progression. Minimum subscale sizes were again set at around twenty-five or fifty patient observations. Missing observations of tumor size, tumor location, T stage, and N stage were replaced in the usual PCM manner, as outlined in section 2.3. Consequently, PCM's ability to improve predictive accuracy relied on indicating via SPSA conversion the underlying shape of each factor's predictive impact (excluding tumor type, because it was dichotomous), together with the selective replacement of missing observations.

A PCM reanalysis of the same 326-patient SR subsample data was then executed. A stepwise multivariate Cox regression analysis with backward elimination was performed. Corresponding UIRI values were substituted for all ten predictors as independent variables. The time in years elapsed between diagnosis/treatment and experiencing the focal event (if it occurred) remained as Cox regression's dependent variable.

UIRIs replacing the same four predictive factors survived PCM's backward elimination. How SPSA converted each factor into its corresponding UIRI is displayed on the next page (see appendix G for raw data coding).

GRAUIRI's optimal scale partitioning and numeric rescaling were as follows.

38/46 IF GRADE=1 ELSE
128/149 IF GRADE=2 ELSE
127/131 IF GRADE=3

NODUIRI's optimal scale partitioning and numeric rescaling were as follows.

74/92 IF N=0 ELSE
178/192 IF N=1 OR N=UNDEFN ELSE (UNDEFN means undefined or missing observation)
41/42 IF N=2

METUIRI's optimal scale partitioning and numeric rescaling were as follows.

271/303 IF M=0 ELSE
22/23 IF M=1

NECUIRI's optimal scale partitioning and numeric rescaling were as follows.

181/205 IF NECROSIS=0 ELSE
53/59 IF NECROSIS=1 ELSE
34/37 IF NECROSIS=2 ELSE
25/25 IF NECROSIS=3

The same procedure outlined in section 5.4 was then repeated to convert the above four UIRIs into corresponding 0/1 dummy variables to drive MRPA. Multivariate logistic regression was again invoked to refine (i.e., to edit selectively) the corresponding dummy variables so as to ensure sufficient separation between successive values of the cure probabilities that would eventually be calculated via Bayesian revision from the results of using these 0/1 dummy variables as independent variables for Cox regression.

The four UIRIs that survived backward elimination were thereby converted into five corresponding 0/1 dummy variables as follows.

DEFINE GRACDV23: 1 IF GRADE>=2 ELSE 0

DEFINE NODCDV1: 1 IF N=1 OR N=UNDEFN ELSE 0
DEFINE NODCDV2: 1 IF N=2 ELSE 0

DEFINE METCDV1: 1 IF M=1 ELSE 0

DEFINE NECCDV23: 1 IF NECROSIS>=2 ELSE 0

C in each dummy variable name indicates that it has been constructed to be an independent variable input to Cox (versus logistic) regression. DV in each name identifies it as a UIRI converted to a corresponding 0/1 dummy variable.

With respect to tumor grade (GRA):

1. grade 1 patients were assigned a value of zero on GRACDV23; and
2. grade 2 and grade 3 patients were assigned a value of one on GRACDV23.
3. There were no missing observations of tumor grade.

With respect to N stage (NOD):

1. N0 patients were assigned zeros on both NODCDV1 and NODCDV2;
2. N1 patients and patients with missing N stage observations were assigned a value of one on NODCDV1 and zero on NODCDV2; and

3. N2 patients were assigned a value of one on NODCDV2 and zero on NODCDV1.

With respect to M stage (MET):

1. M0 patients were assigned a value of zero on METCDV1; and
2. M1 patients were assigned a value of one on METCDV1.
3. There were no missing observations of M stage.

With respect to necrosis (NEC):

1. patients with no necrosis or with spotty necrosis were assigned a value of zero on NECCDV23: and
2. patients with mild necrosis or with severe necrosis were assigned a value of one on NECCDV23.
3. There were no missing observations of necrosis.

Comparing how these five dummy variables were defined for Cox regression with the five dummy variables defined in section 5.4 for logistic regression reveals both similarities and differences.

One similarity is that identical 0/1 dummy variables were constructed for both logistic regression and Cox regression in the case of necrosis (NEC). NECLDV23 and NECCDV23 were identically defined, although NECLDV23 was defined for all 550 intervention patients, while NECCDV23 was defined for only the 326 patients in the SR subsample.

Another similarity is that almost identical 0/1 dummy variables were constructed for both logistic and Cox regression in the case of N stage (NOD). NODLDV2 and NODCDV2 were identically defined, although for different patient sets. NODLDV1 and NODCDV1 were almost identically defined. NODLDV1 grouped patients with missing observations of N stage with N0 patients. NODCDV1 grouped patients with missing observations of N stage with N1 patients.

The main difference is that logistic regression relied on five 0/1 dummy variables constructed from T stage (TUM), N stage (NOD), and necrosis (NEC) as independent variables; while Cox regression relied on five 0/1 dummy variables constructed from tumor grade (GRA), N stage (NOD), M stage (MET), and necrosis (NEC) as independent variables. In each case independent variables were constructed from those factors that survived the respective multivariate logistic regressions of PCM-generated UIRIs with backward elimination.

Results of the dummy-variable Cox regression are shown below and on the next five pages between the horizontal lines. An explicit baseline survival function was produced. It is displayed for comparison next to the standard Kaplan-Meier survival function in the slightly edited computer output. The time unit is one full year.

Likelihood ratio chi-square statistic: 95.236, two-tailed p value: 0.0000.
Score chi-square statistic: 114.814, two-tailed p value: 0.0000.
Wald chi-square statistic: 102.844, two-tailed p value: 0.0000.

All three chi-square statistics are based on 5 degrees of freedom and 326 observations, encompassing 197 distinct focal event times.

INDEPENDENT VARIABLE	REGRESSION COEFFICIENT	STANDARD DEVIATION	CHI-SQUARE (DF = 1)	2-TAIL P VALUE	RELATIVE RISK
GRACDV23	0.4677	0.1814	6.6480	0.0099	1.5962
NODCDV1	0.6267	0.1418	19.5379	0.0000	1.8714
NODCDV2	1.2961	0.2065	39.3797	0.0000	3.6551
METCDV1	0.9139	0.2305	15.7193	0.0001	2.4940
NECCDV23	0.7224	0.1561	21.4272	0.0000	2.0593

COMPARISON OF KAPLAN-MEIER (PRODUCT LIMIT) AND BASELINE SURVIVAL RATES

ELAPSED TIME UNITS	NUMBER OF EVENTS	NUMBER AT RISK	KAPLAN-MEIER SURVIVAL RATE	BASELINE SURVIVAL RATE
0.0000	N/A	326	1.0000	1.0000
0.0821	1	326	0.9969	0.9976
0.0849	2	325	0.9908	0.9927
0.1615	1	323	0.9877	0.9902
0.1670	2	322	0.9816	0.9853
0.1698	1	320	0.9785	0.9828
0.2491	1	319	0.9755	0.9803
0.2519	3	318	0.9663	0.9728
0.3285	1	315	0.9632	0.9703
0.3313	3	314	0.9540	0.9627
0.3340	3	311	0.9448	0.9549
0.4107	1	308	0.9417	0.9523
0.4134	4	307	0.9294	0.9417
0.4189	3	303	0.9202	0.9338
0.4956	1	300	0.9172	0.9311
0.5010	1	299	0.9141	0.9284
0.5804	3	297	0.9049	0.9204
0.5832	1	294	0.9018	0.9177
0.5859	1	293	0.8987	0.9149
0.5887	1	291	0.8956	0.9122
0.6626	2	290	0.8895	0.9066
0.6653	3	288	0.8802	0.8981
0.6680	2	285	0.8740	0.8924
0.6708	1	283	0.8709	0.8896
0.7529	1	282	0.8678	0.8867
0.7557	1	281	0.8647	0.8839
0.8296	1	280	0.8617	0.8810
0.8323	4	279	0.8493	0.8694
0.8351	2	275	0.8431	0.8636
0.8378	3	273	0.8339	0.8548
0.9145	2	270	0.8277	0.8488
0.9172	4	268	0.8153	0.8369
0.9199	2	264	0.8092	0.8309
0.9993	1	262	0.8061	0.8279
1.0815	1	260	0.8030	0.8249
1.0842	3	259	0.7937	0.8158
1.1609	2	256	0.7875	0.8096
1.1663	3	254	0.7782	0.8005
1.1691	2	251	0.7720	0.7944
1.2457	1	249	0.7689	0.7913
1.2485	1	248	0.7658	0.7883
1.2512	4	247	0.7534	0.7760
1.2540	2	243	0.7472	0.7698
1.3306	1	241	0.7441	0.7667

ELAPSED TIME UNITS	NUMBER OF EVENTS	NUMBER AT RISK	KAPLAN-MEIER SURVIVAL RATE	BASELINE SURVIVAL RATE
1.3334	3	240	0.7348	0.7573
1.3361	2	237	0.7286	0.7510
1.4100	1	235	0.7255	0.7478
1.4128	2	234	0.7193	0.7415
1.4182	2	232	0.7131	0.7351
1.4210	2	230	0.7069	0.7288
1.4976	1	228	0.7038	0.7256
1.5004	1	227	0.7007	0.7225
1.5031	1	226	0.6976	0.7193
1.5058	1	225	0.6945	0.7161
1.5798	2	224	0.6883	0.7097
1.5825	2	222	0.6821	0.7033
1.5852	2	220	0.6759	0.6969
1.6619	1	218	0.6728	0.6937
1.6674	2	217	0.6666	0.6872
1.6701	3	215	0.6573	0.6775
1.7468	1	212	0.6542	0.6743
1.7495	3	211	0.6449	0.6646
1.8317	1	208	0.6418	0.6613
1.8344	2	207	0.6356	0.6548
1.8371	1	205	0.6325	0.6515
1.9138	1	204	0.6294	0.6482
1.9165	1	203	0.6263	0.6449
1.9220	1	201	0.6231	0.6416
1.9247	1	200	0.6200	0.6383
1.9987	1	199	0.6169	0.6350
2.0014	3	198	0.6076	0.6248
2.0835	1	193	0.6044	0.6213
2.1629	1	191	0.6012	0.6178
2.1684	2	190	0.5949	0.6108
2.2451	1	188	0.5918	0.6073
2.2478	2	187	0.5854	0.6003
2.2506	2	184	0.5791	0.5932
2.2533	1	182	0.5759	0.5897
2.3300	1	181	0.5727	0.5862
2.3327	1	180	0.5695	0.5827
2.4176	1	179	0.5663	0.5791
2.4203	3	178	0.5568	0.5684
2.4970	1	175	0.5536	0.5647
2.4997	1	174	0.5504	0.5611
2.5024	1	173	0.5472	0.5575
2.5818	1	172	0.5441	0.5538
2.5873	2	171	0.5377	0.5465
2.6667	3	169	0.5282	0.5355
2.6722	1	166	0.5250	0.5318
2.7489	2	165	0.5186	0.5245
2.8337	3	163	0.5091	0.5134
2.8392	1	159	0.5059	0.5096
2.9131	1	158	0.5027	0.5059
2.9159	1	157	0.4995	0.5021
2.9186	2	155	0.4930	0.4946
3.0007	4	153	0.4801	0.4795
3.0829	1	149	0.4769	0.4757
3.1678	2	147	0.4704	0.4682
3.2444	1	145	0.4672	0.4644
3.2526	1	144	0.4639	0.4607

ELAPSED TIME UNITS	NUMBER OF EVENTS	NUMBER AT RISK	KAPLAN-MEIER SURVIVAL RATE	BASELINE SURVIVAL RATE
3.3293	1	142	0.4607	0.4569
3.3348	2	141	0.4541	0.4493
3.4142	2	138	0.4475	0.4416
3.4169	1	136	0.4443	0.4378
3.4196	1	135	0.4410	0.4339
3.4963	2	134	0.4344	0.4260
3.5867	1	132	0.4311	0.4221
3.6715	1	130	0.4278	0.4181
3.7482	3	129	0.4178	0.4062
3.7564	1	126	0.4145	0.4023
3.8303	1	125	0.4112	0.3983
3.8331	1	124	0.4079	0.3943
3.8385	1	122	0.4045	0.3903
3.9152	3	121	0.3945	0.3779
3.9179	1	117	0.3911	0.3737
3.9234	1	116	0.3878	0.3695
4.0001	3	115	0.3776	0.3568
4.0822	1	112	0.3743	0.3525
4.1671	1	111	0.3709	0.3483
4.2465	1	110	0.3675	0.3441
4.2492	1	109	0.3642	0.3399
4.2520	2	108	0.3574	0.3315
4.3341	2	106	0.3507	0.3232
4.3368	1	104	0.3473	0.3191
4.4135	1	103	0.3439	0.3150
4.5011	1	100	0.3405	0.3107
4.5039	1	99	0.3370	0.3064
4.5805	2	96	0.3300	0.2978
4.6654	1	93	0.3265	0.2935
4.7475	1	92	0.3229	0.2891
4.7503	1	91	0.3194	0.2848
4.8324	2	90	0.3123	0.2761
4.8351	1	87	0.3087	0.2718
5.0022	1	85	0.3051	0.2674
5.0843	1	84	0.3014	0.2630
5.0870	1	82	0.2978	0.2587
5.2513	2	80	0.2903	0.2500
5.4211	1	77	0.2865	0.2456
5.5032	1	75	0.2827	0.2412
5.6647	1	73	0.2788	0.2368
5.6702	1	72	0.2750	0.2325
5.8345	1	70	0.2710	0.2280
5.9139	2	68	0.2631	0.2191
5.9166	1	66	0.2591	0.2145
5.9988	2	65	0.2511	0.2056
6.0015	1	62	0.2471	0.2011
6.0782	1	61	0.2430	0.1966
6.0809	1	60	0.2390	0.1920
6.1630	2	59	0.2309	0.1829
6.2534	1	56	0.2267	0.1783
6.4943	1	55	0.2226	0.1738
6.4998	1	54	0.2185	0.1692
6.5025	1	53	0.2144	0.1647
6.5053	1	52	0.2103	0.1601
6.5819	1	51	0.2061	0.1557
6.6641	1	50	0.2020	0.1513

ELAPSED TIME UNITS	NUMBER OF EVENTS	NUMBER AT RISK	KAPLAN-MEIER SURVIVAL RATE	BASELINE SURVIVAL RATE
6.8338	1	49	0.1979	0.1469
7.0008	2	47	0.1895	0.1377
7.1678	2	45	0.1810	0.1286
7.2445	1	43	0.1768	0.1241
7.3321	1	42	0.1726	0.1198
7.4143	3	41	0.1600	0.1069
7.4197	1	38	0.1558	0.1027
7.5867	1	37	0.1516	0.0984
7.6661	1	36	0.1474	0.0943
7.6716	1	35	0.1432	0.0903
7.7483	1	34	0.1389	0.0863
7.7510	1	33	0.1347	0.0824
7.8332	2	32	0.1263	0.0747
8.0850	1	30	0.1221	0.0710
8.1699	1	29	0.1179	0.0673
8.4191	2	28	0.1095	0.0600
8.4985	1	26	0.1053	0.0564
8.7504	1	25	0.1010	0.0529
8.8325	1	24	0.0968	0.0495
8.9174	1	23	0.0926	0.0462
9.7469	1	22	0.0884	0.0430
10.1658	1	21	0.0842	0.0400
10.2507	1	20	0.0800	0.0371
10.2535	1	19	0.0758	0.0343
10.3356	1	18	0.0716	0.0316
10.7518	1	17	0.0674	0.0290
11.3349	1	16	0.0632	0.0264
11.7484	1	15	0.0589	0.0238
11.8332	1	14	0.0547	0.0213
12.1700	1	13	0.0505	0.0189
12.3370	1	12	0.0463	0.0167
12.7477	1	11	0.0421	0.0145
12.8298	1	10	0.0379	0.0123
12.9147	1	9	0.0337	0.0103
13.5828	1	8	0.0295	0.0085
14.9161	1	7	0.0253	0.0068
17.3364	1	6	0.0211	0.0051
17.6622	1	5	0.0168	0.0035
17.6705	1	4	0.0126	0.0023
18.6643	1	3	0.0084	0.0013
20.4193	1	2	0.0042	0.0005
24.2524	1	1	0.0000	0.0000
TOTAL	293			

If the population of elapsed time intervals until an event occurs is assumed to follow an exponential distribution, implying a constant hazard rate throughout every observation subwindow, the maximum likelihood estimate of the ordinary hazard rate is 0.238228, with a standard error of 0.013917.

The assumption of an exponential distribution with a constant hazard rate produces an EXTREMELY GOOD fit with the observed data. The analogue of an unadjusted coefficient of determination (R-squared) would be 0.9972.

An attempt was made to fit a Weibull distribution to the same data. A Weibull distribution permits either an increasing or a decreasing hazard rate over all observation subwindows. This additional flexibility failed to provide a substantially better fit. Consequently, the constant hazard rate assumed by the exponential distribution appears reasonable for this complete observation window.

If the population of elapsed time intervals until an event occurs is assumed to follow an exponential distribution, implying a constant hazard rate throughout every observation subwindow, the maximum likelihood estimate of the BASELINE hazard rate is 0.260039, with a standard error of 0.015192.

The assumption of an exponential distribution with a constant hazard rate produces an EXTREMELY GOOD fit with the observed data. The analogue of an unadjusted coefficient of determination (R-squared) would be 0.9838.

If the population of elapsed time intervals until an event occurs is assumed to follow a Weibull distribution, which permits either an increasing or a decreasing hazard rate over all observation subwindows, the maximum likelihood estimate of the BASELINE intensity parameter (analogous to the constant BASELINE hazard rate parameter characterizing an exponential distribution) is 0.249884, with a standard error of 0.012055. In addition, there appears to be an INCREASING trend in the hazard rate over time. The maximum likelihood estimate of the BASELINE trend parameter is 1.239382, with a standard error of 0.050160.

The assumption of a Weibull distribution with an INCREASING hazard rate produces a better fit with the data, at least in this complete observation window (two-tailed p value: 0.0000). The improved value of the analogue of an unadjusted coefficient of determination (R-squared) is 0.9979, indicating an EXTREMELY GOOD fit.

Once again, successive values of the baseline survival rate estimated by Cox regression tracked very closely the corresponding Kaplan-Meier product-limit values. This means that estimates of each baseline survival rate were based on the "typical" or "average" patient in the 326-patient SR subsample. They were not based on the "null" patient with zero values on all five 0/1 independent dummy variables.

Because of this each patient's individual hazard rate proportionality multiplier (HAZPROP0) must be calculated as the exponentiated (base e) sum of the products of that patient's deviation from the mean value of each 0/1 independent dummy variable (averaged over all 326 patients) multiplied by the regression coefficient generated by Cox regression for the 326 SR patients.

SUMMARY STATISTICS	ATTRIBUTE GRACDV23	ATTRIBUTE NODCDV1	ATTRIBUTE NODCDV2	ATTRIBUTE METCDV1	ATTRIBUTE NECCDV23
n DEFINED	326	326	326	326	326
MINIMUM	0	0	0	0	0
MEDIAN	1	1	0	0	0
MAXIMUM	1	1	1	1	1
MEAN	0.8589	0.5890	0.1288	0.0706	0.1902
STD. DEV.	0.3481	0.4920	0.3350	0.2561	0.3924

DEFINE HAZPROP0:
EXP[.4677*(GRACDV23-.8589)+.6267*(NODCDV1-.5890)+1.2961*(NODCDV2-.1288)+
.9139*(METCDV1-.0706)+.7224*(NECCDV23-.1902)]

SUMMARY STATISTICS	ATTRIBUTE HAZPROP0
n DEFINED	326
MINIMUM	0.3199
MEDIAN	0.9557
MAXIMUM	9.5875
MEAN	1.2655
STD. DEV.	1.0642

5.6 By How Much Did Bayesian Revision Based on Cox Regression Further Improve the Consistency of Cure Probabilities with the Initial Partitioning by Reducing Misclassifications?

We can now calculate an initial Bayesian posterior cure probability (POSTCPR0) for each of the 550 patients in the intervention sample. It is a revised version of that patient's initial prior cure probability (PRECPR0). Her prior probability produced from 0/1 dummy variables generated by the PCM-guided logistic regression is updated by the results produced from 0/1 dummy variables generated by the PCM-guided Cox regression.

Revision (Bayesian updating) is executed by:

1. either assigning a zero posterior cure probability to each patient who experienced the focal event (there were 293 such patients);
2. or evaluating the individually tailored revised cure probability (RCP) formula presented in explanatory note number 6 of section 5.1 for each censored patient (there were 257 censored patients);
3. where each censored patient's survival probability is presumed to be embodied in her individually tailored version of the maximum-likelihood Weibull function obtained from the dummy-variable Cox regression (R-squared = 0.9979); and
4. where each Weibull function is evaluated at the time elapsed since diagnosis and treatment when that patient died or was last seen alive.

DEFINE POSTCPR0: 0 IF DATENEXT#UNDEFN ELSE PRECPR0/{PRECPR0+(1-PRECPR0)*
EXP(-HAZPROP0*[.249884*DATEINT(DATEDIAG,DATELAST)]^1.239382)}

Explanatory Notes:

1. DATENEXT#UNDEFN means that the date of the patient's first evidence of further disease progression following mastectomy and radiation was defined (i.e., not undefined). The patient did experience the focal event.
2. DATEINT(DATEDIAG,DATELAST) computes the time in years elapsed since each patient's initial diagnosis with invasive breast cancer until that patient either died or was last seen alive by a physician.
3. Notice that individually tailored survival probabilities are incorporated.

SUMMARY STATISTICS	ATTRIBUTE POSTCPR0
n DEFINED	550
MINIMUM	0.0000
MEDIAN	0.0000
MAXIMUM	1.0000
MEAN	0.4260
STD. DEV.	0.4693

VALUE OF ATTRIBUTE POSTCPR0	ABSOLUTE FREQUENCIES (COUNTS)	RELATIVE FREQUENCIES (PROPORTIONS)	CUMULATIVE RELATIVE FREQUENCIES
0.00	293	0.5327	0.5327
0.01	1	0.0018	0.5345
0.10	1	0.0018	0.5364
0.15	1	0.0018	0.5382
0.22	1	0.0018	0.5400
0.31	2	0.0036	0.5436
0.37	1	0.0018	0.5455
0.38	1	0.0018	0.5473
0.41	1	0.0018	0.5491
0.43	1	0.0018	0.5509
0.45	1	0.0018	0.5527
0.46	1	0.0018	0.5545
0.49	1	0.0018	0.5564
0.50	1	0.0018	0.5582
0.55	1	0.0018	0.5600
0.57	1	0.0018	0.5618
0.58	1	0.0018	0.5636
0.61	1	0.0018	0.5655
0.64	3	0.0055	0.5709
0.68	2	0.0036	0.5745
0.69	1	0.0018	0.5764
0.71	1	0.0018	0.5782
0.72	3	0.0055	0.5836
0.73	2	0.0036	0.5873
0.74	1	0.0018	0.5891
0.77	1	0.0018	0.5909
0.79	1	0.0018	0.5927
0.80	3	0.0055	0.5982
0.81	1	0.0018	0.6000
0.83	4	0.0073	0.6073
0.84	1	0.0018	0.6091
0.85	1	0.0018	0.6109
0.87	2	0.0036	0.6145
0.88	2	0.0036	0.6182
0.89	3	0.0055	0.6236
0.90	6	0.0109	0.6345
0.91	7	0.0127	0.6473
0.92	5	0.0091	0.6564
0.93	3	0.0055	0.6618
0.94	1	0.0018	0.6636
0.95	16	0.0291	0.6927
0.96	9	0.0164	0.7091
0.97	15	0.0273	0.7364
0.98	25	0.0455	0.7818
0.99	55	0.1000	0.8818
1.00	65	0.1182	1.0000
TOTAL	550	1.0000	

Explanatory Notes:

1. The mean initial posterior cure probability (POSTCPR0) was 0.4260. This is consistent with the horizontal asymptote suggested in figure 7, although 0.4260 is very slightly on the high side of what might have been expected.

2. Zero initial posterior cure probabilities were assigned to the 293 patients who experienced the focal event, including twenty-two of the twenty-three M1 patients.
3. A zero initial posterior cure probability was also assigned to the single censored M1 patient who did not experience the focal event, but who died fairly soon after diagnosis and treatment from a cause unrelated to cancer.
4. The sixty-five POSTCPR0 probabilities reported on the previous page as 1.00 were slightly less than 100 percent. They were at least 0.995 and, therefore, rounded up to two decimal places and represented as 1.00.
5. The thirty-seven long-term survivors were all assigned POSTCPR0 probabilities between 97.34 percent and 100 percent. Their mean probability was 99.62 percent.
6. POSTCPR0 probabilities spanned the entire scale from 0 to 100 percent. A number of individual probabilities were unique. We might characterize them as discriminatingly personalized estimates of each patient's likelihood of having been cured following her mastectomy and radiation.
7. Subsequent iterations of MRPA will attempt to improve the consistency of these estimates relative to subsequent trial partitionings.

An updated misclassification analysis was performed on the ranked sequence of initial posterior cure probabilities (POSTCPR0). The optimum point of vertical separation occurred at a probability of 0.8016. This minimized the number of misclassifications relative to the initial partitioning. A cross tabulation of misclassifications at this optimal separation probability is shown below.

	MR PATIENTS TRANSFORMED TO MINIMAL RISK	SR PATIENTS REMAINING AT SUBSTANTIAL RISK	TOTAL
POSTERIOR CURE PROBABILITY >= 0.8016	218	3	221
POSTERIOR CURE PROBABILITY < 0.8016	6	323	329
TOTAL	224	326	550

MINIMUM NUMBER OF MISCLASSIFICATIONS: 6 + 3 = 9
MINIMUM PERCENTAGE OF MISCLASSIFICATIONS: 9/550 = 1.64 percent
CORRESPONDING AREA UNDER THE ROC CURVE (AUC): 0.9987 = 99.87 percent

Revising the initial prior cure probabilities produced by conventional logistic regression generated more than a tenfold reduction in misclassifications (from 133/550 = 24.18 percent to 9/550 = 1.64 percent). Greater than an order of magnitude improvement qualifies as genuinely noteworthy. Equally noteworthy was the accompanying increase in AUC score from 82.33 to a very high 99.87 percent.

In addition to providing an individually tailored answer to that all-too-familiar patient question posed in section 1.1, the substantial improvement underscores dramatically the benefits of embracing a Bayesian framework. The patient's question, when properly posed in terms of its direction of conditionality, cannot be answered except in Bayesian terms.

All survival probabilities, even when individually tailored, are oppositely directed conditional probabilities. This is not just a question of insufficient accuracy. The issue is more fundamental. It is a logical question of intended meaning, proper directional inference, and valid reasoning.

A survival probability provides a probabilistic estimate of survival time, given that the patient remains at risk of further disease progression (i.e., assuming that the patient has not been cured). It does not address the question of whether or not the patient has been cured. It presumes the absence of cure.

What the patient and the physician really want to know in this context is the reverse conditional probability. Conditional on having survived with no evidence of further disease progression for some given period of time elapsed since undergoing a potentially curative intervention, how likely is it that the intervention was successful and that the patient really was cured?

From a Bayesian analysis, individually tailored posterior cure probability curves may be constructed. They are a function of time elapsed since undergoing a potentially curative treatment without evidence of further disease progression. The likelihood of cure increases monotonically with elapsed time.

For a while following a medical intervention possessing curative potential a cure curve should replace a survival curve both in assessing the patient's progress and in communicating medical conclusions to the patient. Unless or until some event occurs providing indisputable evidence of further disease progression, the cure curve remains relevant. It can provide a basis for both patient management and personal life-planning choices.

Perhaps equally important, at least from the patient's perspective, a curve that continually rises over time depicts a hopeful and optimistic future. Contrast that with the ever-more-depressing future depicted by an always declining, glum-future-projecting survival curve.

If and when the disease reemerges, but only then, must the patient and the physician abandon the cure curve and substitute the patient's individually tailored survival curve. Regrettably, the survival curve has just become the relevant guide. The likelihood of survival then decreases monotonically with further time elapsed, in the absence of subsequent intervention or a spontaneous cure.

How to construct an individually tailored cure curve will be addressed shortly. First, however, we shall attempt to reduce and, perhaps, to eliminate completely the remaining misclassifications. This will be accomplished by executing additional iterations of MRPA.

5.7 Further Reducing Misclassifications: MRPA's Next Iteration

Bayesian revision enabled a large reduction in the number of misclassifications that occurred during the initial partitioning. This was the end result of MRPA's initial iteration.

An obvious way to set up MRPA's next iteration is simply to reclassify the 6 + 3 = 9 patients who were initially misclassified. Just interchange them, as follows, subject to a protection against iteration-to-iteration cycling.

1. Establish a lower bound to the distance separating the posterior probability assigned to a candidate for interchange and the optimum point of vertical separation. A range of five percentage points surrounding the optimum seems appropriate. That means interchange no patients within two and one-half percentage points of the optimum to avoid iteration-to-iteration cycling.
2. Move into the SR subsample as many as appropriate of the six misclassified patients initially included in the MR subsample, but whose posterior cure probabilities ended up being "too small" (i.e., more than two and one-half percentage points below the optimum point of vertical separation that occurred at POSTCPR0 = 0.8016).
3. Four of the six misclassified MR patients satisfied this criterion.

4. Simultaneously, move into the MR subsample as many as appropriate of the three misclassified patients initially included in the SR subsample, but whose posterior cure probabilities were "too large" (i.e., at least two and one-half percentage points above 0.8016).
5. All three misclassified SR patients satisfied this criterion.
6. Check to ensure that none of these seven reclassifications violated the restrictions outlined in section 4.8. In this case, none did.

The reclassifications established a revised partitioning. The total intervention sample of 550 patients now contained an MR subsample of 223 and an SR subsample of 327 patients. The relationship between the initial partitioning (MRSR0) and the revised partitioning (MRSR1) is cross tabulated below.

VALUE OF ATTRIBUTE MRSR0	VALUE OF ATTRIBUTE MRSR1		
	MR	SR	TOTAL
MR	220	4	224
SR	3	323	326
TOTAL	223	327	550

Both the logistic and the Cox regressions were repeated. This time, however, both analyses were guided by the revised partitioning rather than by the initial partitioning. Neither UIRIs nor the corresponding 0/1 dummy variables constructed therefrom were recalculated. Seven reclassifications seemed too few to produce material changes and, therefore, to require their recalculation.

Slightly edited computer output from the repeated logistic regression analysis is presented below between the horizontal lines.

Likelihood ratio chi-square statistic: 218.081, two-tailed p value: 0.0000 (based on 5 degrees of freedom and 550 complete observations).

INDEPENDENT VARIABLE	REGRESSION COEFFICIENT	STANDARD DEVIATION	CHI-SQUARE (DF = 1)	2-TAIL P VALUE	ODDS RATIO
intercept	-1.6868	0.2288	54.3513	0.0000	0.1851
TUMLDV2	1.1459	0.2502	20.9733	0.0000	3.1454
TUMLDV34	2.4722	0.3678	45.1850	0.0000	11.8486
NODLDV1	1.8573	0.2238	68.8893	0.0000	6.4067
NODLDV2	3.5591	1.0416	11.6762	0.0006	35.1300
NECLDV23	0.8233	0.3562	5.3429	0.0208	2.2781

GOODNESS OF STATISTICAL FIT OF LOGISTIC REGRESSION MODEL

Pearson chi-square fit statistic (based on 11 degrees of freedom): 12.678, p value: 0.3149.

Deviance chi-square fit statistic (based on 11 degrees of freedom): 13.675, p value: 0.2515.

Classification improvement index (proportional reduction in the number of wrong classifications enabled by using values of the independent variables): 0.4305.

```
DEFINE PRDVSR1:
EXP(-1.6868+1.1459*TUMLDV2+2.4722*TUMLDV34+1.8573*NODLDV1+3.5591*NODLDV2+
.8233*NECLDV23)/
[1+EXP(-1.6868+1.1459*TUMLDV2+2.4722*TUMLDV34+1.8573*NODLDV1+3.5591*NODLDV2+
.8233*NECLDV23)]

DEFINE PRECPR1: 1-PRDVSR1
```

SUMMARY STATISTICS	ATTRIBUTE PRECPR0	ATTRIBUTE PRECPR1
n DEFINED	550	550
MINIMUM	0.0063	0.0057
MEDIAN	0.4270	0.4298
MAXIMUM	0.8225	0.8438
MEAN	0.4073	0.4055
STD. DEV.	0.2796	0.2900

Slightly edited computer output from the repeated Cox regression analysis is presented below and on the next page between the horizontal lines.

Likelihood ratio chi-square statistic: 96.945, two-tailed p value: 0.0000.
Score chi-square statistic: 116.853, two-tailed p value: 0.0000.
Wald chi-square statistic: 104.450, two-tailed p value: 0.0000.

All three chi-square statistics are based on 5 degrees of freedom and 327 observations, encompassing 197 distinct focal event times.

INDEPENDENT VARIABLE	REGRESSION COEFFICIENT	STANDARD DEVIATION	CHI-SQUARE (DF = 1)	2-TAIL P VALUE	RELATIVE RISK
GRACDV23	0.5873	0.1819	10.4214	0.0012	1.7992
NODCDV1	0.5871	0.1420	17.0917	0.0000	1.7987
NODCDV2	1.2802	0.2072	38.1854	0.0000	3.5974
METCDV1	0.9104	0.2306	15.5854	0.0001	2.4853
NECCDV23	0.7130	0.1560	20.8822	0.0000	2.0400

If the population of elapsed time intervals until an event occurs is assumed to follow an exponential distribution, implying a constant hazard rate throughout every observation subwindow, the maximum likelihood estimate of the ordinary hazard rate is 0.233825, with a standard error of 0.013660.

The assumption of an exponential distribution with a constant hazard rate produces an EXTREMELY GOOD fit with the observed data. The analogue of an unadjusted coefficient of determination (R-squared) would be 0.9975.

An attempt was made to fit a Weibull distribution to the same data. A Weibull distribution permits either an increasing or a decreasing hazard rate over all observation subwindows. This additional flexibility failed to provide a substantially better fit. Consequently, the constant hazard rate assumed by the exponential distribution appears reasonable for this complete observation window.

If the population of elapsed time intervals until an event occurs is assumed to follow an exponential distribution, implying a constant hazard rate throughout every observation subwindow, the maximum likelihood estimate of the BASELINE hazard rate is 0.256330, with a standard error of 0.014975.

The assumption of an exponential distribution with a constant hazard rate produces an EXTREMELY GOOD fit with the observed data. The analogue of an unadjusted coefficient of determination (R-squared) would be 0.9849.

If the population of elapsed time intervals until an event occurs is assumed to follow a Weibull distribution, which permits either an increasing or a decreasing hazard rate over all observation subwindows, the maximum likelihood estimate of the BASELINE intensity parameter (analogous to the constant BASELINE hazard rate parameter characterizing an exponential distribution) is 0.246899, with a standard error of 0.011979. In addition, there appears to be an INCREASING trend in the hazard rate over time. The maximum likelihood estimate of the BASELINE trend parameter is 1.230683, with a standard error of 0.049876.

The assumption of a Weibull distribution with an INCREASING hazard rate produces a better fit with the data, at least in this complete observation window (two-tailed p value: 0.0000). The improved value of the analogue of an unadjusted coefficient of determination (R-squared) is 0.9979, indicating an EXTREMELY GOOD fit.

SUMMARY STATISTICS	ATTRIBUTE GRACDV23	ATTRIBUTE NODCDV1	ATTRIBUTE NODCDV2	ATTRIBUTE METCDV1	ATTRIBUTE NECCDV23
n DEFINED	327	327	327	327	327
MINIMUM	0	0	0	0	0
MEDIAN	1	1	0	0	0
MAXIMUM	1	1	1	1	1
MEAN	0.8532	0.5963	0.1284	0.0703	0.1896
STD. DEV.	0.3539	0.4906	0.3346	0.2557	0.3920

DEFINE HAZPROP1:
EXP[.5873*(GRACDV23-.8532)+.5871*(NODCDV1-.5963)+1.2802*(NODCDV2-.1284)+
.9104*(METCDV1-.0703)+.7130*(NECCDV23-.1896)]

SUMMARY STATISTICS	ATTRIBUTE HAZPROP1
n DEFINED	327
MINIMUM	0.2968
MEDIAN	0.9604
MAXIMUM	9.7384
MEAN	1.2726
STD. DEV.	1.0800

DEFINE POSTCPR1: 0 IF DATENEXT#UNDEFN ELSE PRECPR1/{PRECPR1+(1-PRECPR1)*
EXP(-HAZPROP1*[.246899*DATEINT(DATEDIAG,DATELAST)]^1.230683)}

SUMMARY STATISTICS	ATTRIBUTE POSTCPR0	ATTRIBUTE POSTCPR1
n DEFINED	550	550
MINIMUM	0.0000	0.0000
MEDIAN	0.0000	0.0000
MAXIMUM	1.0000	1.0000
MEAN	0.4260	0.4238
STD. DEV.	0.4693	0.4683

An updated misclassification analysis was performed on the ranked sequence of revised posterior cure probabilities (POSTCPR1). The optimum point of vertical separation occurred at a probability of 0.7718. This minimized the number of misclassifications relative to the revised partitioning. A cross tabulation of misclassifications at this optimal separation probability is shown below.

	MR PATIENTS TRANSFORMED TO MINIMAL RISK	SR PATIENTS REMAINING AT SUBSTANTIAL RISK	TOTAL
POSTERIOR CURE PROBABILITY >= 0.7718	223	2	225
POSTERIOR CURE PROBABILITY < 0.7718	0	325	325
TOTAL	223	327	550

MINIMUM NUMBER OF MISCLASSIFICATIONS: 0 + 2 = 2
MINIMUM PERCENTAGE OF MISCLASSIFICATIONS: 2/550 = 0.36 percent
CORRESPONDING AREA UNDER THE ROC CURVE (AUC): 0.9999 = 99.99 percent

Using the results of Cox regression to revise the next iteration's prior cure probabilities (PRECPR1) generated by logistic regression produced the next iteration's posterior cure probabilities (POSTCPR1). This Bayesian updating enabled an additional 78.05 percent reduction in misclassifications (from 9/550 = 1.64 percent to 2/550 = 0.36 percent). It also raised the AUC score achieved by posterior probabilities from 99.87 percent to 99.99 percent.

Posterior cure probabilities assigned to the two misclassified SR patients were compared with the optimal point of vertical separation (0.7718). Both were around 80 percent, so both patients were moved into the MR subsample for the next iteration. Neither move violated the restrictions outlined in section 4.8. No MR patients were misclassified, so none were moved.

The two reclassifications established a second revised partitioning. The total intervention sample of 550 patients now contained an MR subsample of 225 and an SR subsample of 325 patients. The relationship between the first revised partitioning (MRSR1) and this second revised partitioning (MRSR2) is cross tabulated below.

VALUE OF ATTRIBUTE MRSR1	VALUE OF ATTRIBUTE MRSR2		
	MR	SR	TOTAL
MR	223	0	223
SR	2	325	327
TOTAL	225	325	550

5.8 Eliminating All Misclassifications: MRPA's Final Iteration

Both the logistic and the Cox regressions were repeated. This time, however, both analyses were guided by the second revised partitioning rather than by the first revised partitioning. As before, neither UIRIs nor the corresponding 0/1 dummy variables constructed therefrom were recalculated, since only two additional patients were reclassified.

Slightly edited computer output from the repeated logistic regression analysis is presented on the next page between the horizontal lines.

Likelihood ratio chi-square statistic: 221.861, two-tailed p value: 0.0000 (based on 5 degrees of freedom and 550 complete observations).

INDEPENDENT VARIABLE	REGRESSION COEFFICIENT	STANDARD DEVIATION	CHI-SQUARE (DF = 1)	2-TAIL P VALUE	ODDS RATIO
intercept	-1.7056	0.2299	55.0528	0.0000	0.1817
TUMLDV2	1.1067	0.2510	19.4346	0.0000	3.0243
TUMLDV34	2.4707	0.3688	44.8718	0.0000	11.8304
NODLDV1	1.8973	0.2242	71.5983	0.0000	6.6681
NODLDV2	3.5911	1.0415	11.8893	0.0006	36.2730
NECLDV23	0.8602	0.3572	5.7983	0.0160	2.3636

GOODNESS OF STATISTICAL FIT OF LOGISTIC REGRESSION MODEL

Pearson chi-square fit statistic (based on 11 degrees of freedom): 12.874, p value: 0.3016.

Deviance chi-square fit statistic (based on 11 degrees of freedom): 13.768, p value: 0.2461.

Classification improvement index (proportional reduction in the number of wrong classifications enabled by using values of the independent variables): 0.4444.

DEFINE PRDVSR2:
EXP(-1.7056+1.1067*TUMLDV2+2.4707*TUMLDV34+1.8973*NODLDV1+3.5911*NODLDV2+
.8602*NECLDV23)/
[1+EXP(-1.7056+1.1067*TUMLDV2+2.4707*TUMLDV34+1.8973*NODLDV1+3.5911*NODLDV2+
.8602*NECLDV23)]

DEFINE PRECPR2: 1-PRDVSR2

SUMMARY STATISTICS	ATTRIBUTE PRECPR0	ATTRIBUTE PRECPR1	ATTRIBUTE PRECPR2
n DEFINED	550	550	550
MINIMUM	0.0063	0.0057	0.0054
MEDIAN	0.4270	0.4298	0.4350
MAXIMUM	0.8225	0.8438	0.8463
MEAN	0.4073	0.4055	0.4091
STD. DEV.	0.2796	0.2900	0.2927

Slightly edited computer output from the repeated Cox regression analysis is presented below and on the next page between the horizontal lines.

Likelihood ratio chi-square statistic: 94.880, two-tailed p value: 0.0000.
Score chi-square statistic: 114.151, two-tailed p value: 0.0000.
Wald chi-square statistic: 102.218, two-tailed p value: 0.0000.

All three chi-square statistics are based on 5 degrees of freedom and 325 observations, encompassing 197 distinct focal event times.

INDEPENDENT VARIABLE	REGRESSION COEFFICIENT	STANDARD DEVIATION	CHI-SQUARE (DF = 1)	2-TAIL P VALUE	RELATIVE RISK
GRACDV23	0.5950	0.1818	10.7076	0.0011	1.8130
NODCDV1	0.5636	0.1421	15.7298	0.0001	1.7570
NODCDV2	1.2584	0.2071	36.9148	0.0000	3.5199
METCDV1	0.9065	0.2306	15.4569	0.0001	2.4757
NECCDV23	0.7036	0.1560	20.3443	0.0000	2.0210

If the population of elapsed time intervals until an event occurs is assumed to follow an exponential distribution, implying a constant hazard rate throughout every observation subwindow, the maximum likelihood estimate of the ordinary hazard rate is 0.236055, with a standard error of 0.013790.

The assumption of an exponential distribution with a constant hazard rate produces an EXTREMELY GOOD fit with the observed data. The analogue of an unadjusted coefficient of determination (R-squared) would be 0.9974.

An attempt was made to fit a Weibull distribution to the same data. A Weibull distribution permits either an increasing or a decreasing hazard rate over all observation subwindows. This additional flexibility failed to provide a substantially better fit. The constant hazard rate assumed by the exponential distribution appears reasonable for this complete observation window.

If the population of elapsed time intervals until an event occurs is assumed to follow an exponential distribution, the maximum likelihood estimate of the BASELINE hazard rate is 0.259034, with a standard error of 0.015133.

The assumption of an exponential distribution with a constant hazard rate produces an EXTREMELY GOOD fit with the observed data. The analogue of an unadjusted coefficient of determination (R-squared) would be 0.9849.

If the population of elapsed time intervals until an event occurs is assumed to follow a Weibull distribution, which permits either an increasing or a decreasing hazard rate over all observation subwindows, the maximum likelihood estimate of the BASELINE intensity parameter (analogous to the constant BASELINE hazard rate parameter characterizing an exponential distribution) is 0.249011, with a standard error of 0.012117. In addition, there appears to be an INCREASING trend in the hazard rate over time. The maximum likelihood estimate of the BASELINE trend parameter is 1.228997, with a standard error of 0.049772.

The assumption of a Weibull distribution with an INCREASING hazard rate produces a better fit with the data, at least in this complete observation window (two-tailed p value: 0.0000). The improved value of the analogue of an unadjusted coefficient of determination (R-squared) is 0.9980, indicating an EXTREMELY GOOD fit.

SUMMARY STATISTICS	ATTRIBUTE GRACDV23	ATTRIBUTE NODCDV1	ATTRIBUTE NODCDV2	ATTRIBUTE METCDV1	ATTRIBUTE NECCDV23
n DEFINED	325	325	325	325	325
MINIMUM	0	0	0	0	0
MEDIAN	1	1	0	0	0
MAXIMUM	1	1	1	1	1
MEAN	0.8523	0.6000	0.1292	0.0708	0.1908
STD. DEV.	0.3548	0.4899	0.3355	0.2564	0.3929

DEFINE HAZPROP2:
EXP[.5950*(GRACDV23-.8523)+.5636*(NODCDV1-.6000)+1.2584*(NODCDV2-.1292)+
.9065*(METCDV1-.0708)+.7036*(NECCDV23-.1908)]

SUMMARY STATISTICS	ATTRIBUTE HAZPROP2
n DEFINED	325
MINIMUM	0.2993
MEDIAN	0.9534
MAXIMUM	9.5569
MEAN	1.2666
STD. DEV.	1.0628

DEFINE POSTCPR2: 0 IF DATENEXT#UNDEFN ELSE PRECPR2/{PRECPR2+(1-PRECPR2)*
EXP(-HAZPROP2*[.249011*DATEINT(DATEDIAG,DATELAST)]^1.228997)}

SUMMARY STATISTICS	ATTRIBUTE POSTCPR0	ATTRIBUTE POSTCPR1	ATTRIBUTE POSTCPR2
n DEFINED	550	550	550
MINIMUM	0.0000	0.0000	0.0000
MEDIAN	0.0000	0.0000	0.0000
MAXIMUM	1.0000	1.0000	1.0000
MEAN	0.4260	0.4238	0.4249
STD. DEV.	0.4693	0.4683	0.4693

An updated misclassification analysis was performed on the ranked sequence of
revised posterior cure probabilities (POSTCPR2). The optimum point of vertical
separation occurred at a probability of 0.7850. This minimized the number of
misclassifications relative to the revised partitioning. In fact, it eliminated
all misclassifications. Thanks to the construction of 0/1 dummy variables, the
optimum was unique. It was the only posterior cure probability that, if used to
divide patients into MR and SR subsamples, achieved a perfect separation.

A cross tabulation of misclassifications at this optimal (zero
misclassifications) separation probability is shown below.

	MR PATIENTS TRANSFORMED TO MINIMAL RISK	SR PATIENTS REMAINING AT SUBSTANTIAL RISK	TOTAL
POSTERIOR CURE PROBABILITY >= 0.7850	225	0	225
POSTERIOR CURE PROBABILITY < 0.7850	0	325	325
TOTAL	225	325	550

MINIMUM NUMBER OF MISCLASSIFICATIONS: 0 + 0 = 0
MINIMUM PERCENTAGE OF MISCLASSIFICATIONS: 0/550 = 0.00 percent
CORRESPONDING AREA UNDER THE ROC CURVE (AUC): 1.0000 = 100 percent

Since MRPA converged completely, this was its final iteration. There was no
room for further improvement. Using the results of Cox regression to revise the
final iteration's prior cure probabilities (PRECPR2) generated by logistic
regression produced the final iteration's posterior cure probabilities
(POSTCPR2). This Bayesian updating succeeded in eliminating all
misclassifications. By doing so, it raised the AUC score achieved by posterior
probabilities from 99.99 percent to 100.00 percent.

5.9 Checking the Final Partitioning for Reasonableness

MRPA's final partitioning of the 550 patients in the Turku sample into 225 MR (cured) and 325 SR (at risk) patients may now be checked for reasonableness.

BASIS OF COMPARISON	MR (CURED)	SR (AT RISK)	TWO-TAILED P VALUE
SUBSAMPLE SIZE (patients)	225	325	N/A
MEDIAN TUMOR SIZE (mm.)	20	30	< 0.00005
MEAN TUMOR SIZE (mm.)	25.12	36.45	< 0.00005
MEDIAN LENGTH OF FOLLOW-UP (years)	18.58	3.41	< 0.00005
MEAN LENGTH OF FOLLOW-UP (years)	19.04	4.97	< 0.00005

All differences were highly significant by the median and two-sample t tests.

Following are ten cross tabulations. All but two occur as a pair of tables. The first table contains joint absolute frequencies (counts). The second contains relative frequencies conditional by column to facilitate subsample comparison.

TYPE OF SURGERY PERFORMED	FINAL MRPA-PARTITIONED SUBSAMPLE		
	MR (CURED)	SR (AT RISK)	TOTAL
MODIFIED RADICAL MASTECTOMY	47	78	125
RADICAL MASTECTOMY	178	247	425
TOTAL	225	325	550

TYPE OF SURGERY PERFORMED	FINAL MRPA-PARTITIONED SUBSAMPLE	
	MR (CURED)	SR (AT RISK)
MODIFIED RADICAL MASTECTOMY	0.2089	0.2400
RADICAL MASTECTOMY	0.7911	0.7600
TOTAL	1.0000	1.0000

No significant difference: chi-square two-tailed p value = 0.4517.

TYPE OF BREAST TUMOR	FINAL MRPA-PARTITIONED SUBSAMPLE		
	MR (CURED)	SR (AT RISK)	TOTAL
DUCTAL	183	285	468
LOBULAR	42	40	82
TOTAL	225	325	550

TYPE OF BREAST TUMOR	FINAL MRPA-PARTITIONED SUBSAMPLE	
	MR (CURED)	SR (AT RISK)
DUCTAL	0.8133	0.8769
LOBULAR	0.1867	0.1231
TOTAL	1.0000	1.0000

Not quite significant difference: chi-square two-tailed p value = 0.0528.

T STAGE OF PATIENT	FINAL MRPA-PARTITIONED SUBSAMPLE		
	MR (CURED)	SR (AT RISK)	TOTAL
0 OR 1	101	39	140
2	110	160	270
3	8	72	80
4	4	47	51
TOTAL	223	318	541

T STAGE OF PATIENT	FINAL MRPA-PARTITIONED SUBSAMPLE	
	MR (CURED)	SR (AT RISK)
0 OR 1	0.4529	0.1226
2	0.4933	0.5031
3	0.0359	0.2264
4	0.0179	0.1479
TOTAL	1.0000	1.0000

Significant difference: chi-square two-tailed p value < 0.00005, based on nine missing observations.

N STAGE OF PATIENT	FINAL MRPA-PARTITIONED SUBSAMPLE		
	MR (CURED)	SR (AT RISK)	TOTAL
0	176	88	264
1	46	191	237
2	1	42	43
TOTAL	223	321	544

N STAGE OF PATIENT	FINAL MRPA-PARTITIONED SUBSAMPLE	
	MR (CURED)	SR (AT RISK)
0	0.7892	0.2741
1	0.2063	0.5950
2	0.0045	0.1309
TOTAL	1.0000	1.0000

Significant difference: chi-square two-tailed p value < 0.00005, based on six missing observations.

M STAGE OF PATIENT	FINAL MRPA-PARTITIONED SUBSAMPLE		
	MR (CURED)	SR (AT RISK)	TOTAL
0	225	302	527
1	0	23	23
TOTAL	225	325	550

Statistical test inappropriate (definitional association): zero percent of the MR patients and 7.08 percent of the SR patients were in the M1 stage.

GRADE OF TUMOR	FINAL MRPA-PARTITIONED SUBSAMPLE		
	MR (CURED)	SR (AT RISK)	TOTAL
1	55	48	103
2	115	146	261
3	55	131	186
TOTAL	225	325	550

GRADE OF TUMOR	FINAL MRPA-PARTITIONED SUBSAMPLE	
	MR (CURED)	SR (AT RISK)
1	0.2444	0.1477
2	0.5112	0.4492
3	0.2444	0.4031
TOTAL	1.0000	1.0000

Significant difference: chi-square two-tailed p value = 0.0001.

MITOTIC RATE (PER HPF)	FINAL MRPA-PARTITIONED SUBSAMPLE		
	MR (CURED)	SR (AT RISK)	TOTAL
RARE	98	105	203
2 - 3	98	134	232
> 3	29	86	115
TOTAL	225	325	550

MITOTIC RATE (PER HPF)	FINAL MRPA-PARTITIONED SUBSAMPLE	
	MR (CURED)	SR (AT RISK)
RARE	0.4356	0.3231
2 - 3	0.4356	0.4123
> 3	0.1288	0.2646
TOTAL	1.0000	1.0000

Significant difference: chi-square two-tailed p value = 0.0003.

DEGREE OF NECROSIS	FINAL MRPA-PARTITIONED SUBSAMPLE		
	MR (CURED)	SR (AT RISK)	TOTAL
NONE	179	204	383
SPOTTY	30	59	89
MODERATE	14	37	51
SEVERE	2	25	27
TOTAL	225	325	550

DEGREE OF NECROSIS	FINAL MRPA-PARTITIONED SUBSAMPLE	
	MR (CURED)	SR (AT RISK)
NONE	0.7956	0.6278
SPOTTY	0.1333	0.1815
MODERATE	0.0622	0.1138
SEVERE	0.0089	0.0769
TOTAL	1.0000	1.0000

Significant difference: chi-square two-tailed p value < 0.00005.

RELAPSE OR RECURRENCE EXPERIENCED	FINAL MRPA-PARTITIONED SUBSAMPLE		
	MR (CURED)	SR (AT RISK)	TOTAL
NO	225	198	423
YES	0	127	127
TOTAL	225	325	550

Statistical test inappropriate (definitional association): zero percent of the MR patients and 39.08 percent of the SR patients experienced a relapse or recurrence, which was included among experiences comprising the focal event.

PATIENT STATUS WHEN LAST OBSERVED	FINAL MRPA-PARTITIONED SUBSAMPLE		
	MR (CURED)	SR (AT RISK)	TOTAL
DIED OF BREAST CANCER	0	278	278
DIED OF OTHER CANCER	21	6	27
DIED OF OTHER CAUSE	95	39	134
STILL ALIVE	109	2	111
TOTAL	225	325	550

PATIENT STATUS WHEN LAST OBSERVED	FINAL MRPA-PARTITIONED SUBSAMPLE	
	MR (CURED)	SR (AT RISK)
DIED OF BREAST CANCER	0.0000	0.8553
DIED OF OTHER CANCER	0.0933	0.0185
DIED OF OTHER CAUSE	0.4222	0.1200
STILL ALIVE	0.4845	0.0062
TOTAL	1.0000	1.0000

A statistical test was inappropriate (definitional association).

These results support the conclusion that the total 550-patient intervention sample originally contained a mixture of minimal risk (cured) and still-at-substantial-risk (not cured) patients and that MRPA has successfully partitioned them into two distinct subsamples of 225 MR and 325 SR patients.

No systematic differences were expected between the MR and SR subsamples with respect to either TYPE OF SURGERY PERFORMED (modified radical mastectomy versus radical mastectomy) or TYPE OF BREAST TUMOR (ductal versus lobular). Only the ductal versus lobular subsample difference was close to being significant.

Systematic differences were definitely expected to emerge between the MR and SR subsamples with respect to:

1. MEDIAN AND MEAN TUMOR SIZE (in mm.), where SR tumors were expected to be larger (a known prognostic risk factor);
2. MEDIAN AND MEAN LENGTH OF FOLLOW-UP (in years), where duration of MR follow-up was expected to be longer due to higher SR mortality;
3. T, N, and M STAGE of patient at diagnosis and treatment, where SR patients were expected to be at later stages (known prognostic risk factors);
4. GRADE OF TUMOR, where SR tumors were expected to be higher grade (a known prognostic risk factor);
5. MITOTIC RATE, where SR rates were expected to be higher, indicating more vigorous growth (a known prognostic risk factor);
6. DEGREE OF NECROSIS, where SR degree was expected to be higher (a known prognostic risk factor);
7. RELAPSE OR RECURRENCE EXPERIENCED, since this was guaranteed to be experienced only by SR patients because of the manner in which the focal event was defined and the Bayesian manner in which the partitioning procedure was executed; and
8. PATIENT STATUS WHEN LAST OBSERVED, since death due to breast cancer was guaranteed to be experienced only by SR patients because of the manner in which the focal event was defined and the Bayesian manner in which the partitioning procedure was executed.

All expected differences emerged, all were in the expected direction, and all statistical tests performed produced extremely significant p values.

5.10 A Dramatically Revised Kaplan-Meier Survival Curve: The Apparent
      Disappearance of a Declining Hazard Rate over Time

Since MRPA appears to have been successful in partitioning the Turku intervention sample into 225 MR and 325 SR patients, it is no longer appropriate to submit all 550 patients to a single Kaplan-Meier survival analysis. Now it is only appropriate to do so for the 325 SR patients deemed by MRPA to have remained at substantial risk despite their mastectomy and radiation. The 225 MR (cured) patients were presumed to have been transformed to a state of very low or no (minimal) risk. Including them in the analysis would only serve to contaminate the results and to distort the survival curve.

Annotated computer outputs of a Kaplan-Meier analysis of the 325 SR patients identified in MRPA's final iteration are shown on the next five pages between the horizontal lines. These results may be compared directly with similar results generated in section 4.5 by the same KAPM procedure when it was applied to all 550 intervention patients. The corresponding final Kaplan-Meier survival curve to be presented subsequently in figure 8 may also be compared with the initial survival curve shown in figure 7.

DESCRIPTIVE SUMMARY OF ELAPSED TIME INTERVALS

The set of strictly positive elapsed observation time intervals relating to 325 PATIENTs constitutes the effective sample for the descriptive summary. There are 215 distinct elapsed time intervals in this set. The complete observation window (i.e., the longest elapsed time interval observed) is 24.2524 elapsed time unit(s). The time unit is one full year.

The MINIMUM number of elapsed time units observed is 0.0821.
The MEDIAN number of elapsed time units observed is 2.8125.
The MAXIMUM number of elapsed time units observed is 24.2524.
The MEAN number of elapsed time units observed is 3.8192,
with a STANDARD DEVIATION of 3.6694.

KAPLAN-MEIER ANALYSIS (SURVIVAL RATE ESTIMATED VIA THE PRODUCT-LIMIT METHOD)

The same set of strictly positive elapsed observation time intervals relating to 325 PATIENTs constitutes the effective sample for the Kaplan-Meier analysis. It focuses on the particular subset of 197 distinct intervals that terminate with the occurrence of at least one event. In addition, the analysis considers all truncated-observation intervals that terminate before an event has occurred (censored observations), if any exist. A total of 293 events occur during the observation subwindow that encompasses all events. This observation subwindow spans 24.2524 elapsed time unit(s).

ELAPSED TIME UNITS	NUMBER OF EVENTS	NUMBER AT RISK	HAZARD RATE	CUMULATIVE HAZARD RATE	KAPLAN-MEIER SURVIVAL RATE	STANDARD ERROR
0.0000	N/A	325	N/A	N/A	1.0000	N/A
0.0821	1	325	0.0031	0.0031	0.9969	0.0031
0.0849	2	324	0.0062	0.0092	0.9908	0.0053
0.1615	1	322	0.0031	0.0124	0.9877	0.0061
0.1670	2	321	0.0062	0.0186	0.9815	0.0075
0.1698	1	319	0.0031	0.0217	0.9785	0.0081
0.2491	1	318	0.0031	0.0249	0.9754	0.0086
0.2519	3	317	0.0095	0.0343	0.9662	0.0100
0.3285	1	314	0.0032	0.0375	0.9631	0.0105
0.3313	3	313	0.0096	0.0471	0.9538	0.0116
0.3340	3	310	0.0097	0.0568	0.9446	0.0127
0.4107	1	307	0.0033	0.0600	0.9415	0.0130
0.4134	4	306	0.0131	0.0731	0.9292	0.0142
0.4189	3	302	0.0099	0.0830	0.9200	0.0150
0.4956	1	299	0.0033	0.0864	0.9169	0.0153
0.5010	1	298	0.0034	0.0897	0.9138	0.0156
0.5804	3	296	0.0101	0.0999	0.9046	0.0163
0.5832	1	293	0.0034	0.1033	0.9015	0.0165
0.5859	1	292	0.0034	0.1067	0.8984	0.0168
0.5887	1	290	0.0034	0.1102	0.8953	0.0170
0.6626	2	289	0.0069	0.1171	0.8891	0.0174
0.6653	3	287	0.0105	0.1275	0.8798	0.0181
0.6680	2	284	0.0070	0.1346	0.8736	0.0184
0.6708	1	282	0.0035	0.1381	0.8705	0.0186
0.7529	1	281	0.0036	0.1417	0.8674	0.0188
0.7557	1	280	0.0036	0.1453	0.8643	0.0190
0.8296	1	279	0.0036	0.1488	0.8612	0.0192
0.8323	4	278	0.0144	0.1632	0.8488	0.0199

ELAPSED TIME UNITS	NUMBER OF EVENTS	NUMBER AT RISK	HAZARD RATE	CUMULATIVE HAZARD RATE	KAPLAN-MEIER SURVIVAL RATE	STANDARD ERROR
0.8351	2	274	0.0073	0.1705	0.8426	0.0202
0.8378	3	272	0.0110	0.1816	0.8334	0.0207
0.9145	2	269	0.0074	0.1890	0.8272	0.0210
0.9172	4	267	0.0150	0.2040	0.8148	0.0216
0.9199	2	263	0.0076	0.2116	0.8086	0.0219
0.9993	1	261	0.0038	0.2154	0.8055	0.0220
1.0815	1	259	0.0039	0.2193	0.8024	0.0221
1.0842	3	258	0.0116	0.2309	0.7930	0.0225
1.1609	2	255	0.0078	0.2387	0.7868	0.0228
1.1663	3	253	0.0119	0.2506	0.7775	0.0231
1.1691	2	250	0.0080	0.2586	0.7713	0.0234
1.2457	1	248	0.0040	0.2626	0.7682	0.0235
1.2485	1	247	0.0040	0.2667	0.7650	0.0236
1.2512	4	246	0.0163	0.2829	0.7526	0.0240
1.2540	2	242	0.0083	0.2912	0.7464	0.0242
1.3306	1	240	0.0042	0.2954	0.7433	0.0243
1.3334	3	239	0.0126	0.3079	0.7339	0.0246
1.3361	2	236	0.0085	0.3164	0.7277	0.0248
1.4100	1	234	0.0043	0.3207	0.7246	0.0249
1.4128	2	233	0.0086	0.3293	0.7184	0.0250
1.4182	2	231	0.0087	0.3379	0.7122	0.0252
1.4210	2	229	0.0087	0.3466	0.7060	0.0254
1.4976	1	227	0.0044	0.3510	0.7028	0.0254
1.5004	1	226	0.0044	0.3555	0.6997	0.0255
1.5031	1	225	0.0044	0.3599	0.6966	0.0256
1.5058	1	224	0.0045	0.3644	0.6935	0.0257
1.5798	2	223	0.0090	0.3734	0.6873	0.0258
1.5825	2	221	0.0090	0.3824	0.6811	0.0259
1.5852	2	219	0.0091	0.3915	0.6749	0.0261
1.6619	1	217	0.0046	0.3961	0.6717	0.0261
1.6674	2	216	0.0093	0.4054	0.6655	0.0263
1.6701	3	214	0.0140	0.4194	0.6562	0.0264
1.7468	1	211	0.0047	0.4242	0.6531	0.0265
1.7495	3	210	0.0143	0.4384	0.6438	0.0267
1.8317	1	207	0.0048	0.4433	0.6406	0.0267
1.8344	2	206	0.0097	0.4530	0.6344	0.0268
1.8371	1	204	0.0049	0.4579	0.6313	0.0269
1.9138	1	203	0.0049	0.4628	0.6282	0.0269
1.9165	1	202	0.0050	0.4678	0.6251	0.0270
1.9220	1	200	0.0050	0.4728	0.6220	0.0270
1.9247	1	199	0.0050	0.4778	0.6188	0.0271
1.9987	1	198	0.0051	0.4828	0.6157	0.0271
2.0014	3	197	0.0152	0.4981	0.6063	0.0272
2.0835	1	192	0.0052	0.5033	0.6032	0.0273
2.1629	1	190	0.0053	0.5085	0.6000	0.0273
2.1684	2	189	0.0106	0.5191	0.5937	0.0274
2.2451	1	187	0.0053	0.5245	0.5905	0.0274
2.2478	2	186	0.0108	0.5352	0.5841	0.0275
2.2506	2	183	0.0109	0.5461	0.5778	0.0276
2.2533	1	181	0.0055	0.5517	0.5746	0.0276
2.3300	1	180	0.0056	0.5572	0.5714	0.0276
2.3327	1	179	0.0056	0.5628	0.5682	0.0276
2.4176	1	178	0.0056	0.5684	0.5650	0.0277
2.4203	3	177	0.0169	0.5854	0.5554	0.0277
2.4970	1	174	0.0057	0.5911	0.5522	0.0278
2.4997	1	173	0.0058	0.5969	0.5490	0.0278

ELAPSED TIME UNITS	NUMBER OF EVENTS	NUMBER AT RISK	HAZARD RATE	CUMULATIVE HAZARD RATE	KAPLAN-MEIER SURVIVAL RATE	STANDARD ERROR
2.5024	1	172	0.0058	0.6027	0.5458	0.0278
2.5818	1	171	0.0058	0.6086	0.5426	0.0278
2.5873	2	170	0.0118	0.6203	0.5363	0.0279
2.6667	3	168	0.0179	0.6382	0.5267	0.0279
2.6722	1	165	0.0061	0.6443	0.5235	0.0279
2.7489	2	164	0.0122	0.6565	0.5171	0.0280
2.8337	3	162	0.0185	0.6750	0.5075	0.0280
2.8392	1	158	0.0063	0.6813	0.5043	0.0280
2.9131	1	157	0.0064	0.6877	0.5011	0.0280
2.9159	1	156	0.0064	0.6941	0.4979	0.0280
2.9186	2	154	0.0130	0.7071	0.4914	0.0280
3.0007	4	152	0.0263	0.7334	0.4785	0.0280
3.0829	1	148	0.0068	0.7401	0.4753	0.0280
3.1678	2	146	0.0137	0.7538	0.4687	0.0280
3.2444	1	144	0.0069	0.7608	0.4655	0.0280
3.2526	1	143	0.0070	0.7678	0.4622	0.0280
3.3293	1	141	0.0071	0.7749	0.4590	0.0280
3.3348	2	140	0.0143	0.7892	0.4524	0.0280
3.4142	2	137	0.0146	0.8037	0.4458	0.0279
3.4169	1	135	0.0074	0.8112	0.4425	0.0279
3.4196	1	134	0.0075	0.8186	0.4392	0.0279
3.4963	2	133	0.0150	0.8337	0.4326	0.0279
3.5867	1	131	0.0076	0.8413	0.4293	0.0279
3.6715	1	129	0.0078	0.8490	0.4260	0.0278
3.7482	3	128	0.0234	0.8725	0.4160	0.0278
3.7564	1	125	0.0080	0.8805	0.4126	0.0278
3.8303	1	124	0.0081	0.8885	0.4093	0.0277
3.8331	1	123	0.0081	0.8967	0.4060	0.0277
3.8385	1	121	0.0083	0.9049	0.4026	0.0277
3.9152	3	120	0.0250	0.9299	0.3926	0.0276
3.9179	1	116	0.0086	0.9386	0.3892	0.0276
3.9234	1	115	0.0087	0.9473	0.3858	0.0275
4.0001	3	114	0.0263	0.9736	0.3757	0.0274
4.0822	1	111	0.0090	0.9826	0.3723	0.0274
4.1671	1	110	0.0091	0.9917	0.3689	0.0273
4.2465	1	109	0.0092	1.0008	0.3655	0.0273
4.2492	1	108	0.0093	1.0101	0.3621	0.0272
4.2520	2	107	0.0187	1.0288	0.3553	0.0272
4.3341	2	105	0.0190	1.0478	0.3486	0.0271
4.3368	1	103	0.0097	1.0576	0.3452	0.0270
4.4135	1	102	0.0098	1.0674	0.3418	0.0270
4.5011	1	99	0.0101	1.0775	0.3384	0.0269
4.5039	1	98	0.0102	1.0877	0.3349	0.0268
4.5805	2	95	0.0211	1.1087	0.3279	0.0267
4.6654	1	92	0.0109	1.1196	0.3243	0.0267
4.7475	1	91	0.0110	1.1306	0.3207	0.0266
4.7503	1	90	0.0111	1.1417	0.3172	0.0266
4.8324	2	89	0.0225	1.1642	0.3100	0.0264
4.8351	1	86	0.0116	1.1758	0.3064	0.0264
5.0022	1	84	0.0119	1.1877	0.3028	0.0263
5.0843	1	83	0.0120	1.1997	0.2991	0.0263
5.0870	1	82	0.0122	1.2119	0.2955	0.0262
5.2513	2	80	0.0250	1.2369	0.2881	0.0260
5.4211	1	78	0.0128	1.2498	0.2844	0.0260
5.5032	1	77	0.0130	1.2627	0.2807	0.0259
5.6647	1	75	0.0133	1.2761	0.2770	0.0258

ELAPSED TIME UNITS	NUMBER OF EVENTS	NUMBER AT RISK	HAZARD RATE	CUMULATIVE HAZARD RATE	KAPLAN-MEIER SURVIVAL RATE	STANDARD ERROR
5.6702	1	74	0.0135	1.2896	0.2732	0.0257
5.8345	1	72	0.0139	1.3035	0.2694	0.0257
5.9139	2	71	0.0282	1.3316	0.2618	0.0255
5.9166	1	69	0.0145	1.3461	0.2580	0.0254
5.9988	2	68	0.0294	1.3755	0.2505	0.0252
6.0015	1	66	0.0152	1.3907	0.2467	0.0251
6.0782	1	65	0.0154	1.4061	0.2429	0.0250
6.0809	1	64	0.0156	1.4217	0.2391	0.0249
6.1630	2	63	0.0317	1.4535	0.2315	0.0247
6.2534	1	60	0.0167	1.4701	0.2276	0.0246
6.4943	1	59	0.0169	1.4871	0.2238	0.0245
6.4998	1	58	0.0172	1.5043	0.2199	0.0243
6.5025	1	57	0.0175	1.5219	0.2161	0.0242
6.5053	1	56	0.0179	1.5397	0.2122	0.0241
6.5819	1	55	0.0182	1.5579	0.2083	0.0240
6.6641	1	54	0.0185	1.5764	0.2045	0.0238
6.8338	1	53	0.0189	1.5953	0.2006	0.0237
7.0008	2	51	0.0392	1.6345	0.1928	0.0234
7.1678	2	49	0.0408	1.6753	0.1849	0.0231
7.2445	1	47	0.0213	1.6966	0.1810	0.0229
7.3321	1	46	0.0217	1.7183	0.1770	0.0228
7.4143	3	45	0.0667	1.7850	0.1652	0.0223
7.4197	1	42	0.0238	1.8088	0.1613	0.0221
7.5867	1	41	0.0244	1.8332	0.1573	0.0219
7.6661	1	40	0.0250	1.8582	0.1534	0.0217
7.6716	1	39	0.0256	1.8838	0.1495	0.0215
7.7483	1	38	0.0263	1.9102	0.1455	0.0213
7.7510	1	37	0.0270	1.9372	0.1416	0.0211
7.8332	2	36	0.0556	1.9927	0.1337	0.0206
8.0850	1	34	0.0294	2.0221	0.1298	0.0204
8.1699	1	33	0.0303	2.0525	0.1259	0.0201
8.4191	2	32	0.0625	2.1150	0.1180	0.0196
8.4985	1	30	0.0333	2.1483	0.1141	0.0194
8.7504	1	28	0.0357	2.1840	0.1100	0.0191
8.8325	1	27	0.0370	2.2210	0.1059	0.0188
8.9174	1	26	0.0385	2.2595	0.1019	0.0185
9.7469	1	24	0.0417	2.3012	0.0976	0.0182
10.1658	1	22	0.0455	2.3466	0.0932	0.0179
10.2507	1	21	0.0476	2.3942	0.0887	0.0176
10.2535	1	20	0.0500	2.4442	0.0843	0.0173
10.3356	1	19	0.0526	2.4969	0.0799	0.0169
10.7518	1	18	0.0556	2.5524	0.0754	0.0166
11.3349	1	17	0.0588	2.6112	0.0710	0.0162
11.7484	1	16	0.0625	2.6737	0.0666	0.0158
11.8332	1	14	0.0714	2.7452	0.0618	0.0153
12.1700	1	13	0.0769	2.8221	0.0570	0.0149
12.3370	1	12	0.0833	2.9054	0.0523	0.0144
12.7477	1	11	0.0909	2.9963	0.0475	0.0138
12.8298	1	10	0.1000	3.0963	0.0428	0.0132
12.9147	1	9	0.1111	3.2075	0.0380	0.0126
13.5828	1	8	0.1250	3.3325	0.0333	0.0119
14.9161	1	7	0.1429	3.4753	0.0285	0.0111
17.3364	1	6	0.1667	3.6420	0.0238	0.0102
17.6622	1	5	0.2000	3.8420	0.0190	0.0092
17.6705	1	4	0.2500	4.0920	0.0143	0.0080
18.6643	1	3	0.3333	4.4253	0.0095	0.0066

ELAPSED TIME UNITS	NUMBER OF EVENTS	NUMBER AT RISK	HAZARD RATE	CUMULATIVE HAZARD RATE	KAPLAN-MEIER SURVIVAL RATE	STANDARD ERROR
20.4193	1	2	0.5000	4.9253	0.0048	0.0047
24.2524	1	1	1.0000	5.9253	0.0000	N/A
TOTAL	293					

If the population of elapsed time intervals until an event occurs is assumed to follow an exponential distribution, implying a constant hazard rate throughout every observation subwindow, the maximum likelihood estimate of that hazard rate is 0.2361, with a standard error of 0.013790.

The assumption of an exponential distribution with a constant hazard rate produces an EXTREMELY GOOD fit with the observed data. The analogue of an unadjusted coefficient of determination (R-squared) would be 0.9974.

An attempt was made to fit a Weibull distribution to the same data. A Weibull distribution permits either an increasing or a decreasing hazard rate over all observation subwindows. This additional flexibility failed to provide a substantially better fit. Consequently, the constant hazard rate assumed by the exponential distribution appears reasonable for this complete observation window.

Notice that an exponential function fit the Kaplan-Meier survival estimates for the 325 SR patients extremely closely (R-squared = 0.9974). An exponential survival function implies a constant hazard rate of further disease progression over time. No Weibull function with either an increasing or a decreasing hazard rate could provide a better fit with the same SR patient survival data.

The maximum likelihood estimate of the constant (exponential) hazard rate was 0.2361 focal events per year. Reading from figure 8, the "typical" or "average" SR patient could therefore expect to experience with 50 percent probability some event evidencing further disease progression within approximately 2.91 years following diagnosis and treatment. In stark contrast, MR patients could expect never to experience further disease progression, at least never again from this particular bout with their breast cancer. They were presumed to have been cured following their mastectomy and radiation.

The Kaplan-Meier survival curve for the 325 SR patients is shown in figure 8 on the next page. It differs dramatically from the initial Kaplan-Meier curve for all 550 patients shown in figure 7. In particular:

1. it is almost perfectly exponential;
2. it does not appear to fall toward a limiting survival probability (horizontal asymptote) somewhat below 0.42;
3. instead, it appears to fall toward a limiting survival probability at zero, the way any properly constructed survival curve should;
4. what initially seemed like a sharply decreasing hazard rate over time now appears as a remarkably constant hazard rate over quite a lengthy follow-up period spanning more than twenty-four years; and
5. concluding that there really was no decreasing hazard rate for SR patients reduced dramatically the expectation that a "typical" patient would experience with 50 percent probability some event evidencing further disease progression from within 8.42 years (read from figure 7) to within 2.91 years (read from figure 8) following diagnosis and treatment.

Figure 8

Kaplan-Meier Survival Analysis of 325 SR Patients from Turku, Finland, Initially Diagnosed With Invasive Breast Cancer, Subsequently Given Both Mastectomy and Radiation, but Believed to have Remained at Substantial Risk, Despite Their Treatment

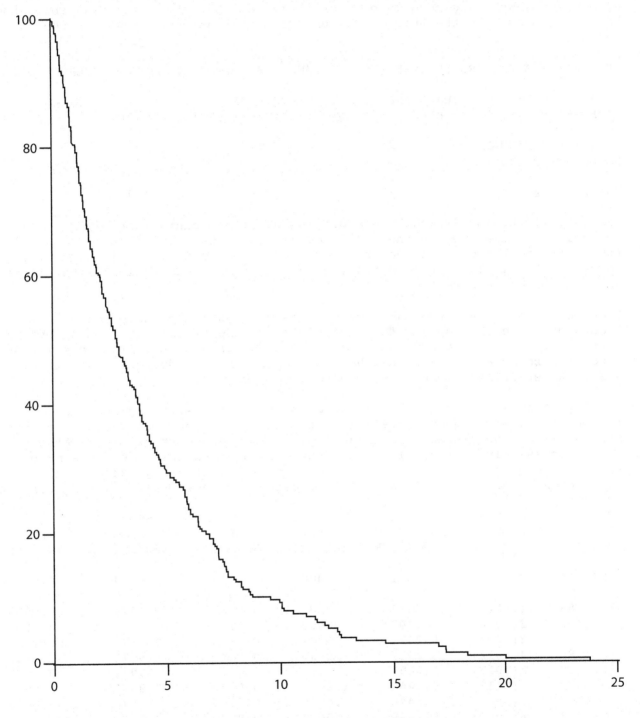

Percentage of Patients Surviving With No Further Disease Progression (%)

Years Elapsed Since Diagnosis/Treatment

The 325 SR patients included thirty-two who had not (yet) experienced the focal event. A search was made for a pattern of cure among their thirty-two censored observations via the KAPM procedure with the CURE option enabled. The CURE option generated a new cross table.

In contrast to the CROSS TABLE OF RESIDUALS presented in section 4.9 (before MRPA had reclassified as MINIMAL RISK 188 of the 220 QUESTIONABLE RISK patients), no remaining evidence of cure was detected in the new cross table. The same 293 patients who experienced the focal event (at 197 distinct focal event times) were included in both cross tables, but the new cross table shown below includes only the thirty-two censored observations drawn from the 325 SR patients.

SEARCH FOR A PATTERN OF CURE (VERY LOW/NO RISK) AMONG CENSORED OBSERVATIONS

CROSS TABLE OF RESIDUALS	EARLY RESIDUAL (KAPM - FITTED)	LATE RESIDUAL (KAPM - FITTED)	TOTAL
POSITIVE RESIDUAL	28	41	69
NEGATIVE RESIDUAL	70	58	128
TOTAL	98	99	197

The data in the above cross table display no significant "lean" in the direction of relatively higher cell counts along the table's major diagonal (top-left and bottom-right cells), compared to its off-diagonal (top-right and bottom-left cells). To the contrary, there is a noticeable "lean," but it is in just the opposite direction.

Even more convincing, the table of successively culled censored observations produced by the CURE option for these 325 SR patients demonstrated a consistent pattern of constant hazard rates (WEIBULL TREND PARAMETER uniformly = 1.0000). Since hazard rates appeared neither to increase nor to decrease over time, all R-SQUARED DIFFERENCE VALUEs were reduced to zero.

Finally, the R-squared value associated with the best-fitting function (exponential) was highest (0.9974) in the top row before culling any censored patients from the Kaplan-Meier analysis. As more and more censored patients were successively culled, all subsequent R-squared values were the same or lower. Consequently, there could be no initially increasing exponential function R-squared values to indicate a pattern of cure. There was no cure.

CENSORED TIME BOUND	NUMBER AND PROPORTION SO CURED	WEIBULL INTENSITY PARAMETER	WEIBULL TREND PARAMETER	R-SQUARED VALUE OF WEIBULL	R-SQUARED VALUE OF EXPONENTIAL	R-SQUARED DIFFERENCE IN VALUE
INFINITE	0(.000)	0.2361	1.0000	0.9974	0.9974	0.0000
11.7484	1(.003)	0.2383	1.0000	0.9974	0.9974	0.0000
9.7469	2(.006)	0.2402	1.0000	0.9973	0.9973	0.0000
8.9174	3(.009)	0.2420	1.0000	0.9972	0.9972	0.0000
8.4985	4(.012)	0.2437	1.0000	0.9971	0.9971	0.0000
6.8338	5(.015)	0.2451	1.0000	0.9971	0.9971	0.0000
6.1630	6(.018)	0.2464	1.0000	0.9970	0.9970	0.0000
5.6702	7(.022)	0.2476	1.0000	0.9970	0.9970	0.0000
5.5032	8(.025)	0.2488	1.0000	0.9970	0.9970	0.0000
5.0870	9(.028)	0.2499	1.0000	0.9970	0.9970	0.0000
4.8351	10(.031)	0.2510	1.0000	0.9969	0.9969	0.0000
4.8324	11(.034)	0.2520	1.0000	0.9969	0.9969	0.0000

CENSORED TIME BOUND	NUMBER AND PROPORTION SO CURED	WEIBULL INTENSITY PARAMETER	WEIBULL TREND PARAMETER	R-SQUARED VALUE OF WEIBULL	R-SQUARED VALUE OF EXPONENTIAL	R-SQUARED DIFFERENCE IN VALUE
4.5805	12(.037)	0.2530	1.0000	0.9969	0.9969	0.0000
4.5039	14(.043)	0.2550	1.0000	0.9968	0.9968	0.0000
4.4135	16(.049)	0.2570	1.0000	0.9967	0.9967	0.0000
3.9152	17(.052)	0.2579	1.0000	0.9967	0.9967	0.0000
3.8331	18(.055)	0.2587	1.0000	0.9967	0.9967	0.0000
3.5867	19(.058)	0.2596	1.0000	0.9966	0.9966	0.0000
3.3348	20(.062)	0.2604	1.0000	0.9966	0.9966	0.0000
3.2526	21(.065)	0.2611	1.0000	0.9966	0.9966	0.0000
3.0829	22(.068)	0.2618	1.0000	0.9966	0.9966	0.0000
2.9159	23(.071)	0.2625	1.0000	0.9966	0.9966	0.0000
2.8337	24(.074)	0.2632	1.0000	0.9965	0.9965	0.0000
2.2478	25(.077)	0.2637	1.0000	0.9965	0.9965	0.0000
2.0835	26(.080)	0.2642	1.0000	0.9965	0.9965	0.0000
2.0014	28(.086)	0.2652	1.0000	0.9965	0.9965	0.0000
1.9165	29(.089)	0.2657	1.0000	0.9965	0.9965	0.0000
0.9993	30(.092)	0.2659	1.0000	0.9965	0.9965	0.0000
0.5859	31(.095)	0.2660	1.0000	0.9965	0.9965	0.0000
0.5010	32(.098)	0.2662	1.0000	0.9966	0.9966	0.0000

5.11 Constructing an Individually Tailored Cure Curve and a Substitutable Survival Curve for a "Typical" Patient, for a High-Risk Patient, and for a Low-Risk Patient

The "average" or "typical" patient is not a real patient. It is an analytical fiction. Nevertheless, it is instructive to construct both a tailored survival curve and a tailored cure curve for this imaginary patient. These may be compared with similar curves constructed for a real high-risk and a real low-risk patient in the intervention sample.

5.11.1 Constructing Tailored Curves for the "Typical" Patient

A baseline survival curve was produced by the final Cox regression analysis described in section 5.8. Values of all three prognostic risk factors (embodied in five independent dummy variables) were entered into the Cox regression in normalized form (i.e., as deviations from their respective dummy variable means). If the "average" or "typical" patient is interpreted to mean the one whose prognostic risk factors all fall exactly at values associated with these five dummy variable means, then the normalized baseline survival curve may be interpreted as the "typical" patient's tailored survival curve.

A graph of the Weibull function that fit this normalized baseline survival curve best (R-squared = 0.9980) is shown in figure 9 on the next page. Points displayed in the figure 9 graph depict survival probabilities at the time of the "typical" patient's mastectomy and radiation (year 0) and at the end of years 1 through 30 following that intervention.

Figure 9

Survival Curve Representing a "Typical" Patient, If Still At Risk Despite Mastectomy and Radiation

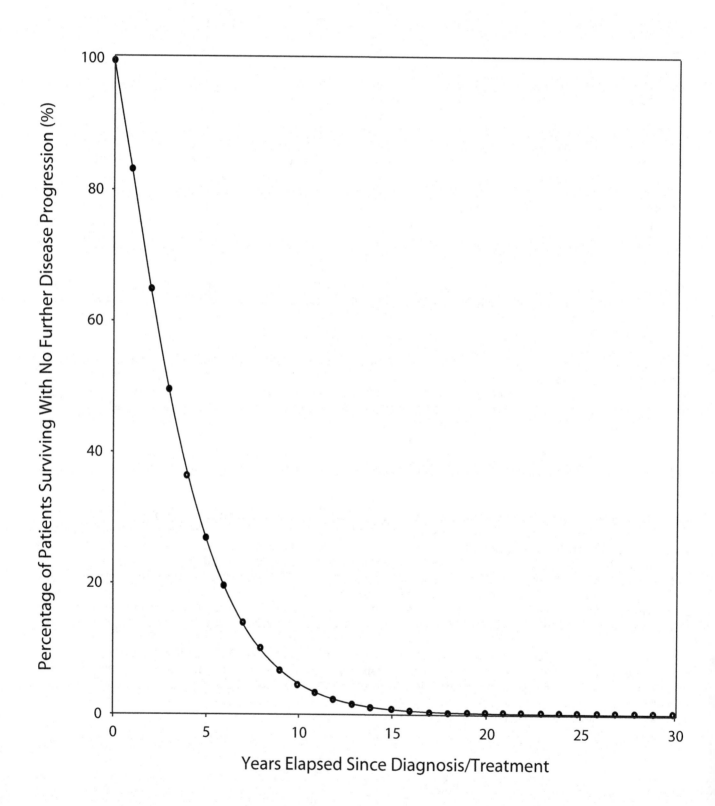

Years Elapsed Since Diagnosis/Treatment

Notice that the survival curve shown in figure 8 and the survival curve shown in figure 9 appear quite similar. They are closely related, but not identical.

Figure 8 depicts the discrete Kaplan-Meier survival curve calculated for the 325 SR patients via the product-limit method. A continuous exponential function with a constant hazard rate over time fit it very closely (R-squared = 0.9974), better than any Weibull function with an increasing or decreasing hazard rate.

Figure 9 displays successive points along a continuous Weibull curve fitted to the discrete normalized baseline survival function produced by Cox regression from the same subsample of 325 SR patients. This Weibull curve fit the normalized baseline survival function very closely (R-squared = 0.9980), but it possessed a slightly increasing (not decreasing) hazard rate over time.

The slight difference between these two curves results primarily from the slightly different concepts they embody and the consequent differences in calculation.

Of much greater import, however, is the dramatic difference between the two of them, considered together, and the initial Kaplan-Meier curve depicted in figure 7. The sharply decreasing hazard rate shown in figure 7 has been completely eliminated by MRPA. It was spurious. This is the important message.

MRPA eliminated the decreasing hazard rate from figure 7 by removing the 225 MR patients from the 550 intervention patients. Assuming that these 225 MR patients really were at little or no risk of further disease progression (cured) following their mastectomy and radiation, their survival curve would have been a horizontal straight line at 100 percent survival probability forever. The only reason figure 7 shows a decreasing hazard rate seems to be because the 225 minimal-risk patients were inadvertently mixed in with the 325 still-at-substantial-risk patients. It was the "apples-and-oranges" mixing together of cured patients with patients who remained still at risk that rendered figure 7 spurious.

A revised (Bayesian posterior) cure probability curve for the same "typical" patient is shown in figure 10 on the next page. It is calculated according to the formula for RCP presented in explanatory note number 6 in section 5.1, where the "typical" prior cure probability (CP) is interpreted as 225 MR (cured) patients out of 550 = 0.4091.

To be comparable with figure 9, points displayed in the figure 10 graph depict successive revised cure probabilities, starting at the time of the "typical" patient's mastectomy and radiation (year 0) and extending through the end of each of the following thirty years. Each successive cure probability represents the likelihood that her mastectomy and radiation succeeded in transforming the "typical" patient from the SR to the MR state (cured her), given that she survived for the indicated number of years following the intervention without any evidence of further disease progression.

Figure 10

Revised Bayesian Posterior Cure Probability
Curve Representing the Same "Typical" Patient

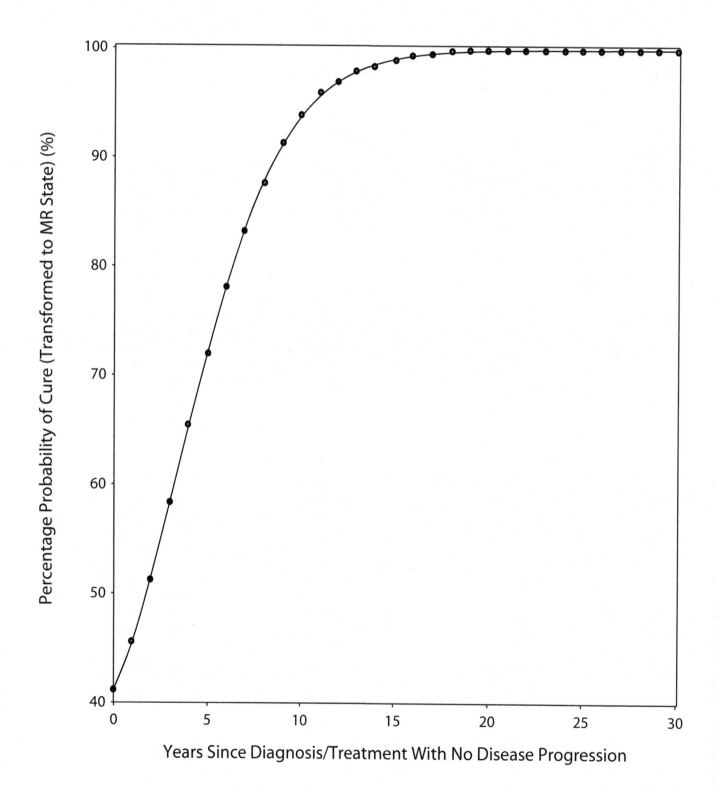

Years Since Diagnosis/Treatment With No Disease Progression

A horizontal survival curve applies to all patients who were transformed from the SR to the MR state (cured). Figure 9 applies to the "typical" patient who was not so transformed (remained still at risk). This suggests a convenient way to use the two curves in practice.

1. The relevant reference curve for a "typical" patient directly following mastectomy and radiation would be her revised cure probability curve. Figure 10 would continue to guide assessing her year-to-year progress without any evidence of further disease progression.
2. The first evidence of disease progression would force a switch. The presumption of cure is no longer tenable. After updating the "typical" survival curve in figure 9 to reflect her elapsed survival time, her consequent increase in age, and any other relevant events that occurred since her mastectomy and radiation, her updated survival curve must be substituted for her revised cure curve to assess her future progress.

5.11.2 Constructing Tailored Curves for High-Risk and Low-Risk Patients

To illustrate the wide range of individual differences in both survival curves and revised cure curves, four additional figures appear in the next four pages.

1. Figure 11 displays the tailored survival curve for the still curable patient with the highest risk of further disease progression (i.e., the patient still in stage M0, but with the least favorable prognosis).
2. Figure 12 displays the corresponding revised (Bayesian posterior) cure curve tailored for the same high-risk patient.
3. Figure 13 displays the tailored survival curve for the patient with the lowest risk of further disease progression (i.e., the patient still in stage M0 with the most favorable prognosis).
4. Figure 14 displays the corresponding revised (Bayesian posterior) cure curve tailored for the same low-risk patient.

Prognostic risk factors for these two extreme patients are tabled below.

PROGNOSTIC RISK FACTOR	PATIENT WITH HIGHEST RISK	PATIENT WITH LOWEST RISK
T STAGE	T4	T1
N STAGE	N2	N0
M STAGE	M0	M0
GRADE OF TUMOR	3	1
DEGREE OF NECROSIS	severe	none
MRPA CLASSIFICATION	at substantial risk (SR)	at minimal risk (MR)

The patient with the highest risk died of breast cancer at age forty-nine, six months after her mastectomy and radiation. Because her risk was so high, her revised cure probability rose quite rapidly (figure 12). However, because she died so quickly, her cure probability had risen only slightly, from an initial (prior) level of 0.0054 to an eventual (revised posterior) level of 0.0073.

The patient with the lowest risk was the longest-surviving of the original thirty-seven long-term survivors. She was last seen alive more than forty-three years after being diagnosed and receiving her mastectomy and radiation. Because her risk was so low, her revised cure probability rose rather slowly (figure 14). It had risen from an initial (prior) level of 0.8463 to an eventual (revised posterior) level of 0.9993 at the time she was last seen. She was then eighty-six years old.

Figure 11

Survival Curve Representing the Highest-Risk Patient,
If Still At Risk Despite Mastectomy and Radiation

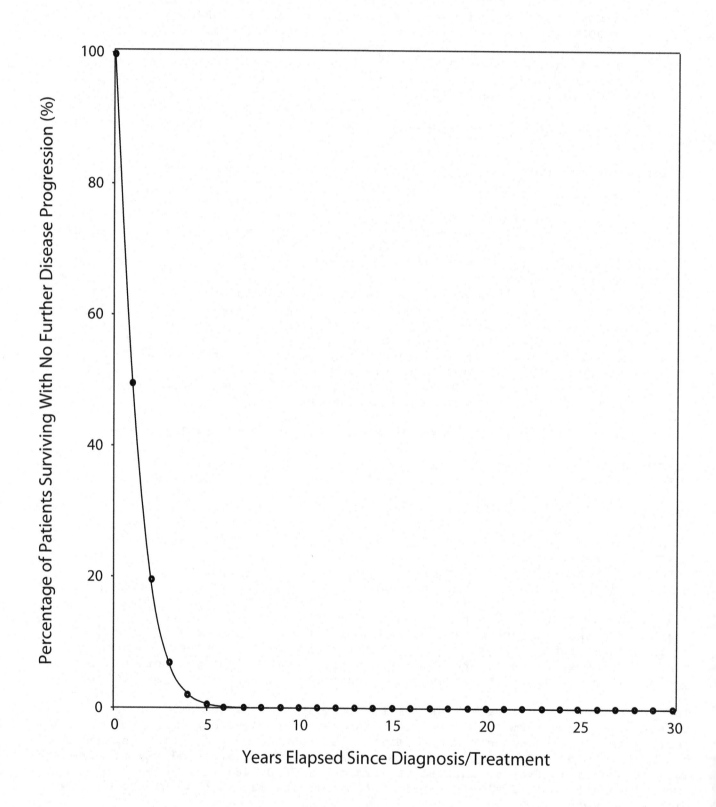

Figure 12

Revised Bayesian Posterior Cure Probability
Curve Representing the Same Highest-Risk Patient

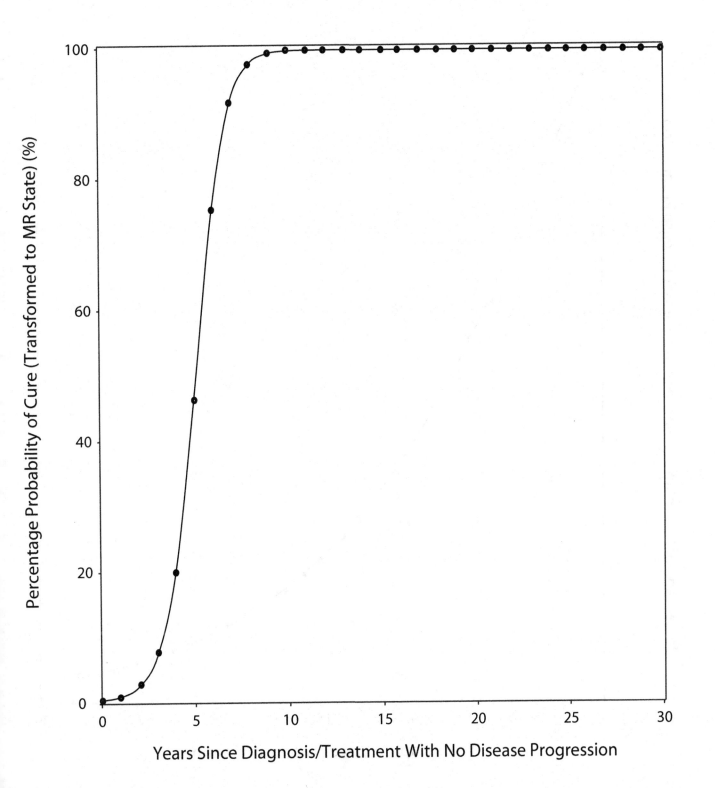

Figure 13

Survival Curve Representing the Lowest-Risk Patient,
If Still At Risk Despite Mastectomy and Radiation

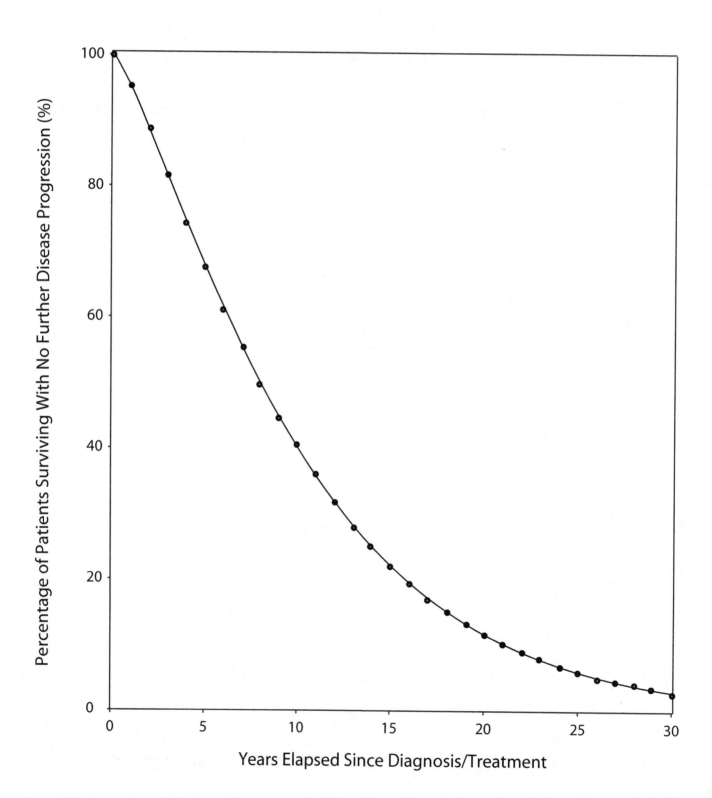

Figure 14

Revised Bayesian Posterior Cure Probability
Curve Representing the Same Lowest-Risk Patient

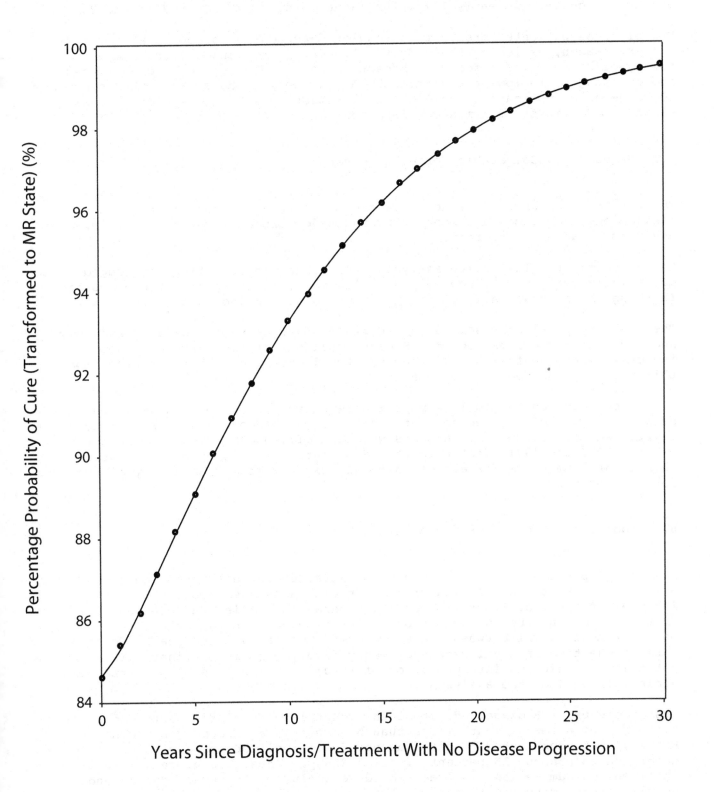

Years Since Diagnosis/Treatment With No Disease Progression

6.0 A SECOND ILLUSTRATIVE ANALYSIS

Medical records of several thousand breast cancer patients were collected between 1975 and 2003 at Guy's Hospital in London, England. Unusually clean and almost complete data for 3,325 of these patients were obtained for analysis. All patients were women diagnosed with some form of breast cancer. The earliest diagnosis occurred in early 1975. The latest diagnosis occurred in mid-2003.

Few of these patients were lost to regularly scheduled follow-up at any time for any reason, excluding their death. The data set spanned more than twenty-eight years. Its focus on breast cancer, its exceptional cleanliness, and its lengthy follow-up rendered the Guy's Hospital data set most appropriate to serve as a replication vehicle for illustrating PCM's method of assessing the curative impact of a medical intervention.

6.1 Selecting a Comparable Target Intervention

The target intervention was again mastectomy (which included lymph node dissection), sometimes accompanied by radiation therapy, but never followed by any form of adjuvant therapy.

As in the first illustrative analysis, the target intervention was judged to be potentially curative. It seemed plausible to expect an appreciable proportion (although by no means all) of the patients so treated to be cured.

The Guy's Hospital data set did not differentiate between radical mastectomy and modified radical mastectomy. Because analysis of the Turku data set indicated little difference between the two in terms of their curative impact, this was not regarded as problematic.

A sufficiently lengthy follow-up period is always required to assess the curative impact of any medical intervention. This second analysis was therefore restricted to include only patients who were diagnosed during the seven years between 1975 and 1981. That permitted a potential follow-up period lasting more than twenty-one years for all of them and slightly more than twenty-eight years for some of them.

6.2 Additional Steps to Homogenize the Second Analysis

A small proportion of the 3,325 Guy's Hospital patients (about 7 percent) experienced breast cancer bilaterally. In all cases there was a distinct interval of time (at least two months) separating the initial diagnosis of breast cancer and the subsequent detection of cancer in the other breast. The median time interval between these two events was about five years. For one patient the time interval exceeded twenty-five years. To eliminate a potentially ambiguous interpretation of results, all bilateral patients were again deleted from the analysis.

Most patients were diagnosed with either ductal or lobular breast cancer. The histology of a few patients (less than 5 percent) was recorded as "other." Exactly what constituted "other" was not specified. Lobular and other patients comprised only about 16 percent of all 3,325 patients. Therefore, the intervention sample was also restricted to include only female ductal and lobular breast cancer patients.

6.3 The Second Intervention Sample

A subsample of 578 patients was selected from the Guy's Hospital data set according to the preceding criteria. All 578 patients shared the following characteristics:

1. women diagnosed with invasive breast cancer (either ductal or lobular) between the beginning of 1975 and the end of 1981 in London, England;
2. no bilaterality (as of the time last observed);
3. received a mastectomy;
4. sometimes, but not always, along with radiation therapy; but
5. never followed by any form of adjuvant therapy; and
6. patient status when last observed was known and properly recorded.

Variable characteristics of these 578 patients are summarized in appendix I.

6.4 Executing an Initial Kaplan-Meier Survival Analysis

The same focal event defined for the 550 Turku patients was adopted for the 578 Guy's Hospital patients. Any patient who experienced either a relapse or recurrence of breast cancer or death due to breast cancer following mastectomy and (sometimes) radiation was clearly not cured by that intervention. Each of these events constituted an unambiguous indication of further disease progression. Each provided indisputable proof that the patient remained at substantial risk (SR) despite the intervention.

The focal event was again defined as whichever of these events (if any) occurred first. Its elapsed time since the patient was originally diagnosed became the focal event time. If none of these events had (yet) occurred when the patient was last observed, the time elapsed between diagnosis and last follow-up alive or the time elapsed to death from a different cause (whichever applied) was treated as a censored observation.

The KAPM procedure was invoked to produce a Kaplan-Meier survival analysis. Outputs of the procedure are shown below and on the next six pages between the horizontal lines. A graphical representation of the KAPM output is then presented in figure 15 as the corresponding Kaplan-Meier survival curve.

DESCRIPTIVE SUMMARY OF ELAPSED TIME INTERVALS

The set of strictly positive elapsed observation time intervals relating to 578 PATIENTs constitutes the effective sample for the descriptive summary. There are 555 distinct elapsed time intervals in this set. The complete observation window (i.e., the longest elapsed time interval observed) is 28.1259 elapsed time unit(s). The time unit is one full year.

The MINIMUM number of elapsed time units observed is 0.0684.
The MEDIAN number of elapsed time units observed is 10.5298.
The MAXIMUM number of elapsed time units observed is 28.1259.
The MEAN number of elapsed time units observed is 12.1674,
with a STANDARD DEVIATION of 9.4352.

KAPLAN-MEIER ANALYSIS (SURVIVAL RATE ESTIMATED VIA THE PRODUCT-LIMIT METHOD)

The same set of strictly positive elapsed observation time intervals relating to 578 PATIENTs constitutes the effective sample for the Kaplan-Meier analysis. It focuses on the particular subset of 247 distinct intervals that terminate with the occurrence of at least one focal event. In addition, the analysis considers all truncated-observation intervals that terminate before a focal event has occurred (censored observations), if any exist. A total of 259 focal events occur during the observation subwindow that encompasses all events. This observation subwindow spans 20.7146 elapsed time unit(s).

ELAPSED TIME UNITS	NUMBER OF EVENTS	NUMBER AT RISK	HAZARD RATE	CUMULATIVE HAZARD RATE	KAPLAN-MEIER SURVIVAL RATE	STANDARD ERROR
0.0000	N/A	578	N/A	N/A	1.0000	N/A
0.1697	1	576	0.0017	0.0017	0.9983	0.0017
0.2738	1	575	0.0017	0.0035	0.9965	0.0025
0.2820	1	574	0.0017	0.0052	0.9948	0.0030
0.3039	1	573	0.0017	0.0070	0.9931	0.0035
0.3559	1	572	0.0017	0.0087	0.9913	0.0039
0.3669	2	571	0.0035	0.0122	0.9878	0.0046
0.3696	1	569	0.0018	0.0140	0.9861	0.0049
0.3806	2	568	0.0035	0.0175	0.9826	0.0054
0.3833	1	566	0.0018	0.0193	0.9809	0.0057
0.3860	1	565	0.0018	0.0210	0.9792	0.0060
0.4435	1	564	0.0018	0.0228	0.9774	0.0062
0.4682	1	562	0.0018	0.0246	0.9757	0.0064
0.4846	1	561	0.0018	0.0264	0.9740	0.0066
0.4956	1	560	0.0018	0.0281	0.9722	0.0068
0.4983	1	559	0.0018	0.0299	0.9705	0.0071
0.5120	1	558	0.0018	0.0317	0.9687	0.0073
0.5147	1	557	0.0018	0.0335	0.9670	0.0074
0.5229	1	556	0.0018	0.0353	0.9653	0.0076
0.5530	1	555	0.0018	0.0371	0.9635	0.0078
0.5613	1	554	0.0018	0.0389	0.9618	0.0080
0.5804	1	553	0.0018	0.0407	0.9600	0.0082
0.5914	1	552	0.0018	0.0426	0.9583	0.0083
0.6105	1	551	0.0018	0.0444	0.9566	0.0085
0.6133	2	550	0.0036	0.0480	0.9531	0.0088
0.6160	1	548	0.0018	0.0498	0.9513	0.0090
0.6297	1	547	0.0018	0.0517	0.9496	0.0091
0.6434	1	546	0.0018	0.0535	0.9479	0.0093
0.6543	1	545	0.0018	0.0553	0.9461	0.0094
0.6708	3	544	0.0055	0.0608	0.9409	0.0098
0.6927	1	541	0.0018	0.0627	0.9392	0.0100
0.7255	1	540	0.0019	0.0645	0.9374	0.0101
0.7283	2	539	0.0037	0.0682	0.9340	0.0104
0.7666	1	537	0.0019	0.0701	0.9322	0.0105
0.7830	1	536	0.0019	0.0720	0.9305	0.0106
0.7885	1	535	0.0019	0.0738	0.9287	0.0107
0.7912	1	534	0.0019	0.0757	0.9270	0.0108
0.8405	1	533	0.0019	0.0776	0.9253	0.0110
0.8487	1	532	0.0019	0.0795	0.9235	0.0111
0.8569	1	531	0.0019	0.0814	0.9218	0.0112
0.8652	1	530	0.0019	0.0832	0.9200	0.0113
0.8788	1	529	0.0019	0.0851	0.9183	0.0114
0.8925	1	528	0.0019	0.0870	0.9166	0.0115
0.9227	2	527	0.0038	0.0908	0.9131	0.0117

ELAPSED TIME UNITS	NUMBER OF EVENTS	NUMBER AT RISK	HAZARD RATE	CUMULATIVE HAZARD RATE	KAPLAN-MEIER SURVIVAL RATE	STANDARD ERROR
0.9391	1	525	0.0019	0.0927	0.9113	0.0119
0.9418	1	524	0.0019	0.0946	0.9096	0.0120
0.9582	1	522	0.0019	0.0966	0.9079	0.0121
0.9747	1	521	0.0019	0.0985	0.9061	0.0122
0.9911	1	520	0.0019	0.1004	0.9044	0.0123
0.9966	1	519	0.0019	0.1023	0.9026	0.0124
1.0157	1	517	0.0019	0.1043	0.9009	0.0125
1.0294	1	516	0.0019	0.1062	0.8991	0.0126
1.0568	1	515	0.0019	0.1081	0.8974	0.0127
1.0732	1	514	0.0019	0.1101	0.8956	0.0127
1.0760	1	513	0.0019	0.1120	0.8939	0.0128
1.1280	1	512	0.0020	0.1140	0.8922	0.0129
1.1417	1	511	0.0020	0.1159	0.8904	0.0130
1.1663	1	510	0.0020	0.1179	0.8887	0.0131
1.1718	1	509	0.0020	0.1199	0.8869	0.0132
1.1855	1	508	0.0020	0.1218	0.8852	0.0133
1.1910	1	507	0.0020	0.1238	0.8834	0.0134
1.2101	1	506	0.0020	0.1258	0.8817	0.0135
1.2266	1	505	0.0020	0.1278	0.8799	0.0136
1.2293	1	504	0.0020	0.1297	0.8782	0.0136
1.2676	1	503	0.0020	0.1317	0.8764	0.0137
1.3498	2	502	0.0040	0.1357	0.8730	0.0139
1.3580	1	500	0.0020	0.1377	0.8712	0.0140
1.3607	1	499	0.0020	0.1397	0.8695	0.0141
1.3799	1	498	0.0020	0.1417	0.8677	0.0141
1.3963	2	497	0.0040	0.1458	0.8642	0.0143
1.4018	1	495	0.0020	0.1478	0.8625	0.0144
1.4182	1	494	0.0020	0.1498	0.8607	0.0144
1.4346	1	492	0.0020	0.1518	0.8590	0.0145
1.4401	1	490	0.0020	0.1539	0.8572	0.0146
1.4538	1	489	0.0020	0.1559	0.8555	0.0147
1.4593	1	487	0.0021	0.1580	0.8537	0.0147
1.4675	1	486	0.0021	0.1600	0.8520	0.0148
1.4702	1	485	0.0021	0.1621	0.8502	0.0149
1.4784	1	484	0.0021	0.1642	0.8484	0.0150
1.5113	1	483	0.0021	0.1662	0.8467	0.0150
1.5496	1	482	0.0021	0.1683	0.8449	0.0151
1.5606	1	481	0.0021	0.1704	0.8432	0.0152
1.5743	1	480	0.0021	0.1725	0.8414	0.0153
1.5825	1	479	0.0021	0.1746	0.8397	0.0153
1.6071	1	477	0.0021	0.1766	0.8379	0.0154
1.6427	1	476	0.0021	0.1787	0.8361	0.0155
1.6482	1	475	0.0021	0.1809	0.8344	0.0155
1.6564	1	474	0.0021	0.1830	0.8326	0.0156
1.6838	1	473	0.0021	0.1851	0.8309	0.0157
1.7084	1	472	0.0021	0.1872	0.8291	0.0157
1.7604	1	471	0.0021	0.1893	0.8273	0.0158
1.7632	1	470	0.0021	0.1914	0.8256	0.0159
1.7659	1	469	0.0021	0.1936	0.8238	0.0159
1.8042	1	468	0.0021	0.1957	0.8221	0.0160
1.8344	1	466	0.0021	0.1979	0.8203	0.0160
1.8754	1	465	0.0022	0.2000	0.8185	0.0161
1.8782	1	464	0.0022	0.2022	0.8168	0.0162
1.8946	1	462	0.0022	0.2043	0.8150	0.0162
1.9521	2	460	0.0043	0.2087	0.8115	0.0163
1.9713	1	458	0.0022	0.2109	0.8097	0.0164

ELAPSED TIME UNITS	NUMBER OF EVENTS	NUMBER AT RISK	HAZARD RATE	CUMULATIVE HAZARD RATE	KAPLAN-MEIER SURVIVAL RATE	STANDARD ERROR
2.0205	1	457	0.0022	0.2131	0.8079	0.0165
2.0616	1	455	0.0022	0.2152	0.8061	0.0165
2.1383	1	454	0.0022	0.2175	0.8044	0.0166
2.1875	2	453	0.0044	0.2219	0.8008	0.0167
2.1958	1	451	0.0022	0.2241	0.7990	0.0168
2.2067	1	450	0.0022	0.2263	0.7973	0.0168
2.2122	1	449	0.0022	0.2285	0.7955	0.0169
2.2669	1	447	0.0022	0.2308	0.7937	0.0169
2.2861	1	446	0.0022	0.2330	0.7919	0.0170
2.3053	1	445	0.0022	0.2353	0.7901	0.0170
2.3080	1	444	0.0023	0.2375	0.7884	0.0171
2.3217	1	443	0.0023	0.2398	0.7866	0.0171
2.3546	1	442	0.0023	0.2420	0.7848	0.0172
2.3737	1	441	0.0023	0.2443	0.7830	0.0173
2.3792	1	440	0.0023	0.2466	0.7812	0.0173
2.3956	1	439	0.0023	0.2489	0.7795	0.0174
2.4695	1	438	0.0023	0.2511	0.7777	0.0174
2.4750	1	437	0.0023	0.2534	0.7759	0.0175
2.4997	1	436	0.0023	0.2557	0.7741	0.0175
2.5270	1	435	0.0023	0.2580	0.7724	0.0176
2.5325	1	434	0.0023	0.2603	0.7706	0.0176
2.5982	1	433	0.0023	0.2626	0.7688	0.0177
2.6475	1	431	0.0023	0.2649	0.7670	0.0177
2.6639	1	430	0.0023	0.2673	0.7652	0.0178
2.6721	1	429	0.0023	0.2696	0.7634	0.0178
2.7844	1	428	0.0023	0.2719	0.7617	0.0178
2.8036	1	427	0.0023	0.2743	0.7599	0.0179
2.8255	1	426	0.0023	0.2766	0.7581	0.0179
2.8392	1	425	0.0024	0.2790	0.7563	0.0180
2.9158	1	424	0.0024	0.2813	0.7545	0.0180
2.9213	1	423	0.0024	0.2837	0.7527	0.0181
2.9322	1	422	0.0024	0.2861	0.7510	0.0181
2.9377	1	421	0.0024	0.2885	0.7492	0.0182
2.9514	1	420	0.0024	0.2908	0.7474	0.0182
2.9706	1	419	0.0024	0.2932	0.7456	0.0183
3.0691	1	416	0.0024	0.2956	0.7438	0.0183
3.1184	1	415	0.0024	0.2980	0.7420	0.0183
3.2170	1	412	0.0024	0.3005	0.7402	0.0184
3.2225	1	411	0.0024	0.3029	0.7384	0.0184
3.3073	1	410	0.0024	0.3053	0.7366	0.0185
3.3429	1	409	0.0024	0.3078	0.7348	0.0185
3.3484	1	408	0.0025	0.3102	0.7330	0.0186
3.3703	1	407	0.0025	0.3127	0.7312	0.0186
3.3730	1	406	0.0025	0.3151	0.7294	0.0186
3.4114	1	405	0.0025	0.3176	0.7276	0.0187
3.5099	1	403	0.0025	0.3201	0.7258	0.0187
3.5291	1	402	0.0025	0.3226	0.7240	0.0188
3.5537	1	400	0.0025	0.3251	0.7222	0.0188
3.5866	1	399	0.0025	0.3276	0.7204	0.0188
3.6194	1	398	0.0025	0.3301	0.7186	0.0189
3.7372	1	397	0.0025	0.3326	0.7168	0.0189
3.7591	1	396	0.0025	0.3351	0.7149	0.0190
4.0082	1	394	0.0025	0.3377	0.7131	0.0190
4.0712	1	393	0.0025	0.3402	0.7113	0.0190
4.1150	1	392	0.0026	0.3428	0.7095	0.0191
4.1780	1	391	0.0026	0.3453	0.7077	0.0191

ELAPSED TIME UNITS	NUMBER OF EVENTS	NUMBER AT RISK	HAZARD RATE	CUMULATIVE HAZARD RATE	KAPLAN-MEIER SURVIVAL RATE	STANDARD ERROR
4.1807	1	390	0.0026	0.3479	0.7059	0.0191
4.1999	1	389	0.0026	0.3505	0.7041	0.0192
4.2190	1	388	0.0026	0.3531	0.7022	0.0192
4.2765	1	387	0.0026	0.3556	0.7004	0.0193
4.3696	1	385	0.0026	0.3582	0.6986	0.0193
4.4326	1	384	0.0026	0.3608	0.6968	0.0193
4.4353	1	383	0.0026	0.3634	0.6950	0.0194
4.4873	1	381	0.0026	0.3661	0.6932	0.0194
4.5038	2	380	0.0053	0.3713	0.6895	0.0195
4.5065	1	378	0.0026	0.3740	0.6877	0.0195
4.5558	1	377	0.0027	0.3766	0.6859	0.0195
4.6899	1	376	0.0027	0.3793	0.6840	0.0196
4.7912	1	374	0.0027	0.3820	0.6822	0.0196
4.8186	1	373	0.0027	0.3846	0.6804	0.0196
4.8706	1	372	0.0027	0.3873	0.6785	0.0197
4.8898	1	371	0.0027	0.3900	0.6767	0.0197
4.9254	1	370	0.0027	0.3927	0.6749	0.0197
5.1280	1	369	0.0027	0.3954	0.6731	0.0198
5.1389	1	368	0.0027	0.3982	0.6712	0.0198
5.1417	1	367	0.0027	0.4009	0.6694	0.0198
5.1745	1	366	0.0027	0.4036	0.6676	0.0199
5.2895	1	364	0.0027	0.4064	0.6657	0.0199
5.3498	1	362	0.0028	0.4091	0.6639	0.0199
5.3607	1	360	0.0028	0.4119	0.6621	0.0199
5.4812	1	358	0.0028	0.4147	0.6602	0.0200
5.6810	1	355	0.0028	0.4175	0.6583	0.0200
5.6865	1	354	0.0028	0.4203	0.6565	0.0200
5.6920	1	353	0.0028	0.4232	0.6546	0.0201
5.8426	1	350	0.0029	0.4260	0.6528	0.0201
6.1355	1	348	0.0029	0.4289	0.6509	0.0201
6.4066	1	345	0.0029	0.4318	0.6490	0.0201
6.6749	1	343	0.0029	0.4347	0.6471	0.0202
6.9240	1	341	0.0029	0.4377	0.6452	0.0202
6.9815	1	340	0.0029	0.4406	0.6433	0.0202
7.0171	1	339	0.0029	0.4435	0.6414	0.0203
7.0582	1	338	0.0030	0.4465	0.6395	0.0203
7.1704	1	337	0.0030	0.4495	0.6376	0.0203
7.4059	1	334	0.0030	0.4525	0.6357	0.0204
7.4579	1	332	0.0030	0.4555	0.6338	0.0204
7.6413	1	331	0.0030	0.4585	0.6319	0.0204
7.8439	1	327	0.0031	0.4616	0.6299	0.0204
7.8741	1	326	0.0031	0.4646	0.6280	0.0205
7.9179	1	325	0.0031	0.4677	0.6261	0.0205
8.1533	1	323	0.0031	0.4708	0.6241	0.0205
8.3888	1	320	0.0031	0.4739	0.6222	0.0206
8.6023	1	318	0.0031	0.4771	0.6202	0.0206
8.6516	1	316	0.0032	0.4802	0.6183	0.0206
9.0979	1	312	0.0032	0.4834	0.6163	0.0206
9.1992	1	310	0.0032	0.4867	0.6143	0.0207
9.2977	1	308	0.0032	0.4899	0.6123	0.0207
9.3169	1	307	0.0033	0.4932	0.6103	0.0207
9.4100	1	304	0.0033	0.4965	0.6083	0.0208
9.7522	1	300	0.0033	0.4998	0.6063	0.0208
9.9849	1	299	0.0033	0.5031	0.6042	0.0208
10.0260	1	298	0.0034	0.5065	0.6022	0.0208
10.1246	1	295	0.0034	0.5099	0.6002	0.0209

ELAPSED TIME UNITS	NUMBER OF EVENTS	NUMBER AT RISK	HAZARD RATE	CUMULATIVE HAZARD RATE	KAPLAN-MEIER SURVIVAL RATE	STANDARD ERROR
10.1355	1	294	0.0034	0.5133	0.5981	0.0209
10.3217	1	291	0.0034	0.5167	0.5961	0.0209
10.3518	1	290	0.0034	0.5202	0.5940	0.0210
10.5298	1	289	0.0035	0.5236	0.5920	0.0210
10.7050	1	287	0.0035	0.5271	0.5899	0.0210
11.2580	1	280	0.0036	0.5307	0.5878	0.0210
11.8111	1	277	0.0036	0.5343	0.5857	0.0211
11.8138	1	276	0.0036	0.5379	0.5836	0.0211
11.8659	1	275	0.0036	0.5415	0.5814	0.0211
12.0465	1	273	0.0037	0.5452	0.5793	0.0212
12.0767	1	272	0.0037	0.5489	0.5772	0.0212
12.6242	1	269	0.0037	0.5526	0.5750	0.0212
12.9774	1	265	0.0038	0.5564	0.5729	0.0213
13.0924	1	264	0.0038	0.5602	0.5707	0.0213
13.1608	1	263	0.0038	0.5640	0.5685	0.0213
13.4839	1	257	0.0039	0.5679	0.5663	0.0213
14.0123	1	253	0.0040	0.5718	0.5641	0.0214
14.0643	1	252	0.0040	0.5758	0.5618	0.0214
14.0999	1	251	0.0040	0.5798	0.5596	0.0214
14.3573	1	250	0.0040	0.5838	0.5574	0.0215
14.5134	1	249	0.0040	0.5878	0.5551	0.0215
14.7954	1	243	0.0041	0.5919	0.5528	0.0215
14.8173	1	242	0.0041	0.5960	0.5505	0.0216
15.0089	1	240	0.0042	0.6002	0.5483	0.0216
15.1814	1	237	0.0042	0.6044	0.5459	0.0216
16.3477	1	229	0.0044	0.6088	0.5436	0.0217
17.0185	1	223	0.0045	0.6133	0.5411	0.0217
17.3470	1	220	0.0045	0.6178	0.5387	0.0217
18.0972	1	212	0.0047	0.6225	0.5361	0.0218
18.1218	1	210	0.0048	0.6273	0.5336	0.0218
18.2067	1	208	0.0048	0.6321	0.5310	0.0219
18.5161	1	203	0.0049	0.6370	0.5284	0.0219
18.8693	1	197	0.0051	0.6421	0.5257	0.0220
18.9624	1	195	0.0051	0.6472	0.5230	0.0220
19.6852	1	187	0.0053	0.6526	0.5202	0.0221
20.7146	1	174	0.0057	0.6583	0.5172	0.0222

| TOTAL | 259 | | | | | |

Estimates of the above KAPLAN-MEIER SURVIVAL RATE(s) and the associated STANDARD ERROR(s) are based on the assumption that both the sample of elapsed focal event time intervals and the sample of truncated-observation (censored) time intervals are randomly and independently drawn from their respective populations and that these two samples are drawn independently of each other.

If the population of elapsed time intervals until an event occurs is assumed to follow an exponential distribution, implying a constant hazard rate throughout every observation subwindow, the maximum likelihood estimate of that hazard rate is 0.0368, with a standard error of 0.002288.

The assumption of an exponential distribution with a constant hazard rate produces a MARGINALLY ACCEPTABLE fit with the observed data. The analogue of an unadjusted coefficient of determination (R-squared) would be 0.4010.

If the population of elapsed time intervals until an event occurs is assumed to follow a Weibull distribution, which permits either an increasing or a decreasing hazard rate over all observation subwindows, the maximum likelihood estimate of the intensity parameter (analogous to the constant hazard rate parameter characterizing an exponential distribution) is 0.0254, with a standard error of 0.003019. In addition, there appears to be a DECREASING trend in the hazard rate over time. The maximum likelihood estimate of the trend parameter is 0.5988, with a standard error of 0.033153.

The assumption of a Weibull distribution with a DECREASING hazard rate produces a better fit with the data, at least in this complete observation window (two-tailed p value: 0.0000). The improved value of the analogue of an unadjusted coefficient of determination (R-squared) is 0.8944, indicating a GOOD fit.

Figure 15

Kaplan-Meier Survival Analysis of 578 Patients from Guy's Hospital
in London, England, Initially Diagnosed With Invasive Breast Cancer
and Subsequently Treated With Mastectomy and (Sometimes) Radiation

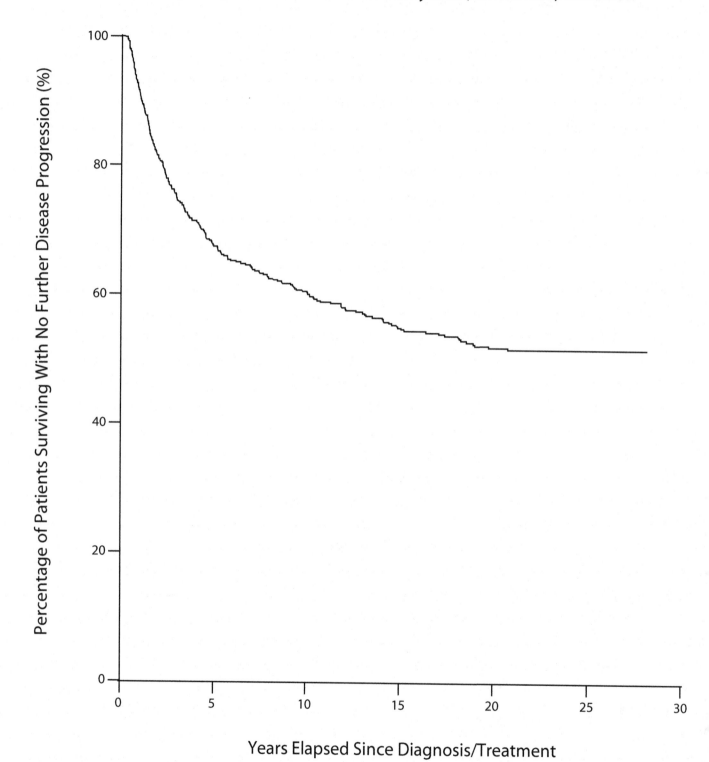

Years Elapsed Since Diagnosis/Treatment

6.5 A Preliminary Interpretation of the Kaplan-Meier Survival Analysis

From figure 15 the single most striking observation is that the curve seems to be falling toward a limiting survival probability (horizontal asymptote). However, that limiting probability is somewhat below 0.52 rather than anywhere near zero. The last focal event occurred after 20.7146 years, yielding an estimated survival probability of 0.5172. After that the curve appears to flatten out (i.e., become virtually horizontal).

The bottom entry in the Kaplan-Meier survival table indicates that 173 other patients were followed up for more than twenty years to a maximum of about twenty-eight years. None of them had yet experienced the focal event when last seen. Because the data suggested the existence of a limiting survival probability (horizontal asymptote), because this probability fell well above zero (somewhat below 0.52), and because enough patients (173) were followed up for a long enough time (more than twenty years) without evidence of further disease progression, it seems quite plausible to suppose that an appreciable proportion of the 578 patients in the intervention sample were actually cured.

Exactly what proportion is not yet clear. The estimate of 0.52 based only on the flattening of the Kaplan-Meier survival curve provides an upper bound. One or more of the 153 survivors among alive censored patients could conceivably still have experienced the focal event, even after a decade or two.

A detailed analysis of the eventual outcomes of the 578 patients in the Guy's Hospital intervention sample yielded the following results.

suffered prior relapse/recurrence and died of breast cancer	235
suffered prior relapse/recurrence but died of something else	16
suffered relapse/recurrence but still alive when last seen	6
suffered no prior relapse/recurrence but died of breast cancer	2
total number of patients who experienced the focal event	259
experienced no relapse/recurrence and died of something else	166
experienced no relapse/recurrence and still alive when last seen	153
total number of censored patients (no focal event when last seen)	319
total number of patients in the Guy's Hospital intervention sample	578
long-term survivors among censored patients	173
other than long-term survivors among censored patients	146
	319
long-term survivors among dead censored patients	27
other than long-term survivors among dead censored patients	139
	166
long-term survivors among alive censored patients	146
other than long-term survivors among alive censored patients	7
	153

These results lend further support to the notion that mastectomy and (sometimes) radiation did cure an appreciable proportion of the 578 patients. Due to the lengthy follow-up, the eventual outcome of 425 patients (almost 75 percent) became clear. Four hundred nineteen had already died (with or without having experienced the focal event), and six had already suffered either a relapse or a recurrence but were still alive when last seen. It was only the 578 - 425 = 153 patients who had suffered neither a relapse nor a recurrence and who were still alive when last seen whose eventual fate remained unclear.

Some way must again be found to partition the total intervention sample into:

1. a cured MR subsample for whom the intervention was successful in altering their state from substantial risk to little or no risk of experiencing further disease progression; and
2. an SR subsample of patients for whom the intervention was not curative and who, therefore, remained at substantial risk of experiencing further disease progression, despite the intervention.

Partitioning the Guy's Hospital patients in this manner will again permit reformulating the traditional Kaplan-Meier paradigm in a Bayesian framework. Combining the results of multiple Cox regression (applied selectively to only the SR subsample) with multiple logistic regression (applied to all patients in the intervention sample) according to Bayes' theorem will again produce a time-phased estimate of each patient's (posterior) cure probability.

Before partitioning the intervention sample into MR and SR subsamples, however, we must again establish that at least some of the 578 Guy's Hospital patients were very likely cured by their mastectomy (and radiation).

6.6   The RISKTEST Simulator

Because the complete history and final outcome of almost 75 percent of the patients were known as of mid-2003, the process of acquiring them, diagnosing them, treating them, and following them up may be simulated. The RISKTEST simulator described in appendix H again accomplished this task.

RISKTEST was tailored to mimic as closely as possible the entire sequence of events occurring between early 1975 and mid-2003.

1. The patient acquisition period spanned seven years between early 1975, when the first of 578 patients was diagnosed and treated, and late 1981, when the last patient was diagnosed and treated.
2. The follow-up period began in early 1982 and ended in mid-2003, spanning 21.1259 years.
3. The focal event was actually experienced by 259 of the 578 patients.
4. An analysis of the 159 patients still alive in mid-2003 disclosed a typically annual follow-up cycle.
5. Simulation of the focal event was based on the results of the Kaplan-Meier analysis of all 578 patients presented in section 6.4. Parameters of the best-fitting Weibull distribution with a significantly decreasing hazard rate over time (R-squared = 0.8944) served as inputs to RISKTEST. The Weibull intensity parameter for the focal event was 0.0254. The corresponding Weibull trend parameter was 0.5988.

6. A second Kaplan-Meier analysis was performed on the same 578-patient data to obtain separate simulation parameters for death due to other causes. In the second analysis, death from other than breast cancer was treated as the focal event, while death due to breast cancer was treated as just another censoring event. The best fit to the data was achieved by a Weibull distribution with a significantly increasing hazard rate over time (R-squared = 0.9890). The Weibull intensity parameter for death from other than breast cancer was 0.0302. The corresponding Weibull trend parameter was 1.4446.

RISKTEST was again used to enable execution of a simulation-based hypothesis test. The null hypothesis was that no patients were cured. All 578 patients were again presumed to have remained at substantial risk (in the SR category) despite their mastectomy (and radiation). The directional alternate hypothesis was that at least some patients were cured.

The test statistic was the simulated number of patients experiencing the focal event. The distribution of this test statistic expected under the null hypothesis was generated by the RISKTEST simulator, fitted to the Guy's Hospital data as described above and on the previous page via maximum likelihood estimation.

RISKTEST executed a simulation run of one hundred thousand trials. Exactly where within the one-hundred-thousand-trial simulated distribution the observed number of 259 patients actually experiencing the focal event fell constituted the test of the hypothesis.

Evidence favoring the null hypothesis was closeness of the observed count of 259 to the middle of the (approximately normal) simulated distribution. Downward displacement of 259 below the middle of the distribution constituted evidence favoring the alternate hypothesis. The exact percentile location in the simulated distribution where 259 fell served as a one-tailed p value.

The run of one hundred thousand trials was made by the RISKTEST simulator guided by the following inputs.

NUMBER OF PATIENTS ACQUIRED: 578
NUMBER OF MR PATIENTS AT VERY LOW/NO RISK: 0
OBSERVED NUMBER OF PATIENTS ACTUALLY EXPERIENCING THE FOCAL EVENT: 259
NUMBER OF YEARS CONSTITUTING PATIENT ACQUISITION PERIOD: 7.0
NUMBER OF YEARS CONSTITUTING PATIENT FOLLOW-UP PERIOD: 21.1259
NUMBER OF YEARS CONSTITUTING PATIENT FOLLOW-UP CYCLE: 1
WEIBULL INTENSITY PARAMETER FOR FOCAL EVENT: 0.0254
WEIBULL TREND PARAMETER FOR FOCAL EVENT: 0.5988
WEIBULL INTENSITY PARAMETER FOR DEATH NOT DUE TO BREAST CANCER: 0.0302
WEIBULL TREND PARAMETER FOR DEATH NOT DUE TO BREAST CANCER: 1.4446

RISKTEST's results are presented on the next three pages. Lightly edited computer output appears between the horizontal lines.

The simulated number of patients experiencing the focal event was less than the target number (259) in 27,875 trials.
The simulated number of patients experiencing the focal event was equal to the target number (259) in 2,877 trials.
The simulated number of patients experiencing the focal event was more than the target number (259) in 69,248 trials.

If interpreted as a statistical test of the goodness of fit of results produced by the simulation model under the null-hypothesized complete absence of cured patients with the target number of 259 patients experiencing the focal event, the null hypothesis cannot be rejected. The directional one-tailed p value was a statistically insignificant 0.30752.

Below are tabled the results of one hundred thousand simulation trials. The second column counts the number of such trials (out of one hundred thousand) in which the number of patients who experience the focal event is as indicated in the first column. The third and fourth columns show these trial counts as equivalent relative and cumulative relative frequencies, respectively.

NUMBER OF PATIENTS WHO EXPERIENCE THE FOCAL EVENT	ABSOLUTE FREQUENCIES (COUNTS)	RELATIVE FREQUENCIES (PROPORTIONS)	CUMULATIVE RELATIVE FREQUENCIES
212	1	0.00001	0.00001
215	1	0.00001	0.00002
217	1	0.00001	0.00003
219	2	0.00002	0.00005
220	1	0.00001	0.00006
221	3	0.00003	0.00009
222	6	0.00006	0.00015
223	10	0.00010	0.00025
224	4	0.00004	0.00029
225	15	0.00015	0.00044
226	14	0.00014	0.00058
227	22	0.00022	0.00080
228	18	0.00018	0.00098
229	27	0.00027	0.00125
230	41	0.00041	0.00166
231	60	0.00060	0.00226
232	63	0.00063	0.00289
233	80	0.00080	0.00369
234	100	0.00100	0.00469
235	154	0.00154	0.00623
236	154	0.00154	0.00777
237	206	0.00206	0.00983
238	248	0.00248	0.01231
239	292	0.00292	0.01523
240	332	0.00332	0.01855
241	386	0.00386	0.02241
242	499	0.00499	0.02740
243	547	0.00547	0.03287
244	703	0.00703	0.03990
245	769	0.00769	0.04759
246	899	0.00899	0.05658
247	1018	0.01018	0.06676
248	1166	0.01166	0.07842
249	1269	0.01269	0.09111

NUMBER OF PATIENTS WHO EXPERIENCE THE FOCAL EVENT	ABSOLUTE FREQUENCIES (COUNTS)	RELATIVE FREQUENCIES (PROPORTIONS)	CUMULATIVE RELATIVE FREQUENCIES
250	1449	0.01449	0.10560
251	1566	0.01566	0.12126
252	1768	0.01768	0.13894
253	1944	0.01944	0.15838
254	2069	0.02069	0.17907
255	2168	0.02168	0.20075
256	2484	0.02484	0.22559
257	2575	0.02575	0.25134
258	2741	0.02741	0.27875
259	2877	0.02877	0.30752
260	3015	0.03015	0.33767
261	3128	0.03128	0.36895
262	3130	0.03130	0.40025
263	3227	0.03227	0.43252
264	3359	0.03359	0.46611
265	3348	0.03348	0.49959
266	3394	0.03394	0.53353
267	3374	0.03374	0.56727
268	3198	0.03198	0.59925
269	3191	0.03191	0.63116
270	3121	0.03121	0.66237
271	2936	0.02936	0.69173
272	2893	0.02893	0.72066
273	2724	0.02724	0.74790
274	2587	0.02587	0.77377
275	2384	0.02384	0.79761
276	2282	0.02282	0.82043
277	2152	0.02152	0.84195
278	1939	0.01939	0.86134
279	1690	0.01690	0.87824
280	1574	0.01574	0.89398
281	1428	0.01428	0.90826
282	1340	0.01340	0.92166
283	1117	0.01117	0.93283
284	1014	0.01014	0.94297
285	958	0.00958	0.95255
286	759	0.00759	0.96014
287	645	0.00645	0.96659
288	595	0.00595	0.97254
289	499	0.00499	0.97753
290	391	0.00391	0.98144
291	356	0.00356	0.98500
292	283	0.00283	0.98783
293	236	0.00236	0.99019
294	190	0.00190	0.99209
295	153	0.00153	0.99362
296	134	0.00134	0.99496
297	98	0.00098	0.99594
298	96	0.00096	0.99690
299	66	0.00066	0.99756
300	53	0.00053	0.99809
301	46	0.00046	0.99855
302	43	0.00043	0.99898
303	17	0.00017	0.99915
304	16	0.00016	0.99931

NUMBER OF PATIENTS WHO EXPERIENCE THE FOCAL EVENT	ABSOLUTE FREQUENCIES (COUNTS)	RELATIVE FREQUENCIES (PROPORTIONS)	CUMULATIVE RELATIVE FREQUENCIES
305	17	0.00017	0.99948
306	15	0.00015	0.99963
307	10	0.00010	0.99973
308	8	0.00008	0.99981
309	1	0.00001	0.99982
310	2	0.00002	0.99984
311	5	0.00005	0.99989
312	4	0.00004	0.99993
313	2	0.00002	0.99995
314	3	0.00003	0.99998
315	1	0.00001	0.99999
318	1	0.00001	1.00000
TOTAL	100000	1.00000	

The 259 patients actually observed to have experienced the focal event were fewer than the most frequently occurring simulated number of 266. This difference is directionally consistent with the notion that some of the 578 patients were cured. Unlike the RISKTEST difference produced from the Turku intervention sample, however, the difference is nowhere near significant.

The apparent convergence of the Kaplan-Meier curve depicted in figure 15 to a horizontal asymptote at slightly below a 0.52 survival probability strongly suggests that we should not consider these simulated results in isolation. Instead, we shall reexecute RISKTEST with different inputs embodying the presumption that at least some of the 578 Guy's Hospital patients were cured by their mastectomy (and radiation) and compare the results of separate simulation runs fitted, respectively, to the competing presumptions of possible versus impossible cure. To accomplish this, we shall again require an estimate of how many and which patients were probably cured.

6.7   A Systematic Search for Evidence of Cure

The Kaplan-Meier survival probabilities tabled in section 6.4 and depicted graphically in figure 15 produced the results summarized below.

1. The focal event (further disease progression) was experienced by 259 of the 578 patients in the Guy's Hospital intervention sample. These were clearly SR patients.
2. The remaining 578 - 259 = 319 patients had not experienced the focal event when they were last observed. These were the censored patients. Any MR patients would have been included among them.
3. The detailed analysis in section 6.5 showed that 166 of these 319 patients were censored because they died of something other than their breast cancer. The remaining 319 - 166 = 153 patients were censored because, when patient follow-up terminated in mid-2003, they had been last seen still alive without evidence of disease progression.
4. The longest focal event time occurred 20.71 years after initial diagnosis.
5. Of the 319 censored patients, 173 were characterized as long-term survivors. Each of them was followed up without evidence of disease

progression for longer than the longest focal event time. Twenty-seven of the 173 eventually died of something other than their breast cancer, and 146 were last seen still alive. These 173 long-term survivors are the most likely candidates for classification as MR patients who were actually cured by their mastectomy (and radiation).

6. The 319 - 173 = 146 censored patients who were not long-term survivors are more difficult to classify. One hundred thirty-nine died of something other than their breast cancer, and seven were last seen still alive without evidence of disease progression. Some of the 146 censored patients were probably cured by their treatment (MR), while others probably remained at substantial risk (SR).

Based on these results, the 578 patients may be divided into the following three risk categories. This is a tentative classification. It follows from the observations just summarized.

PATIENT'S LEVEL OF RISK	ABSOLUTE FREQUENCIES (COUNTS)	RELATIVE FREQUENCIES (PROPORTIONS)	CUMULATIVE RELATIVE FREQUENCIES
CERTAIN RISK (SR)	259	0.4481	0.4481
QUESTIONABLE RISK	146	0.2526	0.7007
MINIMAL RISK (MR)	173	0.2993	1.0000
TOTAL	578	1.0000	

Support for our tentative classification of patients in terms of their risk of disease progression is provided by the following two tables.

PATIENT'S LEVEL OF RISK	T LEVEL OF STAGING				
	T=0	T=1	T=2	T=3 OR 4	TOTAL
CERTAIN RISK (SR)	2	66	154	37	259
QUESTIONABLE RISK	9	48	85	4	146
MINIMAL RISK (MR)	7	88	71	7	173
TOTAL	18	202	310	48	578

PATIENT'S LEVEL OF RISK	N LEVEL OF STAGING				
	N=0	N=1	N=2	N=3	TOTAL
CERTAIN RISK (SR)	117	72	40	30	259
QUESTIONABLE RISK	103	34	9	0	146
MINIMAL RISK (MR)	134	32	6	1	173
TOTAL	354	138	55	31	578

These two tables are quite encouraging. There is a clear tendency in each table for higher levels of patient risk to be associated with later stages of disease progression. The tendency is extremely significant. Based on chi-square tests for the statistical independence of each table's row and column attributes, the associated two-tailed p values were both less than 0.00005.

Including only the 173 long-term survivors would imply that the proportion of patients cured by the intervention was 0.2993. This seems too low. Figure 15 suggests visually a proportion just below 0.52. If there is reasonable evidence that some of the 146 QUESTIONABLE RISK patients were also cured, they need to be reclassified (i.e., moved down into the MR category).

On the other hand, not all QUESTIONABLE RISK patients are reasonable candidates for reclassification. Appendix I shows that no patients were initially diagnosed M1 (as having already experienced a distant metastasis). That was not a problem. Nevertheless, a patient diagnosed N3 and either T3 or T4 in terms of the T/N/M staging criteria might not be curable by mastectomy and radiation alone or by any other kind of strictly locoregional therapy.

Fortunately, there were no such patients in either the QUESTIONABLE RISK or the MINIMAL RISK category. There was only one such patient diagnosed N2 and either T3 or T4. Hence, no restrictions of this nature limiting reclassification of QUESTIONABLE RISK patients into the MINIMAL RISK (MR) category appear necessary.

6.8   Executing the CURE Option of the KAPM Procedure

The KAPM procedure with the CURE option enabled was applied to the Guy's Hospital intervention sample. When enabled, the CURE option makes a systematic search of whatever patient survival data it receives for a time-phased pattern of cure. An edited version of the report it generated is presented below and on the next four pages.

SEARCH FOR A PATTERN OF CURE (VERY LOW/NO RISK) AMONG CENSORED OBSERVATIONS

Patient survival data suggest a pattern of cure if the following conditions are satisfied.

First, the focal event targeted by the Kaplan-Meier analysis must be inherently avoidable. Any evidence of further disease progression does qualify, assuming the possibility of cure.

Second, it must be plausible to expect an appreciable proportion of the patient population from which sample data were obtained to have been cured by virtue of the target intervention. Mastectomy (sometimes with radiation) was preestablished as satisfying this condition (entry 4, "ANNOTATED REFERENCES").

Third, the survival data submitted to the Kaplan-Meier analysis must be tested by the RISKTEST simulator. RISKTEST results must render it at least plausible to reject the null hypothesis of no patients cured despite their mastectomy (and radiation). A one-hundred-thousand-trial run of the RISKTEST simulator provided evidence directionally favorable to the alternate hypothesis. This time, however, the evidence was statistically insignificant.

Fourth, the nature of the progressive disease and the choice of a focal event must be such that patient survival curves are reasonably described by a Weibull distribution. The R-squared value of 0.8944 reported at the end of section 6.4 satisfies this condition.

Fifth, the sequence of Kaplan-Meier survival rates must approach a horizontal asymptote at some decidedly positive survival probability. It must also fit a Weibull distribution with a decreasing trend in hazard rate distinctly better (in terms of comparable R-squared values) than it fits an exponential distribution (each distribution fitted to the same sample data submitted for analysis). The table displayed in section 6.4 and the corresponding survival curve shown directly following it in figure 15 satisfy this condition.

Sixth, analysis of the residuals (fitted Weibull survival probabilities subtracted from corresponding Kaplan-Meier survival rates) must show a statistically significant pattern wherein positive residuals are concentrated among the earlier observations (i.e., survival times of relatively short duration), while negative residuals are concentrated among the later observations (i.e., survival times of relatively long duration). The cross table of residuals analyzed below satisfies this condition.

Seventh, and most compelling, if the preceding six conditions are satisfied, it is worth repeating the Kaplan-Meier analysis a number of times, each successive time with the remaining censored observations of longest duration selectively culled. If the total sample contains a substantial subset of cured patients, such a sequence of analyses should gradually eliminate them.

1. Over the sequence of analyses, the initial advantage of the fitted Weibull model over the fitted exponential model (difference in R-squared values) should initially decline.
2. It should then stabilize at some level, possibly at zero.
3. The sharpness of decrease of the fitted Weibull hazard rate over time should also decline initially and then stabilize at some level, possibly at zero (where the Weibull trend parameter = 1.0).
4. Whichever model (Weibull or exponential) eventually fits the set of Kaplan-Meier survival probability estimates better should have its R-squared statistic increase steadily to a maximum value at a contextually plausible cure rate and then stabilize or decline.

Results bearing on this condition are displayed on the next three pages, following the cross-table analysis immediately below.

CROSS TABLE OF RESIDUALS	EARLY RESIDUAL (KAPM - FITTED)	LATE RESIDUAL (KAPM - FITTED)	TOTAL
POSITIVE RESIDUAL	59	5	64
NEGATIVE RESIDUAL	64	119	183
TOTAL	123	124	247

These data display an extremely significant "lean" in the direction of relatively higher cell counts along the table's major diagonal (top-left and bottom-right cells), compared to its off-diagonal (top-right and bottom-left cells).

A Fisher exact statistical test was performed on this table.

The one-tailed p value (directional alternative to the null hypothesis) is less than 0.00005. The two-tailed p value is also less than 0.00005.

Since positive residuals are relatively heavily concentrated among the earlier observations while negative residuals are heavily concentrated among the later observations, it is quite reasonable to interpret the decreasing hazard rate as at least somewhat spurious. The pattern of residuals may again have been distorted by contaminating the sample with an appreciable proportion of cured patients. We may again be looking at a statistical artifact of the maximum likelihood algorithm's attempt to force fit as closely as possible a Weibull function that must fall asymptotically to zero to a sequence of focal event and censored times whose Kaplan-Meier survival probability appears to approach a horizontal asymptote somewhat below 0.52.

CENSORED TIME BOUND	NUMBER AND PROPORTION SO CURED	WEIBULL INTENSITY PARAMETER	WEIBULL TREND PARAMETER	R-SQUARED VALUE OF WEIBULL	R-SQUARED VALUE OF EXPONENTIAL	R-SQUARED DIFFERENCE IN VALUE
INFINITE	0(.000)	0.0254	0.5988	0.8944	0.4010	0.4934
20.7146	173(.299)	0.0875	0.7876	0.9517	0.8392	0.1125
19.6852	185(.320)	0.0968	0.8150	0.9563	0.8706	0.0857
18.9624	192(.332)	0.1027	0.8321	0.9584	0.8876	0.0708
18.8693	193(.334)	0.1035	0.8346	0.9587	0.8899	0.0687
18.5161	198(.343)	0.1080	0.8476	0.9603	0.9011	0.0593
18.2067	202(.349)	0.1117	0.8584	0.9616	0.9096	0.0520
18.1218	203(.351)	0.1127	0.8612	0.9619	0.9116	0.0503
18.0972	204(.353)	0.1136	0.8640	0.9622	0.9136	0.0486
17.3470	211(.365)	0.1206	0.8843	0.9646	0.9268	0.0378
17.0185	213(.369)	0.1226	0.8903	0.9652	0.9303	0.0349
16.3477	218(.377)	0.1279	0.9054	0.9668	0.9386	0.0282
15.1814	225(.389)	0.1354	0.9267	0.9689	0.9491	0.0198
15.0089	227(.393)	0.1376	0.9325	0.9695	0.9519	0.0176
14.8173	228(.394)	0.1387	0.9354	0.9698	0.9532	0.0166
14.5134	233(.403)	0.1443	0.9502	0.9713	0.9594	0.0119
13.4839	236(.408)	0.1477	0.9584	0.9721	0.9625	0.0096
13.1608	241(.417)	0.1534	0.9719	0.9735	0.9675	0.0060
12.6242	244(.422)	0.1568	0.9796	0.9743	0.9702	0.0042
12.0767	246(.426)	0.1591	0.9844	0.9749	0.9718	0.0031
11.8659	247(.427)	0.1602	0.9866	0.9752	0.9725	0.0026
11.2580	249(.431)	0.1625	0.9910	0.9757	0.9739	0.0017
10.7050	255(.441)	0.1692	1.0000	0.9777	0.9777	0.0000
10.5298	256(.443)	0.1704	1.0000	0.9783	0.9783	0.0000
10.1355	258(.446)	0.1727	1.0000	0.9793	0.9793	0.0000
10.0260	260(.450)	0.1751	1.0000	0.9803	0.9803	0.0000
9.4100	263(.455)	0.1786	1.0000	0.9816	0.9816	0.0000
9.3169	265(.458)	0.1809	1.0000	0.9823	0.9823	0.0000
9.1992	266(.460)	0.1821	1.0000	0.9827	0.9827	0.0000
9.0979	267(.462)	0.1833	1.0000	0.9830	0.9830	0.0000
8.6516	270(.467)	0.1868	1.0000	0.9840	0.9840	0.0000
8.6023	271(.469)	0.1880	1.0000	0.9843	0.9843	0.0000
8.3888	272(.471)	0.1892	1.0000	0.9845	0.9845	0.0000
8.1533	274(.474)	0.1915	1.0000	0.9850	0.9850	0.0000
7.9179	275(.476)	0.1926	1.0000	0.9853	0.9853	0.0000
7.6413	278(.481)	0.1960	1.0000	0.9858	0.9858	0.0000
7.4059	279(.483)	0.1971	1.0000	0.9859	0.9859	0.0000
7.1704	281(.486)	0.1993	1.0000	0.9862	0.9862	0.0000
6.6749	282(.488)	0.2004	1.0000	0.9862	0.9862	0.0000
6.4066	283(.490)	0.2014	1.0000	0.9862	0.9862	0.0000
6.1355	285(.493)	0.2033	1.0000	0.9862	0.9862	0.0000
5.8426	286(.495)	0.2043	1.0000	0.9862	0.9862	0.0000
5.6920	288(.498)	0.2062	1.0000	0.9860	0.9860	0.0000
5.4812	290(.502)	0.2080	1.0000	0.9858	0.9858	0.0000
5.3607	291(.503)	0.2089	1.0000	0.9857	0.9857	0.0000
5.3498	292(.505)	0.2098	1.0000	0.9855	0.9855	0.0000
5.2895	293(.507)	0.2107	1.0000	0.9854	0.9854	0.0000
5.1745	294(.509)	0.2116	1.0000	0.9852	0.9852	0.0000
4.6899	295(.510)	0.2124	1.0000	0.9850	0.9850	0.0000
4.4353	296(.512)	0.2132	1.0000	0.9847	0.9847	0.0000
4.2765	297(.514)	0.2140	1.0000	0.9844	0.9844	0.0000
3.7591	298(.516)	0.2147	1.0000	0.9841	0.9841	0.0000
3.5291	299(.517)	0.2153	1.0000	0.9837	0.9837	0.0000
3.4114	300(.519)	0.2159	1.0000	0.9833	0.9833	0.0000

CENSORED TIME BOUND	NUMBER AND PROPORTION SO CURED	WEIBULL INTENSITY PARAMETER	WEIBULL TREND PARAMETER	R-SQUARED VALUE OF WEIBULL	R-SQUARED VALUE OF EXPONENTIAL	R-SQUARED DIFFERENCE IN VALUE
3.1184	302(.522)	0.2171	1.0000	0.9825	0.9825	0.0000
2.9706	304(.526)	0.2182	1.0000	0.9816	0.9816	0.0000
2.5982	305(.528)	0.2186	1.0000	0.9811	0.9811	0.0000
2.2122	306(.529)	0.2191	1.0000	0.9807	0.9807	0.0000
2.0205	307(.531)	0.2194	1.0000	0.9803	0.9803	0.0000
1.8946	308(.533)	0.2198	1.0000	0.9799	0.9799	0.0000
1.8782	309(.535)	0.2201	1.0000	0.9795	0.9795	0.0000
1.8042	310(.536)	0.2205	1.0000	0.9791	0.9791	0.0000
1.5825	311(.538)	0.2208	1.0000	0.9787	0.9787	0.0000
1.4538	312(.540)	0.2211	1.0000	0.9784	0.9784	0.0000
1.4346	313(.542)	0.2214	0.9990	0.9783	0.9781	0.0002
1.4182	314(.543)	0.2218	0.9979	0.9782	0.9778	0.0004
0.9966	315(.545)	0.2221	0.9969	0.9782	0.9776	0.0005
0.9418	316(.547)	0.2224	0.9960	0.9782	0.9774	0.0007
0.4435	317(.548)	0.2225	0.9953	0.9783	0.9774	0.0008
0.0000	319(.552)	0.2226	0.9949	0.9784	0.9775	0.0009

Explanatory Notes:

1. The top row in the table presumes that no patients in the intervention sample were cured. It recapitulates the results of fitting, first, a Weibull survival function and then an exponential survival function via maximum likelihood to the focal and censored event times, as if all 578 patients remained at risk despite their mastectomy (and radiation).

2. Subsequent rows presume that at least some and successively more censored patients were cured, starting with the 173 long-term survivors who lived without evidence of disease progression longer than the longest focal event time (20.71 years) and ending with all 319 censored patients.

3. Of these 319 censored patients, the shortest-term survivor lived without evidence of disease progression for only a very brief time (virtually zero years as depicted in the bottom row of the table).

4. The ever-expanding subset of patients presumed cured was culled from each successive Kaplan-Meier analysis. The results of successive analyses appear in successive rows of the table.

5. The CENSORED TIME BOUND is the culling criterion. Those censored patients who survived for at least the CENSORED TIME BOUND (in years) with no evidence of further disease progression were deleted from each successive row of the table.

6. The sequence of CENSORED TIME BOUNDs replicated (in reverse order) the sequence of focal event times occurring in the intervention sample.

7. The NUMBER AND PROPORTION SO CURED records the ever-increasing number of patients culled from each successive Kaplan-Meier analysis.

8. The WEIBULL INTENSITY PARAMETER and the WEIBULL TREND PARAMETER are the two parameters fitted via maximum likelihood to the remaining subset of nonculled patients presumed to be at risk in each successive analysis. See appendix C for a description of the Weibull function and its two parameters (LAMBDA, indicating intensity, and DELTA, indicating trend).

9. The R-SQUARED VALUE OF WEIBULL is the unadjusted coefficient of determination associated with the best-fitting (likelihood maximizing) Weibull function. In calculating R-squared, the Kaplan-Meier survival probability estimates produced via the product-limit method are taken to be the "correct" survival probabilities that the best-fitting Weibull function is attempting to reproduce.

10. The R-SQUARED VALUE OF EXPONENTIAL is the unadjusted coefficient of determination associated with the best-fitting exponential function

(Weibull function whose trend parameter is exactly 1.0). In calculating R-squared, the Kaplan-Meier survival probability estimates produced via the product-limit method are taken to be the "correct" survival probabilities that the best-fitting exponential function is attempting to reproduce.

11. The R-SQUARED DIFFERENCE IN VALUE measures the relative improvement in goodness of fit achieved by the best-fitting Weibull function over the best-fitting exponential function. A Weibull survival function must always fit a given data set at least as well as the more restrictive exponential survival function in terms of maximum likelihood. Therefore, an R-squared difference of zero indicates virtually no relative improvement (i.e., that the best-fitting Weibull function is essentially exponential).

This table reflects a striking pattern of cure.

1. All six of the preconditions stated as necessary before producing such a table were satisfied.

2. The compelling pattern of cure specified in the seventh condition was fully realized.

3. The relative improvement in goodness of fit achieved by the best-fitting Weibull function over the best-fitting exponential function, measured by the R-SQUARED DIFFERENCE IN VALUE, declined from an initial value of 0.4934 to a final value of virtually zero.

4. Zero improvement occurred when the longest-surviving 255 of the 319 censored patients were treated as cured and, therefore, removed from the KAPM analysis. The best-fitting Weibull function then became exponential (a Weibull function with trend parameter = 1.0) at a value of R-squared = 0.9777. All 255 patients survived without evidence of further disease progression for at least 10.705 years. This suggests a minimum proportion cured in the neighborhood of 255/578 = 0.441.

5. The exponential function remained best-fitting until 312 of the 319 censored patients were finally removed from the KAPM analysis. That the last seven patients appeared to display a tiny difference in R-squared values between fitting the Weibull and exponential functions is likely due to computer rounding errors.

6. This lends further support to the notion that the initial superiority of the Weibull over the exponential function was spurious. It signified nothing more than a model specification error. A large number of cured MR patients, transformed to a state of minimal risk by virtue of their mastectomy (and radiation), contaminated the remaining sample of SR patients still at risk despite their treatment.

7. The R-squared goodness-of-fit statistic associated with the best-fitting function increased steadily from an initial value of 0.8944, when none of the 578 patients was treated as cured, to a maximum value of 0.9862, when 281/578 = 48.6 percent were treated as cured. All of these 281 censored patients survived without evidence of further disease progression for at least 7.1704 years.

8. The maximum value of R-squared occurred at a cured proportion (0.486) somewhat below the last proportion (0.5172) on the initial Kaplan-Meier curve shown in figure 15, just where the curve became approximately horizontal.

9. Thereafter, R-squared declined gradually, but only very slightly, to 0.9784, when all 319 CENSORED patients (319/578 = 55.2 percent) were treated as cured.

10. The closeness of successive R-squared values between a 0.486 proportion cured (R-squared = 0.9862) and a 0.552 proportion cured (R-squared = 0.9784) again suggests the need for a fine-tuning mechanism to obtain a more precise estimate of the actual proportion cured.

6.9 Fine-Tuning the Initial Estimate of the Actual Proportion Cured

An obvious place to initiate the fine-tuning process is at the CENSORED TIME BOUND that achieved the maximum R-squared value. That occurred at 7.1704 years. There 281 (48.6 percent) of the 578 patients were provisionally regarded as cured (MR). These were the 281 censored patients who survived for at least 7.1704 years after initial diagnosis and treatment without evidence of further disease progression.

Executing the RISKTEST simulator at several smaller and several larger CENSORED TIME BOUNDs will help to produce an appropriate initial estimate of the proportion of the 578 Guy's Hospital patients who were actually cured by their mastectomy (and radiation). It will also help to identify the cured patients.

Notice that each null hypothesis now being tested by RISKTEST will be unique. Each successive simulation run will be initiated by a sequence of inputs specifying some particular number of patients (out of 578) presumed to have been cured. The particular patients are the censored ones who survived at or beyond each successive CENSORED TIME BOUND.

Changing the nature of the null hypothesis has several important implications.

1. Each corresponding alternate hypothesis is now bidirectional. It makes sense to consider either a smaller or a larger number of cured (MR) patients compared to each successive null-hypothesized number. This suggests focusing on two-tailed rather than on one-tailed p values generated by RISKTEST.
2. Each successive CENSORED TIME BOUND provisionally partitions the 578 patients into different MR and SR subsets. Each separate provisional partitioning requires that separate estimates now be made via maximum likelihood of the appropriate parameters of both the focal event and composite censoring event distributions to serve as inputs to successive runs of the RISKTEST simulator.
3. The best-fitting simulation run will be the one whose corresponding set of inputs to RISKTEST center most closely around 259 the simulated distribution of focal events experienced by the particular patients partitioned into the SR subset by that particular CENSORED TIME BOUND.

Nine simulations runs were executed. Each simulation run consisted of ten thousand trials (RISKTEST's default number). Simulation results are shown below and on the next three pages.

Run Number 1

PROVISIONAL NUMBER OF CURED (MR) PATIENTS: 255 (255/578 = 0.4412)
CENSORED TIME BOUND: 10.7050 years
VALUE OF R-SQUARED: 0.9777
RISKTEST INPUTS: 578 255 259 7 21.1259 1 0.1692 1 0.0398 1.1771

RISKTEST OUTPUTS:

The simulated number of patients experiencing the focal event was less than the target number (259) in 555 trials.
The simulated number of patients experiencing the focal event was equal to the target number (259) in 165 trials.
The simulated number of patients experiencing the focal event was more than the target number (259) in 9,280 trials.

If interpreted as a statistical test of the goodness of fit of the simulation model with the observed number of patients experiencing the focal event, these results are consistent with a bidirectional (two-tailed) p value of 0.1440.

Run Number 2

PROVISIONAL NUMBER OF CURED (MR) PATIENTS: 263 (263/578 = 0.4550)
CENSORED TIME BOUND: 9.4100 years
VALUE OF R-SQUARED: 0.9816
RISKTEST INPUTS: 578 263 259 7 21.1259 1 0.1786 1 0.0316 1

RISKTEST OUTPUTS:

The simulated number of patients experiencing the focal event was less than the target number (259) in 1,244 trials.
The simulated number of patients experiencing the focal event was equal to the target number (259) in 326 trials.
The simulated number of patients experiencing the focal event was more than the target number (259) in 8,430 trials.

If interpreted as a statistical test of the goodness of fit of the simulation model with the observed number of patients experiencing the focal event, these results are consistent with a bidirectional (two-tailed) p value of 0.3140.

Run Number 3

PROVISIONAL NUMBER OF CURED (MR) PATIENTS: 267 (267/578 = 0.4619)
CENSORED TIME BOUND: 9.0979 years
VALUE OF R-SQUARED: 0.9830
RISKTEST INPUTS: 578 267 259 7 21.1259 1 0.1833 1 0.0303 1

RISKTEST OUTPUTS:

The simulated number of patients experiencing the focal event was less than the target number (259) in 1,418 trials.
The simulated number of patients experiencing the focal event was equal to the target number (259) in 367 trials.
The simulated number of patients experiencing the focal event was more than the target number (259) in 8,215 trials.

If interpreted as a statistical test of the goodness of fit of the simulation model with the observed number of patients experiencing the focal event, these results are consistent with a bidirectional (two-tailed) p value of 0.3570.

Run Number 4 (highest value of R-squared)

PROVISIONAL NUMBER OF CURED (MR) PATIENTS: 281 (281/578 = 0.4862)
CENSORED TIME BOUND: 7.1704 years
VALUE OF R-SQUARED: 0.9862
RISKTEST INPUTS: 578 281 259 7 21.1259 1 0.1993 1 0.0253 1

RISKTEST OUTPUTS:

The simulated number of patients experiencing the focal event was less than the target number (259) in 2,484 trials.
The simulated number of patients experiencing the focal event was equal to the target number (259) in 593 trials.
The simulated number of patients experiencing the focal event was more than the target number (259) in 6,923 trials.

If interpreted as a statistical test of the goodness of fit of the simulation model with the observed number of patients experiencing the focal event, these results are consistent with a bidirectional (two-tailed) p value of 0.6154.

Run Number 5

PROVISIONAL NUMBER OF CURED (MR) PATIENTS: 288 (288/578 = 0.4983)
CENSORED TIME BOUND: 5.6920 years
VALUE OF R-SQUARED: 0.9860
RISKTEST INPUTS: 578 288 259 7 21.1259 1 0.2062 1 0.0225 1

RISKTEST OUTPUTS:

The simulated number of patients experiencing the focal event was less than the target number (259) in 3,461 trials.
The simulated number of patients experiencing the focal event was equal to the target number (259) in 732 trials.
The simulated number of patients experiencing the focal event was more than the target number (259) in 5,807 trials.

If interpreted as a statistical test of the goodness of fit of the simulation model with the observed number of patients experiencing the focal event, these results are consistent with a bidirectional (two-tailed) p value of 0.8386.

Run Number 6 (best-fitting run)

PROVISIONAL NUMBER OF CURED (MR) PATIENTS: 293 (293/578 = 0.5069)
CENSORED TIME BOUND: 5.2895 years
VALUE OF R-SQUARED: 0.9854
RISKTEST INPUTS: 578 293 259 7 21.1259 1 0.2107 1 0.0204 1

RISKTEST OUTPUTS:

The simulated number of patients experiencing the focal event was less than the target number (259) in 4,634 trials.
The simulated number of patients experiencing the focal event was equal to the target number (259) in 830 trials.
The simulated number of patients experiencing the focal event was more than the target number (259) in 4,536 trials.

If interpreted as a statistical test of the goodness of fit of the simulation model with the observed number of patients experiencing the focal event, these results are consistent with a bidirectional (two-tailed) p value of 1.0000.

Run Number 7

PROVISIONAL NUMBER OF CURED (MR) PATIENTS: 297 (297/578 = 0.5138)
CENSORED TIME BOUND: 4.2765 years
VALUE OF R-SQUARED: 0.9844
RISKTEST INPUTS: 578 297 259 7 21.1259 1 0.2140 1 0.0120 0.7967

RISKTEST OUTPUTS:

The simulated number of patients experiencing the focal event was less than the observed number (259) in 7,374 trials.
The simulated number of patients experiencing the focal event was equal to the observed number (259) in 630 trials.
The simulated number of patients experiencing the focal event was more than the observed number (259) in 1,996 trials.

If interpreted as a statistical test of the goodness of fit of the simulation model with the observed number of patients experiencing the focal event, these results are consistent with a bidirectional (two-tailed) p value of 0.5252.

Run Number 8

PROVISIONAL NUMBER OF CURED (MR) PATIENTS: 300 (300/578 = 0.5190)
CENSORED TIME BOUND: 3.4114 years
VALUE OF R-SQUARED: 0.9833
RISKTEST INPUTS: 578 300 259 7 21.1259 1 0.2159 1 0.0104 0.7804

RISKTEST OUTPUTS:

The simulated number of patients experiencing the focal event was less than the target number (259) in 8,125 trials.
The simulated number of patients experiencing the focal event was equal to the target number (259) in 523 trials.
The simulated number of patients experiencing the focal event was more than the target number (259) in 1,352 trials.

If interpreted as a statistical test of the goodness of fit of the simulation model with the observed number of patients experiencing the focal event, these results are consistent with a bidirectional (two-tailed) p value of 0.3750.

Run Number 9

PROVISIONAL NUMBER OF CURED (MR) PATIENTS: 306 (306/578 = 0.5294)
CENSORED TIME BOUND: 2.2122 years
VALUE OF R-SQUARED: 0.9807
RISKTEST INPUTS: 578 306 259 7 21.1259 1 0.2191 1 0.0077 0.7620

RISKTEST OUTPUTS:

The simulated number of patients experiencing the focal event was less than the target number (259) in 9,312 trials.
The simulated number of patients experiencing the focal event was equal to the target number (259) in 287 trials.
The simulated number of patients experiencing the focal event was more than the target number (259) in 401 trials.

If interpreted as a statistical test of the goodness of fit of the simulation model with the target number of patients experiencing the focal event, these results are consistent with a bidirectional (two-tailed) p value of 0.1376.

On the next page are tabled the results of one hundred thousand simulation trials. Again, the second column counts the number of such trials (out of one hundred thousand) in which the number of patients who experience the focal event is as indicated in the first column.

With one exception, inputs to the best-fitting RISKTEST run (Run Number 6) were replicated precisely to produce this table. The exception was a small increase in the intensity parameter for the focal event from 0.2107 to 0.2110 (to be explained in section 6.10).

NUMBER OF PATIENTS WHO EXPERIENCE THE FOCAL EVENT	ABSOLUTE FREQUENCIES (COUNTS)	RELATIVE FREQUENCIES (PROPORTIONS)	CUMULATIVE RELATIVE FREQUENCIES
235	1	0.00001	0.00001
236	1	0.00001	0.00002
237	1	0.00001	0.00003
238	5	0.00005	0.00008
239	6	0.00006	0.00014
240	17	0.00017	0.00031
241	22	0.00022	0.00053
242	41	0.00041	0.00094
243	87	0.00087	0.00181
244	117	0.00117	0.00298
245	198	0.00198	0.00496
246	314	0.00314	0.00810
247	504	0.00504	0.01314
248	768	0.00768	0.02082
249	1187	0.01187	0.03269
250	1582	0.01582	0.04851
251	2215	0.02215	0.07066
252	3034	0.03034	0.10100
253	3795	0.03795	0.13895
254	4823	0.04823	0.18718
255	5768	0.05768	0.24486
256	6595	0.06595	0.31081
257	7313	0.07313	0.38394
258	7862	0.07862	0.46256
259	8170	0.08170	0.54426
260	8053	0.08053	0.62479
261	7654	0.07654	0.70133
262	6839	0.06839	0.76972
263	6124	0.06124	0.83096
264	4895	0.04895	0.87991
265	3915	0.03915	0.91906
266	2979	0.02979	0.94885
267	1992	0.01992	0.96877
268	1319	0.01319	0.98196
269	831	0.00831	0.99027
270	467	0.00467	0.99494
271	253	0.00253	0.99747
272	130	0.00130	0.99877
273	72	0.00072	0.99949
274	32	0.00032	0.99981
275	8	0.00008	0.99989
276	8	0.00008	0.99997
277	2	0.00002	0.99999
278	1	0.00001	1.00000
TOTAL	100000	1.00000	

6.10 Convincing Confirmation of the Existence of Cure

The distribution of simulated focal event counts tabled on the previous page is close to normal. Its modal value is perfectly centered at 259, the target focal event count actually observed in the 578-patient Guy's Hospital intervention sample. Only a very slight fine-tuning adjustment to the focal event intensity parameter (from 0.2107 to 0.2110) was required to achieve this perfectly centered result. The adjustment moved the center of the simulated distribution up by a single focal event (from 258 to 259).

What rendered it so convincing as confirmation of the existence of cure was that the parameter estimates embodied in the inputs to the best-fitting RISKTEST simulation run were obtained directly from the collected Guy's Hospital sample data in conjunction with a trial-and-error sequence of specific assumptions about how many and just which patients were actually cured by their mastectomy (and radiation).

Consequently, the initial partitioning into MR and SR subsamples will be as follows:

1. number of MR patients cured by mastectomy (and radiation) = 293;
2. MR proportion of patients cured = 293/578 = 0.5069;
3. where all MR patients survived without evidence of further disease progression for at least 5.2895 years after their mastectomy and radiation;
4. where the survival function for 285 SR patients who remained at substantial risk despite their mastectomy (and radiation) was exponential; and
5. where the hazard rate for these 285 SR patients was constant (not decreasing) at 0.2110 focal events per year.

Notice that what originally appeared to be a Weibull survival curve with a decreasing hazard rate over time for the unpartitioned sample of 578 patients turned out to be an exponential survival curve with a constant hazard rate for just the 285 presumed SR patients. The 293 presumed MR patients were not at risk of further disease progression. Their survival curves were forever horizontal at 100 percent survival probability. Purging them from the sample produced the same change in shape of hazard function (and for precisely the same reason) that was demonstrated with the 550 breast cancer patients from Turku in section 4.

7.0 APPLYING MRPA TO THE SECOND ILLUSTRATIVE ANALYSIS

The initial partitioning of the 578 patients in the intervention sample can be refined still further. Refinement will be accomplished via selective reclassification of patients on the basis of various things we know about them that are recorded in the Guy's Hospital data set, in combination with each patient's directly observed posttreatment experience.

The 259 patients who experienced the focal event cannot be reclassified. Their experience provides indisputable proof that they belong in the CERTAIN RISK (hence, SR) category. They were initially and will always remain so classified.

Reclassification of censored patients can only take place between the QUESTIONABLE RISK and the MINIMAL RISK (MR) categories. Selective reclassification will again be implemented by MRPA.

Recall that MRPA operates within a Bayesian framework. Which patients become selectively reclassified will again be based on each patient's individually tailored Bayesian posterior cure probability. Her cure probability may be interpreted as the likelihood that a particular Guy's Hospital patient was actually transformed from the SR state of substantial risk into the MR state of minimal risk of further disease progression following her mastectomy (and radiation).

7.1 Replicating the Bayesian Cure Model

Exactly the same Bayesian cure model developed and tabled in section 5.1 for the 550-patient Turku intervention sample applies equally to the 578-patient Guy's Hospital intervention sample. Neither the tabled model nor its explanatory notes need be reproduced here. Interested readers may find a review of section 5.1 helpful.

When applied to the 578-patient Guy's Hospital data, MRPA again achieved complete convergence. This time, however, MRPA required four iterations rather than three.

7.2 Logistic Regression Analysis (Logit): Obtaining Individually Tailored
     Prior Cure Probabilities from the Fine-Tuned Initial Partitioning of
     Patients into MR and SR Subsamples

A number of individual patient characteristics recorded in the Guy's Hospital data set appeared plausible as prognostic factors that might predict, probabilistically, each patient's membership in the MR and SR subsamples. Annotated values of these candidate factors are summarized in appendix I.

The factors included:

1. age of patient at diagnosis and treatment (in years);
2. size of tumor in millimeters of longest dimension;
3. type of tumor (e.g., lobular);
4. grade of tumor (grade 1, grade 2, or grade 3);
5. number of positive axillary lymph nodes;
6. T stage (T0, T1, T2, T3, or T4);
7. N stage (N0, N1, N2, or N3);
8. M stage (M0 or M1);
9. ER (positive or negative estrogen receptor response); and
10. PR (positive or negative progesterone receptor response).

Age at diagnosis and treatment was again eliminated. Including it would have reflected the same definitional relationship between it and the manner in which the MR and SR subsamples were identified.

M stage at diagnosis was eliminated because all 578 patients were M0. Complete absence of differentiation precluded using it to predict MR and SR subsample membership.

An index was constructed for grade of tumor. The mean of the properly recorded 521 tumor grades was assigned to each of the fifty-seven tumors with missing grade observations.

Strikingly, all fifty-seven missing observations of tumor grade applied to (and only to) the fifty-seven tumors identified as lobular. Because no other tumor characteristics (e.g., tumor size, T stage, and so on) showed the same differential pattern, it seemed possible that there was something unusual about these fifty-seven lobular tumors or something nonobvious about how Guy's Hospital coded tumor type.

In view of this anomaly, it seemed wise to eliminate tumor type as a candidate prognostic factor. It was statistically insignificant as a predictor in the Turku intervention sample, so this may not have been a damaging exclusion.

Eighteen patients had tumor size values of zero. The same eighteen patients were recorded as T stage T0. It was presumed that tumor size observations for these eighteen patients were unavailable (missing data). Consequently, indexes were constructed for both tumor size and T stage at diagnosis. The means of the properly recorded 578 - 18 = 560 tumor sizes and T stages were assigned, respectively, to each of the eighteen patients with presumed missing observations of these two factors.

A separate univariate analysis was then performed on each of the seven remaining factors as the single predictor (independent variable) of logistic regression. The initial partitioning into 293 MR and 285 SR patients served as each dependent variable, which was uniformly coded 0 for MR and 1 for SR.

Coding MR as 0 and SR as 1 ensured that a positive regression coefficient assigned to any prognostic factor would indicate that higher factor values were associated with increasing risk of further disease progression. A negative coefficient would indicate that higher factor values were linked with higher likelihood that a patient was cured following her mastectomy (and radiation).

Results of the seven univariate logistic regression analyses are tabled on the next page. Each analysis was based on the factor or factor index score for the 578 intervention patients. All seven univariate relationships emerged as positive associations.

PROGNOSTIC FACTOR	REGRESSION COEFFICIENT	STANDARD DEVIATION	CHI-SQUARE (DF = 1)	TWO-TAILED P VALUE	ODDS RATIO
SIZ	0.0347	0.0061	32.7865	0.0000	1.0353
GRA	0.4546	0.1403	10.5048	0.0012	1.5756
POS	0.2298	0.0425	29.2689	0.0000	1.2583
TUM	0.7598	0.1341	32.0817	0.0000	2.1378
NOD	0.8331	0.1182	49.6973	0.0000	2.3004
ERP	0.2897	0.1744	2.7601	0.0966	1.3360
PRP	0.1906	0.1701	1.2543	0.2627	1.2099

Explanatory Notes:

1. SIZ was size of tumor in millimeters along its longest dimension, with substituted mean values.
2. GRA was tumor grade, coded 1 for grade 1, 2 for grade 2, 3 for grade 3, and with substituted mean values.
3. POS was number of positive axillary lymph nodes.
4. TUM was T stage, coded 1 for stage T1, 2 for stage T2, and 3.5 for stage T3 or stage T4, and with substituted mean values.
5. NOD was N stage, coded 0 for stage N0, 1 for stage N1, 2 for stage N2, and 3 for stage N3.
6. ERP was estrogen response positivity, coded 1 for positive and 0 for negative.
7. PRP was progesterone response positivity, coded 1 for positive and 0 for negative.
8. Notice that all except ERP and PRP yielded highly significant associations.

Conventional stepwise multivariate logistic regression with backward elimination of the seven prognostic factors produced the following results. Slightly edited computer output is enclosed between the horizontal lines for the four factors that survived backward elimination.

Likelihood ratio chi-square statistic: 97.634, two-tailed p value: 0.0000 (based on 4 degrees of freedom and 578 complete observations).

INDEPENDENT VARIABLE	REGRESSION COEFFICIENT	STANDARD DEVIATION	CHI-SQUARE (DF = 1)	2-TAIL P VALUE	ODDS RATIO
intercept	−3.0125	0.4945	37.1177	0.0000	0.0492
GRA	0.4812	0.1575	9.3395	0.0022	1.6180
TUM	0.6614	0.1422	21.6242	0.0000	1.9375
NOD	0.7535	0.1217	38.3453	0.0000	2.1243
ERP	0.5033	0.1990	6.3966	0.0114	1.6541

Pearson chi-square fit statistic (based on 76 degrees of freedom): 71.966, p value: 0.6098.

Deviance chi-square fit statistic (based on 76 degrees of freedom): 81.073, p value: 0.3240.

Classification improvement index (proportional reduction in the number of wrong classifications enabled by using values of the independent variables): 0.3263

The logistic regression coefficients on the previous page were used to calculate PRMSR0, the initial probability that each of the 578 intervention patients remained in the SR state despite her mastectomy (and radiation).

DEFINE PRMSR0:
EXP(-3.0125+0.4812*GRA+0.6614*TUM+0.7535*NOD+0.5033*ERP)/
[1+EXP(-3.0125+0.4812*GRA+0.6614*TUM+0.7535*NOD+0.5033*ERP)]

SUMMARY STATISTICS	ATTRIBUTE PRMSR0	ATTRIBUTE MRSR0DX
n DEFINED	578	578
MINIMUM	0.1336	0
MEDIAN	0.4442	0
MAXIMUM	0.9710	1
MEAN	0.4931	0.4931
STD. DEV.	0.1978	0.5000

Values of PRMSR0 ranged from a minimum of 13.36 to a maximum of 97.10 percent, with a mean of 49.31 percent. The M in the PRMSR0 attribute name indicates substitution of mean values for missing factor observations wherever appropriate. The 0 indicates MRPA's initial (as opposed to subsequent iteration) partitioning. The mean value of PRMSR0 was the complement of the proportion of patients initially presumed cured (MR = 293/578 = 0.5069).

MRSR0DX (coded 0 for MR and 1 for SR) is a dummy variable encapsulating the initial partitioning. The mean value of MRSR0DX was the proportion of patients initially presumed to have remained in the SR state (SR = 285/578 = 0.4931). Logistic regression ensured identical mean values for PRMSR0 and MRSR0DX.

7.3 By How Much Did PCM Improve the Consistency of the Initial Prior Cure Probabilities with the Initial Partitioning of Patients into MR and SR Subsamples?

The intervention sample size of 578 was again too small to subdivide the patient population into relatively homogeneous strata. However, all seven prognostic factors were converted by SPSA into corresponding UIRIs. Minimum subscale sizes were again uniformly set at twenty-five or fifty patient observations. Missing observations of tumor size, tumor grade, and T stage were replaced in the usual PCM manner, as outlined in section 2.3. Consequently, PCM's ability to improve the consistency of partitioning probabilities relied on indicating via SPSA conversion the underlying shape of each factor's discriminating impact, in combination with its selective replacement of missing observations.

A PCM reanalysis of the same 578-patient intervention sample data was executed. A stepwise multivariate logistic regression analysis with backward elimination was performed. Corresponding UIRI values were substituted for all seven prognostic factors as independent variables. The initial partitioning of the 578 patients into MR and SR subsamples remained as the dependent variable.

UIRIs replacing tumor size, tumor grade, N stage, and estrogen response positivity survived PCM's backward elimination. The manner in which SPSA converted each factor into its corresponding UIRI is shown on the next page. See appendix I for their raw data coding.

SIZUIRI's optimal scale partitioning and numeric rescaling were as follows.

```
14/50 IF TSIZE<12 ELSE
18/59 IF TSIZE>=12 AND TSIZE<20 ELSE
51/120 IF {TSIZE>=20 AND TSIZE<25} OR TSIZE=UNDEFN ELSE
26/55 IF TSIZE=25 ELSE
51/101 IF TSIZE>25 AND TSIZE<35 ELSE
51/92 IF TSIZE>=35 AND TSIZE<45 ELSE
74/101 IF TSIZE>=45
```

GRAUIRI's optimal scale partitioning and numeric rescaling were as follows.

```
16/58 IF GRADE=1 ELSE
131/275 IF GRADE=2 ELSE
102/188 IF GRADE=3 ELSE
36/57 IF GRADE=UNDEFN
```

NODUIRI's optimal scale partitioning and numeric rescaling were as follows.

```
138/354 IF NOD=0 ELSE
77/138 IF NOD=1 ELSE
40/55 IF NOD=2 ELSE
30/31 IF NOD=3
```

ERPUIRI's optimal scale partitioning and numeric rescaling were as follows.

```
92/206 IF ERP=0 ELSE
193/372 IF ERP=1
```

Slightly edited computer output describing the PCM reanalysis is enclosed between the horizontal lines on the following page. It provides a comparison with the corresponding computer output presented in section 7.2.

SPSA enhanced both goodness of statistical fit measures and the classification improvement measure. By converting all four factors to corresponding UIRIs, SPSA also rendered the four odds ratios directly comparable (i.e., no problem with differing underlying factor measurement scales).

SPSA normally accomplishes all of these things. However, the calculation of UIRIs made explicit use of predicted end point values. Classical hypothesis testing and the conventional interpretation of p values was therefore rendered again inapplicable. The underlying reasoning would again have become circular. The reported results should only be interpreted as descriptive, but not as inferential statistics.

Likelihood ratio chi-square statistic: 104.470, two-tailed p value: 0.0000
(based on 4 degrees of freedom and 578 complete observations).

INDEPENDENT VARIABLE	REGRESSION COEFFICIENT	STANDARD DEVIATION	CHI-SQUARE (DF = 1)	2-TAIL P VALUE	ODDS RATIO
intercept	-8.3806	1.5823	28.0522	0.0000	0.0002
SIZUIRI	3.4585	0.7062	23.9819	0.0000	31.7689
GRAUIRI	3.5603	1.1165	10.1692	0.0014	35.1754
NODUIRI	4.1045	0.7118	33.2511	0.0000	60.6129
ERPUIRI	5.8968	2.6761	4.8552	0.0276	363.8602

GOODNESS OF STATISTICAL FIT OF LOGISTIC REGRESSION MODEL

Pearson chi-square fit statistic (based on 138 degrees of freedom): 114.293,
p value: 0.9302.

Deviance chi-square fit statistic (based on 138 degrees of freedom): 137.619,
p value: 0.4931.

Classification improvement index (proportional reduction in the number of wrong
classifications enabled by using values of the independent variables): 0.3474.

Coefficients obtained from the above stepwise multivariate logistic regression
PCM reanalysis with backward elimination were used to calculate PRUSR0. PRUSR0
provides an alternative estimate of the initial probability that each of the
578 intervention patients remained in the SR state despite her mastectomy (and
radiation). The operational definition of PRUSR0 is shown below.

DEFINE PRUSR0:
EXP(-8.3806+3.4585*SIZUIRI+3.5603*GRAUIRI+4.1045*NODUIRI+5.8968*ERPUIRI)/
[1+EXP(-8.3806+3.4585*SIZUIRI+3.5603*GRAUIRI+4.1045*NODUIRI+5.8968*ERPUIRI)]

SUMMARY STATISTICS	ATTRIBUTE PRUSR0	ATTRIBUTE MRSR0DX
n DEFINED	0 578	578
MINIMUM	0.1001	0
MEDIAN	0.4308	0
MAXIMUM	0.9687	1
MEAN	0.4931	0.4931
STD. DEV.	0.2039	0.5000

Values of PRUSR0 ranged from a minimum of 10.01 to a maximum of 96.87 percent,
with a mean of 49.31 percent. The U in the PRUSR0 attribute name indicates
substitution of corresponding UIRIs for prognostic factors in the PCM
reanalysis. The 0 again indicates MRPA's initial partitioning.

MRSR0DX (coded as 0 for MR and 1 for SR) is a dummy variable encapsulating the
initial partitioning. Its mean value was the SR proportion (285/578 = 0.4931)
of patients presumed to be still at risk despite mastectomy (and radiation).
Logistic regression again ensured identical mean values for PRUSR0 and MRSR0DX.

Despite omitting the usual first step of subdividing the patient population into relatively homogeneous strata PCM still achieved a modest and suggestive, but not statistically significant consistency improvement. Matched pairs of individualized patient probabilities of remaining in the SR state (PRMSR0 and PRUSR0) were analyzed for each of the 578 patients. In terms of the accuracy improvement measures outlined in section 1.2, the results were as follows.

1. Conventional methodology (PRMSR0) produced 186 misclassifications. The remaining 578 - 186 = 392 out of 578 = 67.82 percent were correct.
2. PCM-generated discriminations (PRUSR0) produced 180 misclassifications. The remaining 578 - 180 = 398 out of 578 = 68.86 percent were correct.
3. PCM achieved an AUC correct discrimination score of a very modest 0.5 percentage points higher than conventional methodology (0.7307 versus 0.7260).
4. Nevertheless, looking at matched pairs of probabilistic discrimination errors PCM's index of error reduction was a favorable 0.083.
5. According to the Wilcoxon matched-pairs, signed ranks test this reduction generated an equivalent Z value of 1.44, with a two-tailed p value of 0.1487. The error reduction was directionally encouraging, but it was not statistically significant.

7.4 Converting PCM-Generated UIRIs into Dummy Variables to Drive MRPA

Section 5.4 outlined a procedure to convert all PCM-generated UIRIs used as independent variable inputs to both logistic and Cox regression into corresponding 0/1 dummy variables. The purpose of conversion was to eliminate ambiguity in discriminating between MR and SR patients. The same procedure was applied to the Guy's Hospital data.

Ambiguity arises from nonuniqueness in the misclassification-minimizing posterior cure probabilities that drive successive iterations of MRPA. The conversion procedure tends to reduce ambiguity. Selective editing of the converted dummy variables can then discriminate even more sharply between MR and SR patients in refined versions of both logistic and Cox regression.

The four UIRIs identified in section 7.3 as having survived backward elimination were converted into corresponding 0/1 dummy variables as follows.

```
DEFINE SIZLDV20: 1 IF [TSIZE>=20 AND TSIZE<25.25] OR TSIZE=UNDEFN ELSE 0
DEFINE SIZLDV25: 1 IF TSIZE>=25.25 AND TSIZE<45 ELSE 0
DEFINE SIZLDV45: 1 IF TSIZE>=45 ELSE 0

DEFINE GRALDV2: 1 IF GRADE=2 ELSE 0
DEFINE GRALDV3: 1 IF GRADE=3 OR GRADE=UNDEFN ELSE 0

DEFINE NODLDV1: 1 IF NOD=1 ELSE 0
DEFINE NODLDV2: 1 IF NOD=2 ELSE 0
DEFINE NODLDV3: 1 IF NOD=3 ELSE 0

DEFINE ERPLDV1: 1 IF ERP=1 ELSE 0
```

L in each dummy variable name indicates that it has been constructed to be an independent variable input to logistic (versus Cox) regression. DV in each name identifies it as a UIRI converted to a corresponding 0/1 dummy variable.

With respect to tumor size (SIZ):

1. patients whose tumors were less than 20 millimeters along their longest dimension were assigned zeros on SIZLDV20, SIZLDV25, and SIZLDV45;
2. patients whose tumor size fell between 20 and 25.25 millimeters or whose tumor size was not recorded were assigned a value of one on SIZLDV20 and zero on SIZLDV25 and SIZLDV45;
3. patients whose tumor size fell between 25.25 and 45 millimeters were assigned a value of one on SIZLDV25 and zero on SIZLDV20 and SIZLDV45; and
4. patients whose tumor size equaled or exceeded 45 millimeters were assigned a value of one on SIZLDV45 and zero on SIZLDV20 and SIZLDV25.

With respect to tumor grade (GRA):

1. grade 1 patients were assigned zeros on GRALDV2 and GRALDV3;
2. grade 2 patients were assigned a value of one on GRALDV2 and zero on GRALDV3; and
3. grade 3 patients and patients whose tumor grade was not recorded were assigned a value of one on GRALDV3 and zero on GRALDV2.

With respect to N stage (NOD):

1. N0 patients were assigned zeros on NODLDV1, NODLDV2, and NODLDV3;
2. N1 patients were assigned a value of one on NODLDV1 and zero on NODLDV2 and NODLDV3;
3. N2 patients were assigned a value of one on NODLDV2 and zero on NODLDV1 and NODLDV3; and
4. N3 patients were assigned a value of one on NODLDV3 and zero on NODLDV1 and NODLDV2.

With respect to estrogen receptor positivity (ERP):

1. estrogen receptor positive patients were assigned a value of one on ERPLDV1; and
2. estrogen receptor negative patients were assigned a value of zero on ERPLDV1.

A multivariate logistic regression analysis was executed with these nine dummy variables as its discriminating factor inputs and with the initial partitioning of patients into MR and SR subsamples as its end point. Slightly edited computer output is displayed below and on the next page between the horizontal lines.

Likelihood ratio chi-square statistic: 106.685, two-tailed p value: 0.0000 (based on 9 degrees of freedom and 578 complete observations).

INDEPENDENT VARIABLE	REGRESSION COEFFICIENT	STANDARD DEVIATION	CHI-SQUARE (DF = 1)	2-TAIL P VALUE	ODDS RATIO
intercept	−2.1960	0.4025	29.7619	0.0000	0.1113
SIZLDV20	0.6672	0.2745	5.9060	0.0151	1.9487
SIZLDV25	0.8906	0.2694	10.9307	0.0009	2.4366
SIZLDV45	1.5672	0.3290	22.6953	0.0000	4.7934
GRALDV2	0.6217	0.3314	3.5203	0.0606	1.8621
GRALDV3	1.0039	0.3407	8.6812	0.0032	2.7290

INDEPENDENT VARIABLE	REGRESSION COEFFICIENT	STANDARD DEVIATION	CHI-SQUARE (DF = 1)	2-TAIL P VALUE	ODDS RATIO
NODLDV1	0.5693	0.2148	7.0274	0.0080	1.7670
NODLDV2	1.1815	0.3348	12.4526	0.0004	3.2592
NODLDV3	3.5137	1.0297	11.6435	0.0006	33.5734
ERPLDV1	0.4926	0.1988	6.1374	0.0132	1.6365

GOODNESS OF STATISTICAL FIT OF LOGISTIC REGRESSION MODEL

Pearson chi-square fit statistic (based on 67 degrees of freedom): 53.746, p value: 0.8794.

Deviance chi-square fit statistic (based on 67 degrees of freedom): 55.649, p value: 0.8374.

Classification improvement index (proportional reduction in the number of wrong classifications enabled by using values of the independent variables): 0.3404.

Each set of dummy variables associated, respectively, with each separate discriminating factor fell in an ascending sequence with respect to its estimated REGRESSION COEFFICIENTs. There were no inversions to eliminate. Each set of dummy variables also displayed clear separation (one-tailed p values consistently below 0.05). Consequently, no replacement dummy variables needed to be defined and substituted. The REGRESSION COEFFICIENTS displayed above were used to define PRDVSR0.

DEFINE PRDVSR0:
EXP(-2.1960+.6672*SIZLDV20+.8906*SIZLDV25+1.5672*SIZLDV45+.6217*GRALDV2+
1.0039*GRALDV3+.5693*NODLDV1+1.1815*NODLDV2+3.5137*NODLDV3+.4926*ERPLDV1)/
[1+EXP(-2.1960+.6672*SIZLDV20+.8906*SIZLDV25+1.5672*SIZLDV45+.6217*GRALDV2+
1.0039*GRALDV3+.5693*NODLDV1+1.1815*NODLDV2+3.5137*NODLDV3+.4926*ERPLDV1)]

Values of PRDVSR0 served as individually tailored probabilities that each of the 578 intervention patients would fall into the SR subsample of the initial partitioning.

In terms of matched pairs of probabilistic discrimination errors PRDVSR0's index of error reduction achieved a favorable value of 0.0727 compared to PRMSR0. This was directionally favorable, but the error reduction was not statistically significant (two-tailed p value = 0.1709). PRDVSR0 also achieved an AUC correct discrimination score of 0.7305 compared to 0.7260 for PRMSR0.

Prior cure probabilities for the initial partitioning (PRECPR0) were then defined as the complement of the calculated PRDVSR0 probabilities.

DEFINE PRECPR0: 1-PRDVSR0

SUMMARY STATISTICS	ATTRIBUTE PRECPR0
n DEFINED	578
MINIMUM	0.0124
MEDIAN	0.5476
MAXIMUM	0.8999
MEAN	0.5069
STD. DEV.	0.2033

Values of PRECPR0 ranged from a minimum of 1.24 to a maximum of 89.99 percent, with a mean of 50.69 percent. The PRE in the PRECPR0 attribute name indicates a prior distribution of probabilities produced from logistic regression in such a manner as to be suitable for subsequent Bayesian revision via corresponding survival probabilities generated from Cox regression. CPR stands for cure probability. The 0 indicates MRPA's initial partitioning.

Notice that logistic regression again ensured identical values for the mean of PRECPR0 (50.69 percent) and the percentage of intervention patients estimated to have fallen into the MR subsample of the initial partitioning (293/578).

A cross tabulation of prior cure probabilities with the initial partitioning was again encouraging. The first table below displays absolute frequencies (counts). The second table displays corresponding relative frequencies (proportions).

VALUE OF PRECPR0	MR	SR	TOTAL
0% < PRIOR CURE PROBABILITY =< 25%	8	55	63
25% < PRIOR CURE PROBABILITY =< 50%	62	112	174
50% < PRIOR CURE PROBABILITY =< 75%	187	110	297
75% < PRIOR CURE PROBABILITY =< 100%	36	8	44
TOTAL	293	285	578

VALUE OF PRECPR0	MR	SR	TOTAL
0% < PRIOR CURE PROBABILITY =< 25%	0.1270	0.8730	1.0000
25% < PRIOR CURE PROBABILITY =< 50%	0.3563	0.6437	1.0000
50% < PRIOR CURE PROBABILITY =< 75%	0.6296	0.3704	1.0000
75% < PRIOR CURE PROBABILITY =< 100%	0.8182	0.1818	1.0000

7.5 Cox Regression Analysis (Cox): Survival Given the Initial Partitioning

Eight univariate Cox regression analyses were performed. All analyses were based on the same patient attributes included in the Guy's Hospital data set. The same factor indexes constructed by grouping values and by substituting mean values were used again. This time, however, each factor was reinterpreted as a candidate predictor (independent variable) to produce a univariate patient survival function. The end point (dependent variable) of each Cox regression was the time in years elapsed from diagnosis and treatment to the first evidence (if any) of further disease progression (Cox regression's focal event time).

Each patient's age at diagnosis was reinstated as a candidate predictive factor. The dependent variable in Cox regression was no longer defined in terms of a minimum time elapsed since treatment without evidence of disease progression. M stage was again excluded, since all patients were M0. Tumor type was also excluded for the same reasons as before.

Each analysis was restricted to the 285 SR patients initially presumed to have remained at substantial risk of further disease progression despite their mastectomy (and radiation). The remaining 293 MR patients were presumed to be at little or no such risk and, therefore, were excluded from consideration.

Results of the eight univariate Cox regression analyses are displayed below.

PROGNOSTIC FACTOR	REGRESSION COEFFICIENT	STANDARD DEVIATION	CHI-SQUARE (DF = 1)	TWO-TAILED P VALUE	RELATIVE RISK
AGE	0.0029	0.0058	0.2439	0.6214	1.0029
SIZ	0.0106	0.0036	8.5418	0.0035	1.0106
GRA	0.6448	0.1142	31.8671	0.0000	1.9056
POS	0.0375	0.0064	33.9213	0.0000	1.0382
TUM	0.1852	0.0852	4.7244	0.0297	1.2034
NOD	0.3716	0.0602	38.0830	0.0000	1.4500
ERP	-0.1842	0.1335	1.9044	0.1676	0.8318
PRP	-0.0707	0.1271	0.3092	0.5781	0.9318

Explanatory Notes:

1. AGE was patient age at diagnosis and treatment (in years).
2. SIZ was size of tumor in millimeters along its longest dimension, with substituted mean values.
3. GRA was tumor grade, coded 1 for grade 1, 2 for grade 2, 3 for grade 3, and with substituted mean values.
4. POS was number of positive axillary lymph nodes.
5. TUM was T stage, coded 1 for stage T1, 2 for stage T2, and 3.5 for stage T3 or stage T4, and with substituted mean values.
6. NOD was N stage, coded 0 for stage N0, 1 for stage N1, 2 for stage N2, and 3 for stage N3.
7. ERP was estrogen response positivity, coded 1 for positive and 0 for negative.
8. PRP was progesterone response positivity, coded 1 for positive and 0 for negative.
9. Notice that all except AGE, ERP, and PRP yielded significant associations in the proper direction.

From a conventional stepwise multivariate Cox regression of these eight factor indexes with backward elimination, tumor size (SIZ), tumor grade (GRA), and N stage (NOD) emerged as the significant independent predictors of time elapsed until experiencing the focal event. Slightly edited computer output showing these results is enclosed below between the horizontal lines.

Likelihood ratio chi-square statistic: 78.392, two-tailed p value: 0.0000.
Score chi-square statistic: 80.657, two-tailed p value: 0.0000.
Wald chi-square statistic: 77.231, two-tailed p value: 0.0000.

All three chi-square statistics are based on 3 degrees of freedom and 285 observations, encompassing 247 distinct focal event times.

INDEPENDENT VARIABLE	REGRESSION COEFFICIENT	STANDARD DEVIATION	CHI-SQUARE (DF = 1)	2-TAIL P VALUE	RELATIVE RISK
SIZ	0.0085	0.0038	4.8516	0.0276	1.0085
GRA	0.7328	0.1195	37.5740	0.0000	2.0808
NOD	0.3939	0.0608	41.9509	0.0000	1.4828

The SR subsample size of 285 was too small to subdivide the patient population into relatively homogeneous strata. However, all eight predictive factors were converted by SPSA into corresponding UIRIs. This time the end point used by SPSA to generate UIRIs was whether or not each of the 285 SR patients had experienced any kind of disease progression. Minimum subscale sizes were again set at around twenty-five or fifty patient observations. Missing observations of tumor size, tumor grade, and T stage were replaced in the usual PCM manner, as outlined in section 2.3. PCM's ability to improve predictive accuracy therefore relied on indicating via SPSA the underlying shape of each factor's actual impact, together with the selective replacement of missing observations.

A PCM reanalysis of the same 285-patient SR subsample data was then executed. A stepwise multivariate Cox regression analysis with backward elimination was performed. Corresponding UIRI values were substituted for all eight predictors as independent variables. The time in years elapsed between diagnosis/treatment and experiencing the focal event (if it occurred) remained as Cox regression's dependent variable.

UIRIs replacing the same three predictive factors survived PCM's backward elimination. How SPSA converted each factor into its corresponding UIRI is displayed below (see appendix I for raw data coding).

SIZUIRI's optimal scale partitioning and numeric rescaling were as follows.

```
28/32 IF TSIZE<20 ELSE
71/80 IF [TSIZE>=20 AND TSIZE<30] OR TSIZE=UNDEFN ELSE
98/109 IF TSIZE>=30 AND TSIZE<50 ELSE
30/32 IF TSIZE>=50 AND TSIZE<60 ELSE
32/32 IF TSIZE>=60
```

GRAUIRI's optimal scale partitioning and numeric rescaling were as follows.

```
13/16 IF GRADE=1 ELSE
117/131 IF GRADE=2 ELSE
95/102 IF GRADE=3 ELSE
34/36 IF GRADE=UNDEFN
```

NODUIRI's optimal scale partitioning and numeric rescaling were as follows.

```
117/138 IF NOD=0 ELSE
72/77 IF NOD=1 ELSE
70/70 IF NOD>=2
```

The same procedure outlined in section 5.4 was then repeated to convert the three surviving UIRIs into corresponding 0/1 dummy variables to drive MRPA. Multivariate logistic regression was again invoked to refine (i.e., edit selectively) the corresponding dummy variables so as to ensure sufficient separation between successive values of the cure probabilities that would eventually be calculated via Bayesian revision from the results of using these 0/1 dummy variables as independent variables for Cox regression.

The three UIRIs that survived backward elimination were thereby converted into five corresponding 0/1 dummy variables as follows.

```
DEFINE SIZCDV60: 1 IF TSIZE>=60 ELSE 0

DEFINE GRACDV2: 1 IF GRADE=2 ELSE 0
DEFINE GRACDV3: 1 IF GRADE=3 OR GRADE=UNDEFN ELSE 0

DEFINE NODCDV1: 1 IF NOD=1 ELSE 0
DEFINE NODCDV2: 1 IF NOD>=2 ELSE 0
```

C in each dummy variable name indicates that it has been constructed to be an independent variable input to Cox (versus logistic) regression. DV in each name identifies it as a UIRI converted to a corresponding 0/1 dummy variable.

With respect to tumor size (SIZ):

1. patients with tumors less than 60 millimeters and patients whose tumor size was not recorded were assigned a value of zero on SIZCDV60; and
2. patients with tumors at least 60 millimeters were assigned a value of one on SIZCDV60.

With respect to tumor grade (GRA):

1. grade 1 patients were assigned zeros on both GRACDV2 and GRACDV3;
2. grade 2 patients were assigned a value of one on GRACDV2 and zero on GRACDV3; and
3. grade 3 patients and patients whose tumor grade was not recorded were assigned a value of one on GRACDV3 and zero on GRACDV2.

With respect to N stage (NOD):

1. N0 patients were assigned zeros on both NODCDV1 and NODCDV2;
2. N1 patients were assigned a value of one on NODCDV1 and zero on NODCDV2; and
3. N2 patients and N3 patients were assigned a value of one on NODCDV2 and zero on NODCDV1.
4. There were no missing observations of N stage.

Results of the dummy-variable Cox regression are shown below and on the next five pages between the horizontal lines. An explicit baseline survival function was produced. It is displayed for comparison next to the standard Kaplan-Meier survival function in the slightly edited computer output. The time unit is one full year.

Likelihood ratio chi-square statistic: 66.261, two-tailed p value: 0.0000.
Score chi-square statistic: 68.268, two-tailed p value: 0.0000.
Wald chi-square statistic: 64.807, two-tailed p value: 0.0000.

All three chi-square statistics are based on 5 degrees of freedom and 285 observations, encompassing 247 distinct focal event times.

INDEPENDENT VARIABLE	REGRESSION COEFFICIENT	STANDARD DEVIATION	CHI-SQUARE (DF = 1)	2-TAIL P VALUE	RELATIVE RISK
SIZCDV60	0.4965	0.1943	6.5262	0.0106	1.6429
GRACDV2	0.9864	0.3136	9.8919	0.0017	2.6817
GRACDV3	1.3471	0.3142	18.3878	0.0000	3.8464
NODCDV1	0.5564	0.1533	13.1754	0.0003	1.7443
NODCDV2	0.8552	0.1562	29.9663	0.0000	2.3519

COMPARISON OF KAPLAN-MEIER (PRODUCT LIMIT) AND BASELINE SURVIVAL RATES

ELAPSED TIME UNITS	NUMBER OF EVENTS	NUMBER AT RISK	KAPLAN-MEIER SURVIVAL RATE	BASELINE SURVIVAL RATE
0.0000	N/A	285	1.0000	1.0000

ELAPSED TIME UNITS	NUMBER OF EVENTS	NUMBER AT RISK	KAPLAN-MEIER SURVIVAL RATE	BASELINE SURVIVAL RATE
0.1697	1	283	0.9965	0.9969
0.2738	1	282	0.9929	0.9939
0.2820	1	281	0.9894	0.9908
0.3039	1	280	0.9859	0.9877
0.3559	1	279	0.9823	0.9846
0.3669	2	278	0.9753	0.9784
0.3696	1	276	0.9717	0.9753
0.3806	2	275	0.9647	0.9690
0.3833	1	273	0.9611	0.9659
0.3860	1	272	0.9576	0.9627
0.4435	1	271	0.9541	0.9596
0.4682	1	269	0.9505	0.9564
0.4846	1	268	0.9470	0.9532
0.4956	1	267	0.9434	0.9500
0.4983	1	266	0.9399	0.9468
0.5120	1	265	0.9363	0.9436
0.5147	1	264	0.9328	0.9404
0.5229	1	263	0.9292	0.9372
0.5530	1	262	0.9257	0.9340
0.5613	1	261	0.9221	0.9307
0.5804	1	260	0.9186	0.9275
0.5914	1	259	0.9150	0.9242
0.6105	1	258	0.9115	0.9209
0.6133	2	257	0.9044	0.9144
0.6160	1	255	0.9009	0.9111
0.6297	1	254	0.8973	0.9078
0.6434	1	253	0.8938	0.9045
0.6543	1	252	0.8902	0.9012
0.6708	3	251	0.8796	0.8911
0.6927	1	248	0.8760	0.8877
0.7255	1	247	0.8725	0.8844
0.7283	2	246	0.8654	0.8777
0.7666	1	244	0.8618	0.8743
0.7830	1	243	0.8583	0.8709
0.7885	1	242	0.8548	0.8675
0.7912	1	241	0.8512	0.8641
0.8405	1	240	0.8477	0.8607
0.8487	1	239	0.8441	0.8573
0.8569	1	238	0.8406	0.8539
0.8652	1	237	0.8370	0.8505
0.8788	1	236	0.8335	0.8470
0.8925	1	235	0.8299	0.8436
0.9227	2	234	0.8228	0.8367
0.9391	1	232	0.8193	0.8333
0.9418	1	231	0.8157	0.8298
0.9582	1	229	0.8122	0.8263
0.9747	1	228	0.8086	0.8229
0.9911	1	227	0.8051	0.8194
0.9966	1	226	0.8015	0.8159
1.0157	1	224	0.7979	0.8124
1.0294	1	223	0.7943	0.8089
1.0568	1	222	0.7908	0.8053
1.0732	1	221	0.7872	0.8018
1.0760	1	220	0.7836	0.7982
1.1280	1	219	0.7800	0.7946
1.1417	1	218	0.7764	0.7911

ELAPSED TIME UNITS	NUMBER OF EVENTS	NUMBER AT RISK	KAPLAN-MEIER SURVIVAL RATE	BASELINE SURVIVAL RATE
1.1663	1	217	0.7729	0.7875
1.1718	1	216	0.7693	0.7839
1.1855	1	215	0.7657	0.7803
1.1910	1	214	0.7621	0.7767
1.2101	1	213	0.7586	0.7731
1.2266	1	212	0.7550	0.7695
1.2293	1	211	0.7514	0.7658
1.2676	1	210	0.7478	0.7622
1.3498	2	209	0.7407	0.7550
1.3580	1	207	0.7371	0.7514
1.3607	1	206	0.7335	0.7478
1.3799	1	205	0.7299	0.7442
1.3963	2	204	0.7228	0.7370
1.4018	1	202	0.7192	0.7334
1.4182	1	201	0.7156	0.7298
1.4346	1	199	0.7120	0.7262
1.4401	1	197	0.7084	0.7225
1.4538	1	196	0.7048	0.7189
1.4593	1	194	0.7012	0.7152
1.4675	1	193	0.6975	0.7115
1.4702	1	192	0.6939	0.7079
1.4784	1	191	0.6903	0.7042
1.5113	1	190	0.6866	0.7005
1.5496	1	189	0.6830	0.6967
1.5606	1	188	0.6794	0.6930
1.5743	1	187	0.6757	0.6892
1.5825	1	186	0.6721	0.6854
1.6071	1	184	0.6684	0.6815
1.6427	1	183	0.6648	0.6777
1.6482	1	182	0.6611	0.6738
1.6564	1	181	0.6575	0.6700
1.6838	1	180	0.6538	0.6661
1.7084	1	179	0.6502	0.6623
1.7604	1	178	0.6465	0.6584
1.7632	1	177	0.6429	0.6545
1.7659	1	176	0.6392	0.6506
1.8042	1	175	0.6356	0.6468
1.8344	1	173	0.6319	0.6429
1.8754	1	172	0.6282	0.6390
1.8782	1	171	0.6245	0.6351
1.8946	1	169	0.6209	0.6312
1.9521	2	167	0.6134	0.6233
1.9713	1	165	0.6097	0.6193
2.0205	1	164	0.6060	0.6153
2.0616	1	162	0.6022	0.6113
2.1383	1	161	0.5985	0.6073
2.1875	2	160	0.5910	0.5994
2.1958	1	158	0.5873	0.5954
2.2067	1	157	0.5835	0.5913
2.2122	1	156	0.5798	0.5873
2.2669	1	154	0.5760	0.5833
2.2861	1	153	0.5723	0.5793
2.3053	1	152	0.5685	0.5752
2.3080	1	151	0.5647	0.5711
2.3217	1	150	0.5610	0.5671
2.3546	1	149	0.5572	0.5630

ELAPSED TIME UNITS	NUMBER OF EVENTS	NUMBER AT RISK	KAPLAN-MEIER SURVIVAL RATE	BASELINE SURVIVAL RATE
2.3737	1	148	0.5534	0.5589
2.3792	1	147	0.5497	0.5548
2.3956	1	146	0.5459	0.5508
2.4695	1	145	0.5421	0.5467
2.4750	1	144	0.5384	0.5426
2.4997	1	143	0.5346	0.5385
2.5270	1	142	0.5309	0.5344
2.5325	1	141	0.5271	0.5302
2.5982	1	140	0.5233	0.5261
2.6475	1	138	0.5195	0.5219
2.6639	1	137	0.5157	0.5177
2.6721	1	136	0.5119	0.5135
2.7844	1	135	0.5082	0.5093
2.8036	1	134	0.5044	0.5051
2.8255	1	133	0.5006	0.5009
2.8392	1	132	0.4968	0.4966
2.9158	1	131	0.4930	0.4924
2.9213	1	130	0.4892	0.4882
2.9322	1	129	0.4854	0.4840
2.9377	1	128	0.4816	0.4797
2.9514	1	127	0.4778	0.4755
2.9706	1	126	0.4740	0.4713
3.0691	1	123	0.4702	0.4670
3.1184	1	122	0.4663	0.4627
3.2170	1	119	0.4624	0.4583
3.2225	1	118	0.4585	0.4539
3.3073	1	117	0.4546	0.4494
3.3429	1	116	0.4506	0.4450
3.3484	1	115	0.4467	0.4406
3.3703	1	114	0.4428	0.4362
3.3730	1	113	0.4389	0.4318
3.4114	1	112	0.4350	0.4274
3.5099	1	110	0.4310	0.4230
3.5291	1	109	0.4271	0.4186
3.5537	1	107	0.4231	0.4142
3.5866	1	106	0.4191	0.4097
3.6194	1	105	0.4151	0.4052
3.7372	1	104	0.4111	0.4008
3.7591	1	103	0.4071	0.3963
4.0082	1	101	0.4031	0.3918
4.0712	1	100	0.3990	0.3874
4.1150	1	99	0.3950	0.3829
4.1780	1	98	0.3910	0.3785
4.1807	1	97	0.3870	0.3740
4.1999	1	96	0.3829	0.3696
4.2190	1	95	0.3789	0.3652
4.2765	1	94	0.3749	0.3607
4.3696	1	92	0.3708	0.3562
4.4326	1	91	0.3667	0.3517
4.4353	1	90	0.3626	0.3472
4.4873	1	88	0.3585	0.3426
4.5038	2	87	0.3503	0.3333
4.5065	1	85	0.3462	0.3287
4.5558	1	84	0.3420	0.3241
4.6899	1	83	0.3379	0.3194
4.7912	1	81	0.3337	0.3147

ELAPSED TIME UNITS	NUMBER OF EVENTS	NUMBER AT RISK	KAPLAN-MEIER SURVIVAL RATE	BASELINE SURVIVAL RATE
4.8186	1	80	0.3296	0.3100
4.8706	1	79	0.3254	0.3053
4.8898	1	78	0.3212	0.3005
4.9254	1	77	0.3171	0.2958
5.1280	1	76	0.3129	0.2911
5.1389	1	75	0.3087	0.2865
5.1417	1	74	0.3045	0.2818
5.1745	1	73	0.3004	0.2772
5.2895	1	71	0.2961	0.2725
5.3498	1	70	0.2919	0.2679
5.3607	1	69	0.2877	0.2633
5.4812	1	68	0.2834	0.2587
5.6810	1	67	0.2792	0.2541
5.6865	1	66	0.2750	0.2495
5.6920	1	65	0.2708	0.2450
5.8426	1	64	0.2665	0.2405
6.1355	1	63	0.2623	0.2359
6.4066	1	62	0.2581	0.2314
6.6749	1	61	0.2538	0.2268
6.9240	1	60	0.2496	0.2223
6.9815	1	59	0.2454	0.2178
7.0171	1	58	0.2411	0.2133
7.0582	1	57	0.2369	0.2088
7.1704	1	56	0.2327	0.2043
7.4059	1	55	0.2284	0.1999
7.4579	1	54	0.2242	0.1955
7.6413	1	53	0.2200	0.1910
7.8439	1	52	0.2158	0.1866
7.8741	1	51	0.2115	0.1822
7.9179	1	50	0.2073	0.1778
8.1533	1	49	0.2031	0.1735
8.3888	1	48	0.1988	0.1692
8.6023	1	47	0.1946	0.1649
8.6516	1	46	0.1904	0.1607
9.0979	1	45	0.1861	0.1565
9.1992	1	44	0.1819	0.1524
9.2977	1	43	0.1777	0.1484
9.3169	1	42	0.1734	0.1444
9.4100	1	41	0.1692	0.1404
9.7522	1	40	0.1650	0.1366
9.9849	1	39	0.1608	0.1327
10.0260	1	38	0.1565	0.1288
10.1246	1	37	0.1523	0.1249
10.1355	1	36	0.1481	0.1211
10.3217	1	35	0.1438	0.1170
10.3518	1	34	0.1396	0.1127
10.5298	1	33	0.1354	0.1085
10.7050	1	32	0.1311	0.1043
11.2580	1	31	0.1269	0.1001
11.8111	1	30	0.1227	0.0958
11.8138	1	29	0.1185	0.0914
11.8659	1	28	0.1142	0.0871
12.0465	1	27	0.1100	0.0828
12.0767	1	26	0.1058	0.0787
12.6242	1	25	0.1015	0.0745
12.9774	1	24	0.0973	0.0705

ELAPSED TIME UNITS	NUMBER OF EVENTS	NUMBER AT RISK	KAPLAN-MEIER SURVIVAL RATE	BASELINE SURVIVAL RATE
13.0924	1	23	0.0931	0.0665
13.1608	1	22	0.0888	0.0625
13.4839	1	21	0.0846	0.0587
14.0123	1	20	0.0804	0.0550
14.0643	1	19	0.0761	0.0515
14.0999	1	18	0.0719	0.0479
14.3573	1	17	0.0677	0.0442
14.5134	1	16	0.0635	0.0405
14.7954	1	15	0.0592	0.0370
14.8173	1	14	0.0550	0.0335
15.0089	1	13	0.0508	0.0300
15.1814	1	12	0.0465	0.0267
16.3477	1	11	0.0423	0.0236
17.0185	1	10	0.0381	0.0206
17.3470	1	9	0.0338	0.0174
18.0972	1	8	0.0296	0.0140
18.1218	1	7	0.0254	0.0107
18.2067	1	6	0.0212	0.0077
18.5161	1	5	0.0169	0.0050
18.8693	1	4	0.0127	0.0026
18.9624	1	3	0.0085	0.0012
19.6852	1	2	0.0042	0.0003
20.7146	1	1	0.0000	0.0000
TOTAL	259			

If the population of elapsed time intervals until an event occurs is assumed to follow an exponential distribution, implying a constant hazard rate throughout every observation subwindow, the maximum likelihood estimate of the ordinary hazard rate is 0.210709, with a standard error of 0.013093.

The assumption of an exponential distribution with a constant hazard rate produces an EXTREMELY GOOD fit with the observed data. The analogue of an unadjusted coefficient of determination (R-squared) would be 0.9854.

An attempt was made to fit a Weibull distribution to the same data. The additional flexibility provided failed to produce a substantially better fit. Consequently, the constant hazard rate assumed by the exponential distribution appears reasonable for this complete observation window.

If the population of elapsed time intervals until an event occurs is assumed to follow an exponential distribution, implying a constant hazard rate throughout every observation subwindow, the maximum likelihood estimate of the BASELINE hazard rate is 0.227116, with a standard error of 0.014112.

The assumption of an exponential distribution with a constant hazard rate produces an EXTREMELY GOOD fit with the observed data. The analogue of an unadjusted coefficient of determination (R-squared) would be 0.9922.

An attempt was made to fit a Weibull distribution to the same data. The additional flexibility provided again failed to produce a substantially better fit. Consequently, the constant hazard rate assumed by the exponential distribution appears reasonable for this complete observation window.

Once again, successive values of the baseline survival rate estimated by Cox regression tracked very closely the corresponding Kaplan-Meier product-limit values. This means that estimates of each baseline survival rate were based on the "typical" or "average" patient in the 285-patient SR subsample. They were not based on the "null" patient with zero values on all five 0/1 independent dummy variables.

Because of this, each patient's individual hazard rate proportionality multiplier (HAZPROP0) must be calculated as the exponentiated (base e) sum of the products of that patient's deviation from the mean value of each 0/1 independent dummy variable (averaged over all 285 patients) multiplied by the regression coefficient generated by Cox regression for the 285 SR patients.

SUMMARY STATISTICS	ATTRIBUTE SIZCDV60	ATTRIBUTE GRACDV2	ATTRIBUTE GRACDV3	ATTRIBUTE NODCDV1	ATTRIBUTE NODCDV2
n DEFINED	285	285	285	285	285
MINIMUM	0	0	0	0	0
MEDIAN	0	0	0	0	0
MAXIMUM	1	1	1	1	1
MEAN	0.1123	0.4596	0.4842	0.2702	0.2456
STD. DEV.	0.3157	0.4984	0.4998	0.4441	0.4305

DEFINE HAZPROP0:
EXP[.4965*(SIZCDV60-.1123)+.9864*(GRACDV2-.4596)+1.3471*(GRACDV3-.4842)+.5564*(NODCDV1-.2702)+.8552*(NODCDV2-.2456)]

SUMMARY STATISTICS	ATTRIBUTE HAZPROP0
n DEFINED	285
MINIMUM	0.2183
MEDIAN	1.0212
MAXIMUM	3.2447
MEAN	1.1529
STD. DEV.	0.6296

7.6 By How Much Did Bayesian Revision Based on Cox Regression Further Improve the Consistency of Cure Probabilities with the Initial Partitioning by Reducing Misclassifications?

We can now calculate an initial Bayesian posterior cure probability (POSTCPR0) for each of the 578 patients in the intervention sample. It is a revised version of that patient's initial prior cure probability (PRECPR0). Her prior probability produced from 0/1 dummy variables generated by the PCM-guided logistic regression is updated by the results produced from 0/1 dummy variables generated by the PCM-guided Cox regression.

Revision (Bayesian updating) is executed by:

1. either assigning a zero posterior cure probability to each patient who experienced the focal event (there were 259 such patients);
2. or evaluating the individually tailored revised cure probability (RCP) formula presented in explanatory note number 6 of section 5.1 for each censored patient (there were 319 censored patients);
3. where each censored patient's survival probability is presumed to be embodied in her individually tailored version of the maximum-likelihood

exponential function obtained from the dummy-variable Cox regression
(R-squared = 0.9922); and
4. where each exponential function is evaluated at the time elapsed since
diagnosis and treatment when that patient died or was last seen alive.

DEFINE POSTCPR0: 0 IF NEXTIME#UNDEFN ELSE PRECPR0/{PRECPR0+(1-PRECPR0)*
EXP(-HAZPROP0*[.227116*LASTIME])}

Explanatory Notes:

1. NEXTIME#UNDEFN means that the time elapsed between the patient's initial
   diagnosis and treatment and that patient's first evidence of further disease
   progression (NEXTIME) was defined (i.e., not undefined). In other words,
   that patient did actually experience the focal event.
2. LASTIME is the time in years elapsed since each patient's initial diagnosis
   with invasive breast cancer until that patient either died or was last seen
   alive by a physician.
3. Notice that individually tailored survival probabilities were best described
   by an exponential distribution instead of by a Weibull distribution. Unlike
   the Turku patients, there was no significant indication of an increasing
   hazard rate associated with the Guy's Hospital patients' BASELINE survival
   function.

SUMMARY STATISTICS	ATTRIBUTE POSTCPR0
n DEFINED	578
MINIMUM	0.0000
MEDIAN	0.7634
MAXIMUM	1.0000
MEAN	0.5082
STD. DEV.	0.4658

VALUE OF ATTRIBUTE POSTCPR0	ABSOLUTE FREQUENCIES (COUNTS)	RELATIVE FREQUENCIES (PROPORTIONS)	CUMULATIVE RELATIVE FREQUENCIES
0.00	259	0.4481	0.4481
0.38	1	0.0017	0.4498
0.40	1	0.0017	0.4516
0.41	1	0.0017	0.4533
0.48	1	0.0017	0.4550
0.51	1	0.0017	0.4567
0.53	1	0.0017	0.4585
0.54	1	0.0017	0.4602
0.55	3	0.0052	0.4654
0.60	1	0.0017	0.4671
0.62	2	0.0035	0.4706
0.63	1	0.0017	0.4723
0.65	1	0.0017	0.4740
0.66	2	0.0035	0.4775
0.67	1	0.0017	0.4792
0.69	1	0.0017	0.4810
0.70	1	0.0017	0.4827
0.71	2	0.0035	0.4862
0.73	3	0.0052	0.4913
0.74	2	0.0035	0.4948
0.75	2	0.0035	0.4983
0.76	2	0.0035	0.5017

VALUE OF ATTRIBUTE POSTCPR0	ABSOLUTE FREQUENCIES (COUNTS)	RELATIVE FREQUENCIES (PROPORTIONS)	CUMULATIVE RELATIVE FREQUENCIES
0.77	3	0.0052	0.5069
0.78	3	0.0052	0.5121
0.79	2	0.0035	0.5156
0.81	2	0.0035	0.5190
0.82	2	0.0035	0.5225
0.83	5	0.0087	0.5311
0.84	4	0.0069	0.5381
0.85	5	0.0087	0.5467
0.86	6	0.0104	0.5571
0.87	7	0.0121	0.5692
0.88	7	0.0121	0.5813
0.89	9	0.0156	0.5969
0.90	4	0.0069	0.6038
0.91	4	0.0069	0.6107
0.92	1	0.0017	0.6125
0.93	8	0.0138	0.6263
0.94	12	0.0208	0.6471
0.95	12	0.0208	0.6678
0.96	16	0.0277	0.6955
0.97	23	0.0398	0.7353
0.98	39	0.0675	0.8028
0.99	59	0.1021	0.9048
1.00	55	0.0952	1.0000
TOTAL	578	1.0000	

Explanatory Notes:

1. The mean initial posterior cure probability (POSTCPR0) was 0.5082. This is consistent with the horizontal asymptote suggested in figure 15.
2. Initial posterior cure probabilities = 0 were assigned to the 259 patients who experienced the focal event.
3. The fifty-five POSTCPR0 probabilities reported as 1.00 were slightly less than 100 percent. They were at least 0.995 and, therefore, rounded up to two decimal places and represented as 1.00.
4. The 173 long-term survivors were all assigned POSTCPR0 probabilities between 84.16 percent and 100 percent. Their mean probability was 97.77 percent.
5. POSTCPR0 probabilities spanned the entire scale from 0 to 100 percent. A number of individual probabilities were unique. We might characterize them as discriminatingly personalized estimates of each patient's likelihood of having been cured following her mastectomy (and radiation).
6. Subsequent iterations of MRPA will attempt to improve the consistency of these estimates relative to subsequent trial partitionings.

An updated misclassification analysis was performed on the ranked sequence of initial posterior cure probabilities (POSTCPR0). The optimum point of vertical separation occurred at a probability of 0.7388. This minimized the number of misclassifications relative to the initial partitioning. A cross tabulation of misclassifications at this optimal separation probability is shown on the next page.

	MR PATIENTS TRANSFORMED TO MINIMAL RISK	SR PATIENTS REMAINING AT SUBSTANTIAL RISK	TOTAL
POSTERIOR CURE PROBABILITY >= 0.7388	287	5	292
POSTERIOR CURE PROBABILITY < 0.7388	6	280	286
TOTAL	293	285	578

MINIMUM NUMBER OF MISCLASSIFICATIONS: 6 + 5 = 11
MINIMUM PERCENTAGE OF MISCLASSIFICATIONS: 11/578 = 1.90 percent
CORRESPONDING AREA UNDER THE ROC CURVE (AUC): 0.9982 = 99.82 percent

Revising the initial prior cure probabilities produced by conventional logistic regression (the complement of PRMSR0) generated a 94.09 percent reduction in misclassifications (from 186/578 = 32.18 percent to 11/578 = 1.90 percent). Such dramatic improvement again qualifies as noteworthy. Equally noteworthy were the accompanying increase in AUC score from 72.60 to 99.82 percent and the very high AUC score achieved.

In addition to providing an individually tailored answer to that all-too-familiar patient question posed in section 1.1, this improvement again underscores the benefits of embracing a Bayesian framework. Only in such a framework can the patient's question be conveniently formulated and answered quantitatively.

Now we shall attempt to reduce and, hopefully, eliminate completely the remaining misclassifications. This will be accomplished by executing additional iterations of MRPA.

7.7 Further Reducing Misclassifications: MRPA's Second Iteration

An obvious way to set up MRPA's second iteration is simply to reclassify the 6 + 5 = 11 patients who were initially misclassified. Just interchange them, subject to the same protection against iteration-to-iteration cycling adopted in analyzing the Turku patients.

1. Establish the same lower bound to the distance separating the posterior probability assigned to a candidate for interchange and the optimum point of vertical separation. That means interchange no patients within two and one-half percentage points of the optimum to avoid iteration-to-iteration cycling.
2. Move into the SR subsample as many as appropriate of the six misclassified patients initially included in the MR subsample, but whose posterior cure probabilities ended up being "too small" (i.e., more than two and one-half percentage points below the optimum point of vertical separation that occurred at POSTCPR0 = 0.7388).
3. Five of the six misclassified MR patients satisfied this criterion.
4. Simultaneously, move into the MR subsample as many as appropriate of the five misclassified patients initially included in the SR subsample, but whose posterior cure probabilities were "too large" (i.e., at least two and one-half percentage points above 0.7388).
5. All five misclassified SR patients satisfied this criterion.

The reclassifications established a revised partitioning. The total intervention sample of 578 patients still contained an MR subsample of 293 and an SR subsample of 285 patients, but ten patients were interchanged. The relationship between the initial partitioning (MRSR0) and the revised partitioning (MRSR1) is cross tabulated below.

VALUE OF ATTRIBUTE MRSR0	VALUE OF ATTRIBUTE MRSR1		
	MR	SR	TOTAL
MR	288	5	293
SR	5	280	285
TOTAL	293	285	578

Both the logistic and the Cox regressions were repeated. This time, however, both analyses were guided by the revised partitioning rather than by the initial partitioning. Neither UIRIs nor the corresponding 0/1 dummy variables constructed therefrom were recalculated. Ten reclassifications seemed too few to produce material changes and, therefore, to require their recalculation.

Slightly edited computer output from the repeated logistic regression analysis is presented below between the horizontal lines.

Likelihood ratio chi-square statistic: 123.195, two-tailed p value: 0.0000 (based on 8 degrees of freedom and 578 complete observations).

INDEPENDENT VARIABLE	REGRESSION COEFFICIENT	STANDARD DEVIATION	CHI-SQUARE (DF = 1)	2-TAIL P VALUE	ODDS RATIO
intercept	-1.9588	0.3023	41.9749	0.0000	0.1410
SIZ20LDV	0.8827	0.2835	9.6934	0.0018	2.4174
SIZ25LDV	1.1288	0.2782	16.4615	0.0000	3.0918
SIZ45LDV	1.9659	0.3415	33.1318	0.0000	7.1412
GRA3LDV	0.5186	0.1948	7.0865	0.0078	1.6796
NOD1LDV	0.6344	0.2172	8.5317	0.0035	1.8858
NOD2LDV	1.4368	0.3509	16.7661	0.0000	4.2073
NOD3LDV	3.5868	1.0324	12.0698	0.0005	36.1173
ERP1LDV	0.5137	0.2024	6.4444	0.0111	1.6715

GOODNESS OF STATISTICAL FIT OF LOGISTIC REGRESSION MODEL

Pearson chi-square fit statistic (based on 52 degrees of freedom): 50.067, p value: 0.5502.

Deviance chi-square fit statistic (based on 52 degrees of freedom): 50.557, p value: 0.5308.

Classification improvement index (proportional reduction in the number of wrong classifications enabled by using values of the independent variables): 0.3544.

```
DEFINE PRDVSR1:
EXP(-1.9588+.8827*SIZ20LDV+1.1288*SIZ25LDV+1.9659*SIZ45LDV+.5186*GRA3LDV+
.6344*NOD1LDV+1.4368*NOD2LDV+3.5868*NOD3LDV+.5137*ERP1LDV)/[1+
EXP(-1.9588+.8827*SIZ20LDV+1.1288*SIZ25LDV+1.9659*SIZ45LDV+.5186*GRA3LDV+
.6344*NOD1LDV+1.4368*NOD2LDV+3.5868*NOD3LDV+.5137*ERP1LDV)]
```

DEFINE PRECPR1: 1-PRDVSR1

SUMMARY STATISTICS	ATTRIBUTE PRECPR0	ATTRIBUTE PRECPR1
n DEFINED	578	578
MINIMUM	0.0124	0.0097
MEDIAN	0.5476	0.5773
MAXIMUM	0.8999	0.8764
MEAN	0.5069	0.5069
STD. DEV.	0.2033	0.2183

Slightly edited computer output from the repeated Cox regression analysis is presented below and on the next page between the horizontal lines.

Likelihood ratio chi-square statistic: 64.547, two-tailed p value: 0.0000.
Score chi-square statistic: 65.916, two-tailed p value: 0.0000.
Wald chi-square statistic: 62.747, two-tailed p value: 0.0000.

All three chi-square statistics are based on 5 degrees of freedom and 285 observations, encompassing 247 distinct focal event times.

INDEPENDENT VARIABLE	REGRESSION COEFFICIENT	STANDARD DEVIATION	CHI-SQUARE (DF = 1)	2-TAIL P VALUE	RELATIVE RISK
SIZCDV60	0.5315	0.1941	7.4975	0.0062	1.7014
GRACDV2	0.9778	0.3135	9.7281	0.0018	2.6587
GRACDV3	1.3663	0.3142	18.9149	0.0000	3.9208
NODCDV1	0.5491	0.1536	12.7778	0.0004	1.7316
NODCDV2	0.8032	0.1557	26.6211	0.0000	2.2327

If the population of elapsed time intervals until an event occurs is assumed to follow an exponential distribution, implying a constant hazard rate throughout every observation subwindow, the maximum likelihood estimate of the ordinary hazard rate is 0.206668, with a standard error of 0.012842.

The assumption of an exponential distribution with a constant hazard rate produces an EXTREMELY GOOD fit with the observed data. The analogue of an unadjusted coefficient of determination (R-squared) would be 0.9835.

An attempt was made to fit a Weibull distribution to the same data. A Weibull distribution permits either an increasing or a decreasing hazard rate over all observation subwindows. This additional flexibility failed to provide a substantially better fit. Consequently, the constant hazard rate assumed by the exponential distribution appears reasonable for this complete observation window.

If the population of elapsed time intervals until an event occurs is assumed to follow an exponential distribution, implying a constant hazard rate throughout every observation subwindow, the maximum likelihood estimate of the BASELINE hazard rate is 0.225400, with a standard error of 0.014006.

The assumption of an exponential distribution with a constant hazard rate produces an EXTREMELY GOOD fit with the observed data. The analogue of an unadjusted coefficient of determination (R-squared) would be 0.9924.

An attempt was made to fit a Weibull distribution to the same data. A Weibull distribution permits either an increasing or a decreasing hazard rate over all observation subwindows. This additional flexibility failed to provide a substantially better fit. Consequently, the constant hazard rate assumed by the exponential distribution appears reasonable for this complete observation window.

SUMMARY STATISTICS	ATTRIBUTE SIZCDV60	ATTRIBUTE GRACDV2	ATTRIBUTE GRACDV3	ATTRIBUTE NODCDV1	ATTRIBUTE NODCDV2
n DEFINED	285	285	285	285	285
MINIMUM	0	0	0	0	0
MEDIAN	0	0	0	0	0
MAXIMUM	1	1	1	1	1
MEAN	0.1123	0.4596	0.4877	0.2737	0.2526
STD. DEV.	0.3157	0.4984	0.4998	0.4458	0.4345

DEFINE HAZPROP1:
EXP[.5315*(SIZCDV60-.1123)+.9778*(GRACDV2-.4596)+1.3663*(GRACDV3-.4877)+
.5491*(NODCDV1-.2737)+.8032*(NODCDV2-.2526)]

SUMMARY STATISTICS	ATTRIBUTE HAZPROP1
n DEFINED	285
MINIMUM	0.2168
MEDIAN	0.9982
MAXIMUM	3.2294
MEAN	1.1451
STD. DEV.	0.6136

DEFINE POSTCPR1: 0 IF NEXTIME#UNDEFN ELSE PRECPR1/{PRECPR1+(1-PRECPR1)*
EXP(-HAZPROP1*[.225400*LASTIME])}

SUMMARY STATISTICS	ATTRIBUTE POSTCPR0	ATTRIBUTE POSTCPR1
n DEFINED	578	578
MINIMUM	0.0000	0.0000
MEDIAN	0.7634	0.7438
MAXIMUM	1.0000	1.0000
MEAN	0.5082	0.5046
STD. DEV.	0.4658	0.4639

An updated misclassification analysis was performed on the ranked sequence of revised posterior cure probabilities (POSTCPR1). The optimum point of vertical separation occurred at a probability of 0.6787. This minimized the number of misclassifications relative to the revised partitioning. A cross tabulation of misclassifications at this optimal separation probability is shown on the next page.

	MR PATIENTS TRANSFORMED TO MINIMAL RISK	SR PATIENTS REMAINING AT SUBSTANTIAL RISK	TOTAL
POSTERIOR CURE PROBABILITY >= 0.6787	291	5	296
POSTERIOR CURE PROBABILITY < 0.6787	2	280	282
TOTAL	293	285	578

MINIMUM NUMBER OF MISCLASSIFICATIONS: 2 + 5 = 7
MINIMUM PERCENTAGE OF MISCLASSIFICATIONS: 7/578 = 1.21 percent
CORRESPONDING AREA UNDER THE ROC CURVE (AUC): 0.9994 = 99.94 percent

Using the results of the second iteration's Cox regression to revise its prior cure probabilities generated by its logistic regression produced the second iteration's posterior cure probabilities. This Bayesian updating enabled an additional 36.36 percent reduction in misclassifications (from 11/578 = 1.90 percent to 7/578 = 1.21 percent). It also raised the AUC score achieved by posterior probabilities from 99.82 percent to 99.94 percent.

7.8   Further Reducing Misclassifications: MRPA's Third Iteration

Posterior cure probabilities assigned to the two misclassified MR patients were compared with the optimal point of vertical separation (67.87 percent). Only one (60.06 percent) was sufficiently below the optimal point of vertical separation to warrant reclassification. That patient was moved into the SR subsample.

All five misclassified SR patients were assigned posterior cure probabilities sufficiently greater than the optimal point of vertical separation. All five were moved into the MR subsample.

These six reclassifications established a second revised partitioning. The total intervention sample of 578 patients now contained an MR subsample of 297 and an SR subsample of 281 patients. The relationship between the first revised partitioning (MRSR1) and this second revised partitioning (MRSR2) is cross tabulated below.

VALUE OF ATTRIBUTE MRSR1	VALUE OF ATTRIBUTE MRSR2		
	MR	SR	TOTAL
MR	292	1	293
SR	5	280	285
TOTAL	297	281	578

Both the logistic and the Cox regressions were repeated. This time, however, both analyses were guided by the second revised partitioning rather than by the first revised partitioning. As before, neither UIRIs nor the corresponding 0/1 dummy variables constructed therefrom were recalculated, since only six additional patients were reclassified.

Slightly edited computer output from the repeated logistic regression analysis is presented on the next page between the horizontal lines.

Likelihood ratio chi-square statistic: 130.765, two-tailed p value: 0.0000
(based on 8 degrees of freedom and 578 complete observations).

INDEPENDENT VARIABLE	REGRESSION COEFFICIENT	STANDARD DEVIATION	CHI-SQUARE (DF = 1)	2-TAIL P VALUE	ODDS RATIO
intercept	-2.0590	0.3063	45.1775	0.0000	0.1276
SIZ20LDV	0.8195	0.2857	8.2296	0.0041	2.2693
SIZ25LDV	1.1100	0.2797	15.7435	0.0001	3.0342
SIZ45LDV	1.9702	0.3435	32.9009	0.0000	7.1720
GRA3LDV	0.5632	0.1965	8.2176	0.0041	1.7562
NOD1LDV	0.7236	0.2182	10.9917	0.0009	2.0618
NOD2LDV	1.5030	0.3521	18.2207	0.0000	4.4952
NOD3LDV	3.6470	1.0329	12.4659	0.0004	38.3594
ERP1LDV	0.5831	0.2047	8.1146	0.0044	1.7915

GOODNESS OF STATISTICAL FIT OF LOGISTIC REGRESSION MODEL

Pearson chi-square fit statistic (based on 52 degrees of freedom): 49.600,
p value: 0.5688.

Deviance chi-square fit statistic (based on 52 degrees of freedom): 49.990,
p value: 0.5533.

Classification improvement index (proportional reduction in the number of wrong
classifications enabled by using values of the independent variables): 0.3808.

DEFINE PRDVSR2:
EXP(-2.0590+.8195*SIZ20LDV+1.1100*SIZ25LDV+1.9702*SIZ45LDV+.5632*GRA3LDV+
.7236*NOD1LDV+1.5030*NOD2LDV+3.6470*NOD3LDV+.5831*ERP1LDV)/[1+
EXP(-2.0590+.8195*SIZ20LDV+1.1100*SIZ25LDV+1.9702*SIZ45LDV+.5632*GRA3LDV+
.7236*NOD1LDV+1.5030*NOD2LDV+3.6470*NOD3LDV+.5831*ERP1LDV)]

DEFINE PRECPR2: 1-PRDVSR2

SUMMARY STATISTICS	ATTRIBUTE PRECPR0	ATTRIBUTE PRECPR1	ATTRIBUTE PRECPR2
n DEFINED	578	578	578
MINIMUM	0.0124	0.0097	0.0090
MEDIAN	0.5476	0.5773	0.5905
MAXIMUM	0.8999	0.8764	0.8868
MEAN	0.5069	0.5069	0.5138
STD. DEV.	0.2033	0.2183	0.2250

Slightly edited computer output from the repeated Cox regression analysis is
presented on the next page between the horizontal lines.

Likelihood ratio chi-square statistic: 64.182, two-tailed p value: 0.0000.
Score chi-square statistic: 64.759, two-tailed p value: 0.0000.
Wald chi-square statistic: 61.453, two-tailed p value: 0.0000.

All three chi-square statistics are based on 5 degrees of freedom and 281
observations, encompassing 247 distinct focal event times.

INDEPENDENT VARIABLE	REGRESSION COEFFICIENT	STANDARD DEVIATION	CHI-SQUARE (DF = 1)	2-TAIL P VALUE	RELATIVE RISK
SIZCDV60	0.5233	0.1941	7.2714	0.0070	1.6876
GRACDV2	1.0406	0.3124	11.0942	0.0009	2.8308
GRACDV3	1.4202	0.3134	20.5401	0.0000	4.1379
NODCDV1	0.5194	0.1539	11.3908	0.0007	1.6810
NODCDV2	0.7846	0.1557	25.3867	0.0000	2.1916

If the population of elapsed time intervals until an event occurs is assumed to
follow an exponential distribution, implying a constant hazard rate throughout
every observation subwindow, the maximum likelihood estimate of the ordinary
hazard rate is 0.207509, with a standard error of 0.012894.

The assumption of an exponential distribution with a constant hazard rate
produces an EXTREMELY GOOD fit with the observed data. The analogue of an
unadjusted coefficient of determination (R-squared) would be 0.9815.

An attempt was made to fit a Weibull distribution to the same data. A Weibull
distribution permits either an increasing or a decreasing hazard rate over all
observation subwindows. This additional flexibility failed to provide a
substantially better fit. Consequently, the constant hazard rate assumed by the
exponential distribution appears reasonable for this complete observation
window.

If the population of elapsed time intervals until an event occurs is assumed to
follow an exponential distribution, implying a constant hazard rate throughout
every observation subwindow, the maximum likelihood estimate of the BASELINE
hazard rate is 0.227587, with a standard error of 0.014142.

The assumption of an exponential distribution with a constant hazard rate
produces an EXTREMELY GOOD fit with the observed data. The analogue of an
unadjusted coefficient of determination (R-squared) would be 0.9920.

An attempt was made to fit a Weibull distribution to the same data. A Weibull
distribution permits either an increasing or a decreasing hazard rate over all
observation subwindows. This additional flexibility failed to provide a
substantially better fit. Consequently, the constant hazard rate assumed by the
exponential distribution appears reasonable for this complete observation
window.

Calculating mean values for the five 0/1 dummy variables just used in Cox
regression, combining these means with the five Cox regression coefficients to
calculate HAZPROP2, and using HAZPROP2 to calculate POSTCPR2 are carried out on
the next page.

SUMMARY STATISTICS	ATTRIBUTE SIZCDV60	ATTRIBUTE GRACDV2	ATTRIBUTE GRACDV3	ATTRIBUTE NODCDV1	ATTRIBUTE NODCDV2
n DEFINED	281	281	281	281	281
MINIMUM	0	0	0	0	0
MEDIAN	0	0	0	0	0
MAXIMUM	1	1	1	1	1
MEAN	0.1139	0.4520	0.4911	0.2811	0.2562
STD. DEV.	0.3177	0.4977	0.4999	0.4496	0.4365

DEFINE HAZPROP2:
EXP[.5233*(SIZCDV60-.1139)+1.0406*(GRACDV2-.4520)+1.4202*(GRACDV3-.4911)+
.5194*(NODCDV1-.2811)+.7846*(NODCDV2-.2562)]

SUMMARY STATISTICS	ATTRIBUTE HAZPROP2
n DEFINED	281
MINIMUM	0.2071
MEDIAN	0.9857
MAXIMUM	3.1700
MEAN	1.1432
STD. DEV.	0.6016

DEFINE POSTCPR2: 0 IF NEXTIME#UNDEFN ELSE PRECPR2/{PRECPR2+(1-PRECPR2)*
EXP(-HAZPROP2*[.227587*LASTIME])}

SUMMARY STATISTICS	ATTRIBUTE POSTCPR0	ATTRIBUTE POSTCPR1	ATTRIBUTE POSTCPR2
n DEFINED	578	578	578
MINIMUM	0.0000	0.0000	0.0000
MEDIAN	0.7634	0.7438	0.7496
MAXIMUM	1.0000	1.0000	1.0000
MEAN	0.5082	0.5046	0.5061
STD. DEV.	0.4658	0.4639	0.4651

An updated misclassification analysis was performed on the ranked sequence of
revised posterior cure probabilities (POSTCPR2). The optimum point of vertical
separation occurred at a probability of 0.6753. This minimized the number of
misclassifications relative to the revised partitioning. A cross tabulation of
misclassifications at this optimal separation probability is shown below.

	MR PATIENTS TRANSFORMED TO MINIMAL RISK	SR PATIENTS REMAINING AT SUBSTANTIAL RISK	TOTAL
POSTERIOR CURE PROBABILITY >= 0.6753	296	1	297
POSTERIOR CURE PROBABILITY < 0.6753	1	280	281
TOTAL	297	281	578

MINIMUM NUMBER OF MISCLASSIFICATIONS: 1 + 1 = 2
MINIMUM PERCENTAGE OF MISCLASSIFICATIONS: 2/578 = 0.35 percent
CORRESPONDING AREA UNDER THE ROC CURVE (AUC): 0.9999 = 99.99 percent

Using the third iteration of Cox regression results to revise its prior cure
probabilities generated by logistic regression produced the third iteration
posterior cure probabilities. Bayesian updating enabled an additional 71.43

percent reduction in misclassifications (7/578 = 1.21 percent to 2/578 = 0.35 percent) and raised the posterior probability AUC from 99.94 to 99.99 percent.

7.9 Eliminating All Misclassifications: MRPA's Final Iteration

Posterior cure probabilities assigned to the two misclassified patients were compared with the optimal point of vertical separation (67.53 percent). Both were sufficiently far removed to permit reclassification. Hence, each patient was moved into the other subsample (i.e., the two patients were interchanged).

These two reclassifications established a third revised partitioning. Because of the balanced interchange, the total intervention sample of 578 patients still contained an MR subsample of 297 and an SR subsample of 281 patients. The relationship between the second revised partitioning (MRSR2) and this third revised partitioning (MRSR3) is cross tabulated below.

VALUE OF ATTRIBUTE MRSR2	VALUE OF ATTRIBUTE MRSR3		
	MR	SR	TOTAL
MR	296	1	297
SR	1	280	281
TOTAL	297	281	578

Both the logistic and the Cox regressions were repeated. Both analyses were guided by the third revised partitioning rather than by the second revised partitioning. As before, neither UIRIs nor the corresponding 0/1 dummy variables constructed therefrom were recalculated, since only two additional patients were reclassified.

Slightly edited computer output from the repeated logistic regression analysis is presented below and on the next page between the horizontal lines.

Likelihood ratio chi-square statistic: 134.521, two-tailed p value: 0.0000 (based on 8 degrees of freedom and 578 complete observations).

INDEPENDENT VARIABLE	REGRESSION COEFFICIENT	STANDARD DEVIATION	CHI-SQUARE (DF = 1)	2-TAIL P VALUE	ODDS RATIO
intercept	-2.0703	0.3072	45.4055	0.0000	0.1262
SIZ20LDV	0.7926	0.2865	7.6557	0.0057	2.2091
SIZ25LDV	1.1298	0.2803	16.2433	0.0001	3.0950
SIZ45LDV	1.9651	0.3441	32.6062	0.0000	7.1354
GRA3LDV	0.5637	0.1971	8.1780	0.0042	1.7572
NOD1LDV	0.7338	0.2184	11.2878	0.0008	2.0831
NOD2LDV	1.6261	0.3606	20.3352	0.0000	5.0841
NOD3LDV	3.6596	1.0330	12.5510	0.0004	38.8464
ERP1LDV	0.5845	0.2054	8.0953	0.0044	1.7941

GOODNESS OF STATISTICAL FIT OF LOGISTIC REGRESSION MODEL

Pearson chi-square fit statistic (based on 52 degrees of freedom): 51.500, p value: 0.4935.

Deviance chi-square fit statistic (based on 52 degrees of freedom): 50.901, p value: 0.5171.

Classification improvement index (proportional reduction in the number of wrong classifications enabled by using values of the independent variables): 0.3879.

DEFINE PRDVSR3:
EXP(-2.0703+.7926*SIZ20LDV+1.1298*SIZ25LDV+1.9651*SIZ45LDV+.5637*GRA3LDV+
.7338*NOD1LDV+1.6261*NOD2LDV+3.6596*NOD3LDV+.5845*ERP1LDV)/[1+
EXP(-2.0703+.7926*SIZ20LDV+1.1298*SIZ25LDV+1.9651*SIZ45LDV+.5637*GRA3LDV+
.7338*NOD1LDV+1.6261*NOD2LDV+3.6596*NOD3LDV+.5845*ERP1LDV)]

DEFINE PRECPR3: 1-PRDVSR3

SUMMARY STATISTICS	ATTRIBUTE PRECPR0	ATTRIBUTE PRECPR1	ATTRIBUTE PRECPR2	ATTRIBUTE PRECPR3
n DEFINED	578	578	578	578
MINIMUM	0.0124	0.0097	0.0090	0.0090
MEDIAN	0.5476	0.5773	0.5905	0.5881
MAXIMUM	0.8999	0.8764	0.8868	0.8880
MEAN	0.5069	0.5069	0.5138	0.5138
STD. DEV.	0.2033	0.2183	0.2250	0.2281

Slightly edited computer output from the repeated Cox regression analysis is presented below and on the next page between the horizontal lines.

Likelihood ratio chi-square statistic: 66.796, two-tailed p value: 0.0000.
Score chi-square statistic: 65.679, two-tailed p value: 0.0000.
Wald chi-square statistic: 62.258, two-tailed p value: 0.0000.

All three chi-square statistics are based on 5 degrees of freedom and 281 observations, encompassing 247 distinct focal event times.

INDEPENDENT VARIABLE	REGRESSION COEFFICIENT	STANDARD DEVIATION	CHI-SQUARE (DF = 1)	2-TAIL P VALUE	RELATIVE RISK
SIZCDV60	0.5314	0.1940	7.5002	0.0062	1.7013
GRACDV2	1.1719	0.3123	14.0853	0.0002	3.2281
GRACDV3	1.5525	0.3126	24.6584	0.0000	4.7234
NODCDV1	0.5184	0.1540	11.3353	0.0008	1.6793
NODCDV2	0.7608	0.1559	23.8122	0.0000	2.1400

If the population of elapsed time intervals until an event occurs is assumed to follow an exponential distribution, implying a constant hazard rate throughout every observation subwindow, the maximum likelihood estimate of the ordinary hazard rate is 0.205033, with a standard error of 0.012740.

The assumption of an exponential distribution with a constant hazard rate produces an EXTREMELY GOOD fit with the observed data. The analogue of an unadjusted coefficient of determination (R-squared) would be 0.9798.

An attempt was made to fit a Weibull distribution to the same data. A Weibull distribution permits either an increasing or a decreasing hazard rate over all observation subwindows. This additional flexibility failed to provide a significantly better fit. Consequently, the constant hazard rate assumed by the exponential distribution appears reasonable for this complete observation window.

If the population of elapsed time intervals until an event occurs is assumed to follow an exponential distribution, implying a constant hazard rate throughout every observation subwindow, the maximum likelihood estimate of the BASELINE hazard rate is 0.225648, with a standard error of 0.014021.

The assumption of an exponential distribution with a constant hazard rate produces an EXTREMELY GOOD fit with the observed data. The analogue of an unadjusted coefficient of determination (R-squared) would be 0.9919.

An attempt was made to fit a Weibull distribution to the same data. A Weibull distribution permits either an increasing or a decreasing hazard rate over all observation subwindows. This additional flexibility failed to provide a substantially better fit. Consequently, the constant hazard rate assumed by the exponential distribution appears reasonable for this complete observation window.

SUMMARY STATISTICS	ATTRIBUTE SIZCDV60	ATTRIBUTE GRACDV2	ATTRIBUTE GRACDV3	ATTRIBUTE NODCDV1	ATTRIBUTE NODCDV2
n DEFINED	281	281	281	281	281
MINIMUM	0	0	0	0	0
MEDIAN	0	0	0	0	0
MAXIMUM	1	1	1	1	1
MEAN	0.1139	0.4484	0.4911	0.2811	0.2598
STD. DEV.	0.3177	0.4973	0.4999	0.4496	0.4385

DEFINE HAZPROP3:
EXP[.5314*(SIZCDV60-.1139)+1.1719*(GRACDV2-.4484)+1.5525*(GRACDV3-.4911)+ .5184*(NODCDV1-.2811)+.7608*(NODCDV2-.2598)]

SUMMARY STATISTICS	ATTRIBUTE HAZPROP3
n DEFINED	281
MINIMUM	0.1842
MEDIAN	0.9984
MAXIMUM	3.1674
MEAN	1.1477
STD. DEV.	0.6021

DEFINE POSTCPR3: 0 IF NEXTIME#UNDEFN ELSE PRECPR3/{PRECPR3+(1-PRECPR3)* EXP(-HAZPROP3*[.225648*LASTIME])}

SUMMARY STATISTICS	ATTRIBUTE POSTCPR0	ATTRIBUTE POSTCPR1	ATTRIBUTE POSTCPR2	ATTRIBUTE POSTCPR3
n DEFINED	578	578	578	578
MINIMUM	0.0000	0.0000	0.0000	0.0000
MEDIAN	0.7634	0.7438	0.7496	0.7379
MAXIMUM	1.0000	1.0000	1.0000	1.0000
MEAN	0.5082	0.5046	0.5061	0.5051
STD. DEV.	0.4658	0.4639	0.4651	0.4646

An updated misclassification analysis was performed on the ranked sequence of revised posterior cure probabilities (POSTCPR3). The optimum point of vertical separation occurred at a probability of 0.6804. This eliminated all misclassifications relative to the revised partitioning. A cross tabulation of misclassifications at this optimal separation probability is shown below.

	MR PATIENTS TRANSFORMED TO MINIMAL RISK	SR PATIENTS REMAINING AT SUBSTANTIAL RISK	TOTAL
POSTERIOR CURE PROBABILITY >= 0.6804	297	0	297
POSTERIOR CURE PROBABILITY < 0.6804	0	281	281
TOTAL	297	281	578

MINIMUM NUMBER OF MISCLASSIFICATIONS: 0 + 0 = 0
MINIMUM PERCENTAGE OF MISCLASSIFICATIONS: 0/578 = 0.00 percent
CORRESPONDING AREA UNDER THE ROC CURVE (AUC): 1.0000 = 100 percent

Since MRPA converged completely, this was its final iteration. There was no room for further improvement. Using the results of Cox regression to revise the final iteration's prior cure probabilities (PRECPR3) generated by logistic regression produced the final iteration's posterior cure probabilities (POSTCPR3). The final Bayesian updating succeeded in eliminating all misclassifications. By doing so it raised the AUC score achieved by posterior cure probabilities from 99.99 percent to 100.00 percent.

7.10 Checking the Final Partitioning for Reasonableness

MRPA's final partitioning of the 578 Guy's Hospital patients into 297 MR (cured) and 281 SR (at risk) patients may now be checked for reasonableness.

BASIS OF COMPARISON	MR (CURED)	SR (AT RISK)	TWO-TAILED P VALUE
SUBSAMPLE SIZE (patients)	297	281	N/A
MEDIAN TUMOR SIZE (mm.)	20	30	< 0.00005
MEAN TUMOR SIZE (mm.)	24.62	34.80	< 0.00005
MEDIAN LENGTH OF FOLLOW-UP (years)	21.87	5.41	< 0.00005
MEAN LENGTH OF FOLLOW-UP (years)	19.43	7.45	< 0.00005

All differences were highly significant by the median and two-sample t tests.

Following are eight cross tabulations. All but two occur as a pair of tables. The first table in each pair contains joint absolute frequencies (counts). The second contains relative frequencies conditional by column to facilitate subsample comparison.

T STAGE OF PATIENT	FINAL MRPA-PARTITIONED SUBSAMPLE		
	MR (CURED)	SR (AT RISK)	TOTAL
T1	134	68	202
T2	138	172	310
T3/T4	10	38	48
TOTAL	282	278	560

T STAGE OF PATIENT	FINAL MRPA-PARTITIONED SUBSAMPLE	
	MR (CURED)	SR (AT RISK)
T1	0.4752	0.2446
T2	0.4893	0.6187
T3/T4	0.0355	0.1367
TOTAL	1.0000	1.0000

Significant difference: chi-square two-tailed p value < 0.00005, where eighteen observations originally coded as T0 were treated as missing data.

N STAGE OF PATIENT	FINAL MRPA-PARTITIONED SUBSAMPLE		
	MR (CURED)	SR (AT RISK)	TOTAL
N0	225	129	354
N1	59	79	138
N2	12	43	55
N3	1	30	31
TOTAL	297	281	578

N STAGE OF PATIENT	FINAL MRPA-PARTITIONED SUBSAMPLE	
	MR (CURED)	SR (AT RISK)
N0	0.7575	0.4591
N1	0.1987	0.2811
N2	0.0404	0.1530
N3	0.0034	0.1068
TOTAL	1.0000	1.0000

Significant difference: chi-square two-tailed p value < 0.00005.

M STAGE OF PATIENT	FINAL MRPA-PARTITIONED SUBSAMPLE		
	MR (CURED)	SR (AT RISK)	TOTAL
M0	297	281	578
TOTAL	297	281	578

No statistical test was appropriate (all 578 patients M0).

GRADE OF TUMOR	FINAL MRPA-PARTITIONED SUBSAMPLE		
	MR (CURED)	SR (AT RISK)	TOTAL
1	41	17	58
2	149	126	275
3	86	102	188
TOTAL	276	245	521

GRADE OF TUMOR	FINAL MRPA-PARTITIONED SUBSAMPLE	
	MR (CURED)	SR (AT RISK)
1	0.1486	0.0694
2	0.5398	0.5143
3	0.3116	0.4163
TOTAL	1.0000	1.0000

Significant difference: chi-square two-tailed p value = 0.0033, based on fifty-seven missing observations (all recorded as indicating lobular tumors).

ESTROGEN RECEPTOR (ER) POSITIVITY	FINAL MRPA-PARTITIONED SUBSAMPLE		
	MR (CURED)	SR (AT RISK)	TOTAL
NEGATIVE	117	89	206
POSITIVE	180	192	372
TOTAL	297	281	578

ESTROGEN RECEPTOR (ER) POSITIVITY	FINAL MRPA-PARTITIONED SUBSAMPLE	
	MR (CURED)	SR (AT RISK)
NEGATIVE	0.3939	0.3167
POSITIVE	0.6061	0.6833
TOTAL	1.0000	1.0000

Suggestive, but not quite significant difference: chi-square two-tailed p value = 0.0643.

PROGESTERONE RECEPTOR (PR) POSITIVITY	FINAL MRPA-PARTITIONED SUBSAMPLE		
	MR (CURED)	SR (AT RISK)	TOTAL
NEGATIVE	186	162	348
POSITIVE	111	119	230
TOTAL	297	281	578

PROGESTERONE RECEPTOR (PR) POSITIVITY	FINAL MRPA-PARTITIONED SUBSAMPLE	
	MR (CURED)	SR (AT RISK)
NEGATIVE	0.6263	0.5765
POSITIVE	0.3737	0.4235
TOTAL	1.0000	1.0000

Slightly suggestive, but far from significant difference: chi-square two-tailed p value = 0.2558.

RELAPSE OR RECURRENCE EXPERIENCED	FINAL MRPA-PARTITIONED SUBSAMPLE		
	MR (CURED)	SR (AT RISK)	TOTAL
NO	297	22	319
YES	0	259	259
TOTAL	297	281	578

Statistical test inappropriate (definitional association): zero percent of the MR patients and 92.17 percent of the SR patients had either experienced a relapse or a recurrence or died of their breast cancer when last seen, which constituted having experienced the focal event.

PATIENT STATUS WHEN LAST OBSERVED	FINAL MRPA-PARTITIONED SUBSAMPLE		
	MR (CURED)	SR (AT RISK)	TOTAL
STILL ALIVE	153	6	159
DIED OF BREAST CANCER	0	237	237
DIED OF OTHER CAUSE (DISTANT METS)	0	13	13
DIED OF OTHER CAUSE (NO DISTANT METS)	144	25	169
TOTAL	297	281	578

PATIENT STATUS WHEN LAST OBSERVED	FINAL MRPA-PARTITIONED SUBSAMPLE	
	MR (CURED)	SR (AT RISK)
STILL ALIVE	0.5152	0.0214
DIED OF BREAST CANCER	0.0000	0.8433
DIED OF OTHER CAUSE (DISTANT METS)	0.0000	0.0463
DIED OF OTHER CAUSE (NO DISTANT METS)	0.4848	0.0890
TOTAL	1.0000	1.0000

A statistical test was inappropriate (definitional association).

These results support the conclusion that the total 578-patient intervention sample originally contained a mixture of minimal risk (cured) and still-at-substantial-risk (not cured) patients and that MRPA has successfully partitioned them into two distinct subsamples of 297 MR and 281 SR patients.

Systematic differences were definitely expected to emerge between the MR and SR subsamples with respect to:

1. MEDIAN AND MEAN TUMOR SIZE (in mm.), where SR tumors were expected to be larger (a known prognostic risk factor);
2. MEDIAN AND MEAN LENGTH OF FOLLOW-UP (in years), where duration of MR follow-up was expected to be longer due to higher SR mortality;
3. T and N STAGE of patient at diagnosis and treatment, where SR patients were expected to be at later stages (known prognostic risk factors);
4. GRADE OF TUMOR, where SR tumors were expected to be higher grade (a known prognostic risk factor);
5. RELAPSE OR RECURRENCE EXPERIENCED, since this was guaranteed to be experienced only by SR patients because of the manner in which the focal event was defined and the Bayesian manner in which the partitioning procedure was executed; and

6. PATIENT STATUS WHEN LAST OBSERVED, since death due to breast cancer was guaranteed to be experienced only by SR patients because of the manner in which the focal event was defined and the Bayesian manner in which the partitioning procedure was executed.

All expected differences emerged, all were in the expected direction, and all statistical tests performed produced highly significant p values.

In addition, systematic differences were expected to emerge between the MR and SR subsamples with respect to estrogen receptor (ER) and progesterone receptor (PR) positivity. Both differences occurred in the expected direction. A higher percentage of SR patients tended to be both ER and PR positive compared to MR patients. However, both differences were only suggestive (not statistically significant).

7.11 A Dramatically Revised Kaplan-Meier Survival Curve: The Apparent Disappearance of a Declining Hazard Rate over Time

MRPA appears to have been successful in partitioning the Guy's Hospital intervention sample into 297 MR and 281 SR patients. It is no longer appropriate to submit all 578 patients to a single Kaplan-Meier survival analysis. It is only appropriate to do so for the 281 SR patients deemed by MRPA to have remained at substantial risk despite their mastectomy (and radiation). Once again, including the 297 MR patients deemed by MRPA to have been transformed into a state of little or no risk of further disease progression would serve only to contaminate the analysis and to distort the survival curve.

Annotated computer outputs of a Kaplan-Meier analysis of the 281 SR patients identified in MRPA's final iteration are shown below and on the next five pages between the horizontal lines. These results may be compared directly with similar results generated in section 6.4 by the same KAPM procedure when it was applied to all 578 Guy's Hospital patients. The corresponding final Kaplan-Meier survival curve to be presented subsequently in figure 16 may also be compared with the initial survival curve shown in figure 15.

DESCRIPTIVE SUMMARY OF ELAPSED TIME INTERVALS

The set of strictly positive elapsed observation time intervals relating to 281 PATIENTs constitutes the effective sample for the descriptive summary. There are 268 distinct elapsed time intervals in this set. The complete observation window (i.e., the longest elapsed time interval observed) is 20.7146 elapsed time unit(s). The time unit is one full year.

The MINIMUM number of elapsed time units observed is 0.0684.
The MEDIAN number of elapsed time units observed is 2.6407.
The MAXIMUM number of elapsed time units observed is 20.7146.
The MEAN number of elapsed time units observed is 4.4954,
with a STANDARD DEVIATION of 4.6900.

KAPLAN-MEIER ANALYSIS (SURVIVAL RATE ESTIMATED VIA THE PRODUCT-LIMIT METHOD)

The same set of strictly positive elapsed observation time intervals relating to 281 PATIENTs constitutes the effective sample for the Kaplan-Meier analysis. It focuses on the particular subset of 247 distinct intervals that terminate with the occurrence of at least one focal event. In addition, the analysis considers all truncated-observation intervals that terminate before a focal event has occurred (censored observations), if any exist. A total of 259 focal events occur during the observation subwindow that encompasses all events. This observation subwindow spans 20.7146 elapsed time unit(s).

ELAPSED TIME UNITS	NUMBER OF EVENTS	NUMBER AT RISK	HAZARD RATE	CUMULATIVE HAZARD RATE	KAPLAN-MEIER SURVIVAL RATE	STANDARD ERROR
0.0000	N/A	281	N/A	N/A	1.0000	N/A
0.1697	1	279	0.0036	0.0036	0.9964	0.0036
0.2738	1	278	0.0036	0.0072	0.9928	0.0051
0.2820	1	277	0.0036	0.0108	0.9892	0.0062
0.3039	1	276	0.0036	0.0144	0.9857	0.0071
0.3559	1	275	0.0036	0.0181	0.9821	0.0079
0.3669	2	274	0.0073	0.0254	0.9749	0.0094
0.3696	1	272	0.0037	0.0290	0.9713	0.0100
0.3806	2	271	0.0074	0.0364	0.9642	0.0111
0.3833	1	269	0.0037	0.0401	0.9606	0.0117
0.3860	1	268	0.0037	0.0439	0.9570	0.0121
0.4435	1	267	0.0037	0.0476	0.9534	0.0126
0.4682	1	265	0.0038	0.0514	0.9498	0.0131
0.4846	1	264	0.0038	0.0552	0.9462	0.0135
0.4956	1	263	0.0038	0.0590	0.9426	0.0139
0.4983	1	262	0.0038	0.0628	0.9390	0.0143
0.5120	1	261	0.0038	0.0666	0.9354	0.0147
0.5147	1	260	0.0038	0.0705	0.9318	0.0151
0.5229	1	259	0.0039	0.0743	0.9282	0.0155
0.5530	1	258	0.0039	0.0782	0.9246	0.0158
0.5613	1	257	0.0039	0.0821	0.9210	0.0162
0.5804	1	256	0.0039	0.0860	0.9174	0.0165
0.5914	1	255	0.0039	0.0899	0.9138	0.0168
0.6105	1	254	0.0039	0.0939	0.9102	0.0171
0.6133	2	253	0.0079	0.1018	0.9030	0.0177
0.6160	1	251	0.0040	0.1057	0.8994	0.0180
0.6297	1	250	0.0040	0.1097	0.8958	0.0183
0.6434	1	249	0.0040	0.1138	0.8922	0.0186
0.6543	1	248	0.0040	0.1178	0.8886	0.0189
0.6708	3	247	0.0121	0.1299	0.8779	0.0196
0.6927	1	244	0.0041	0.1340	0.8743	0.0199
0.7255	1	243	0.0041	0.1381	0.8707	0.0201
0.7283	2	242	0.0083	0.1464	0.8635	0.0206
0.7666	1	240	0.0042	0.1506	0.8599	0.0208
0.7830	1	239	0.0042	0.1548	0.8563	0.0210
0.7885	1	238	0.0042	0.1590	0.8527	0.0212
0.7912	1	237	0.0042	0.1632	0.8491	0.0215
0.8405	1	236	0.0042	0.1674	0.8455	0.0217
0.8487	1	235	0.0043	0.1717	0.8419	0.0219
0.8569	1	234	0.0043	0.1760	0.8383	0.0221
0.8652	1	233	0.0043	0.1802	0.8347	0.0223
0.8788	1	232	0.0043	0.1846	0.8311	0.0225
0.8925	1	231	0.0043	0.1889	0.8275	0.0227
0.9227	2	230	0.0087	0.1976	0.8203	0.0230

ELAPSED TIME UNITS	NUMBER OF EVENTS	NUMBER AT RISK	HAZARD RATE	CUMULATIVE HAZARD RATE	KAPLAN-MEIER SURVIVAL RATE	STANDARD ERROR
0.9391	1	228	0.0044	0.2020	0.8167	0.0232
0.9418	1	227	0.0044	0.2064	0.8131	0.0234
0.9582	1	226	0.0044	0.2108	0.8095	0.0235
0.9747	1	225	0.0044	0.2152	0.8059	0.0237
0.9911	1	224	0.0045	0.2197	0.8023	0.0239
0.9966	1	223	0.0045	0.2242	0.7987	0.0240
1.0157	1	221	0.0045	0.2287	0.7951	0.0242
1.0294	1	220	0.0045	0.2333	0.7915	0.0244
1.0568	1	219	0.0046	0.2378	0.7879	0.0245
1.0732	1	218	0.0046	0.2424	0.7842	0.0247
1.0760	1	217	0.0046	0.2470	0.7806	0.0248
1.1280	1	216	0.0046	0.2516	0.7770	0.0250
1.1417	1	215	0.0047	0.2563	0.7734	0.0251
1.1663	1	214	0.0047	0.2610	0.7698	0.0253
1.1718	1	213	0.0047	0.2657	0.7662	0.0254
1.1855	1	212	0.0047	0.2704	0.7626	0.0255
1.1910	1	211	0.0047	0.2751	0.7589	0.0257
1.2101	1	210	0.0048	0.2799	0.7553	0.0258
1.2266	1	209	0.0048	0.2847	0.7517	0.0259
1.2293	1	208	0.0048	0.2895	0.7481	0.0260
1.2676	1	207	0.0048	0.2943	0.7445	0.0262
1.3498	2	206	0.0097	0.3040	0.7373	0.0264
1.3580	1	204	0.0049	0.3089	0.7336	0.0265
1.3607	1	203	0.0049	0.3138	0.7300	0.0266
1.3799	1	202	0.0050	0.3188	0.7264	0.0268
1.3963	2	201	0.0100	0.3287	0.7192	0.0270
1.4018	1	199	0.0050	0.3338	0.7156	0.0271
1.4182	1	198	0.0051	0.3388	0.7120	0.0272
1.4346	1	197	0.0051	0.3439	0.7084	0.0273
1.4401	1	196	0.0051	0.3490	0.7047	0.0274
1.4538	1	195	0.0051	0.3541	0.7011	0.0275
1.4593	1	194	0.0052	0.3593	0.6975	0.0276
1.4675	1	193	0.0052	0.3645	0.6939	0.0277
1.4702	1	192	0.0052	0.3697	0.6903	0.0278
1.4784	1	191	0.0052	0.3749	0.6867	0.0278
1.5113	1	190	0.0053	0.3802	0.6831	0.0279
1.5496	1	189	0.0053	0.3855	0.6794	0.0280
1.5606	1	188	0.0053	0.3908	0.6758	0.0281
1.5743	1	187	0.0053	0.3961	0.6722	0.0282
1.5825	1	186	0.0054	0.4015	0.6686	0.0283
1.6071	1	184	0.0054	0.4069	0.6650	0.0283
1.6427	1	183	0.0055	0.4124	0.6613	0.0284
1.6482	1	182	0.0055	0.4179	0.6577	0.0285
1.6564	1	181	0.0055	0.4234	0.6541	0.0286
1.6838	1	180	0.0056	0.4290	0.6504	0.0286
1.7084	1	179	0.0056	0.4346	0.6468	0.0287
1.7604	1	178	0.0056	0.4402	0.6432	0.0288
1.7632	1	177	0.0056	0.4458	0.6395	0.0288
1.7659	1	176	0.0057	0.4515	0.6359	0.0289
1.8042	1	175	0.0057	0.4572	0.6323	0.0290
1.8344	1	173	0.0058	0.4630	0.6286	0.0290
1.8754	1	172	0.0058	0.4688	0.6250	0.0291
1.8782	1	171	0.0058	0.4747	0.6213	0.0291
1.8946	1	169	0.0059	0.4806	0.6176	0.0292
1.9521	2	167	0.0120	0.4926	0.6102	0.0293
1.9713	1	165	0.0061	0.4986	0.6065	0.0294

ELAPSED TIME UNITS	NUMBER OF EVENTS	NUMBER AT RISK	HAZARD RATE	CUMULATIVE HAZARD RATE	KAPLAN-MEIER SURVIVAL RATE	STANDARD ERROR
2.0205	1	164	0.0061	0.5047	0.6028	0.0294
2.0616	1	163	0.0061	0.5109	0.5991	0.0295
2.1383	1	162	0.0062	0.5170	0.5954	0.0295
2.1875	2	161	0.0124	0.5295	0.5880	0.0296
2.1958	1	159	0.0063	0.5357	0.5843	0.0297
2.2067	1	158	0.0063	0.5421	0.5806	0.0297
2.2122	1	157	0.0064	0.5484	0.5769	0.0297
2.2669	1	156	0.0064	0.5549	0.5732	0.0298
2.2861	1	155	0.0065	0.5613	0.5695	0.0298
2.3053	1	154	0.0065	0.5678	0.5658	0.0299
2.3080	1	153	0.0065	0.5743	0.5621	0.0299
2.3217	1	152	0.0066	0.5809	0.5584	0.0299
2.3546	1	151	0.0066	0.5875	0.5547	0.0300
2.3737	1	150	0.0067	0.5942	0.5510	0.0300
2.3792	1	149	0.0067	0.6009	0.5474	0.0300
2.3956	1	148	0.0068	0.6077	0.5437	0.0300
2.4695	1	147	0.0068	0.6145	0.5400	0.0301
2.4750	1	146	0.0068	0.6213	0.5363	0.0301
2.4997	1	145	0.0069	0.6282	0.5326	0.0301
2.5270	1	144	0.0069	0.6352	0.5289	0.0301
2.5325	1	143	0.0070	0.6422	0.5252	0.0301
2.5982	1	142	0.0070	0.6492	0.5215	0.0301
2.6475	1	140	0.0071	0.6563	0.5177	0.0302
2.6639	1	139	0.0072	0.6635	0.5140	0.0302
2.6721	1	138	0.0072	0.6708	0.5103	0.0302
2.7844	1	137	0.0073	0.6781	0.5066	0.0302
2.8036	1	136	0.0074	0.6854	0.5028	0.0302
2.8255	1	135	0.0074	0.6928	0.4991	0.0302
2.8392	1	134	0.0075	0.7003	0.4954	0.0302
2.9158	1	133	0.0075	0.7078	0.4917	0.0302
2.9213	1	132	0.0076	0.7154	0.4879	0.0302
2.9322	1	131	0.0076	0.7230	0.4842	0.0302
2.9377	1	130	0.0077	0.7307	0.4805	0.0302
2.9514	1	129	0.0078	0.7385	0.4768	0.0302
2.9706	1	128	0.0078	0.7463	0.4730	0.0302
3.0691	1	126	0.0079	0.7542	0.4693	0.0302
3.1184	1	125	0.0080	0.7622	0.4655	0.0302
3.2170	1	123	0.0081	0.7704	0.4617	0.0302
3.2225	1	122	0.0082	0.7786	0.4580	0.0301
3.3073	1	121	0.0083	0.7868	0.4542	0.0301
3.3429	1	120	0.0083	0.7951	0.4504	0.0301
3.3484	1	119	0.0084	0.8036	0.4466	0.0301
3.3703	1	118	0.0085	0.8120	0.4428	0.0301
3.3730	1	117	0.0085	0.8206	0.4390	0.0301
3.4114	1	116	0.0086	0.8292	0.4353	0.0300
3.5099	1	115	0.0087	0.8379	0.4315	0.0300
3.5291	1	114	0.0088	0.8467	0.4277	0.0300
3.5537	1	112	0.0089	0.8556	0.4239	0.0300
3.5866	1	111	0.0090	0.8646	0.4200	0.0299
3.6194	1	110	0.0091	0.8737	0.4162	0.0299
3.7372	1	109	0.0092	0.8829	0.4124	0.0299
3.7591	1	108	0.0093	0.8921	0.4086	0.0298
4.0082	1	107	0.0093	0.9015	0.4048	0.0298
4.0712	1	106	0.0094	0.9109	0.4010	0.0298
4.1150	1	105	0.0095	0.9204	0.3971	0.0297
4.1780	1	104	0.0096	0.9300	0.3933	0.0297

ELAPSED TIME UNITS	NUMBER OF EVENTS	NUMBER AT RISK	HAZARD RATE	CUMULATIVE HAZARD RATE	KAPLAN-MEIER SURVIVAL RATE	STANDARD ERROR
4.1807	1	103	0.0097	0.9398	0.3895	0.0296
4.1999	1	102	0.0098	0.9496	0.3857	0.0296
4.2190	1	101	0.0099	0.9595	0.3819	0.0296
4.2765	1	100	0.0100	0.9695	0.3780	0.0295
4.3696	1	99	0.0101	0.9796	0.3742	0.0295
4.4326	1	98	0.0102	0.9898	0.3704	0.0294
4.4353	1	97	0.0103	1.0001	0.3666	0.0293
4.4873	1	95	0.0105	1.0106	0.3627	0.0293
4.5038	2	94	0.0213	1.0319	0.3550	0.0292
4.5065	1	92	0.0109	1.0427	0.3512	0.0291
4.5558	1	91	0.0110	1.0537	0.3473	0.0290
4.6899	1	90	0.0111	1.0648	0.3434	0.0290
4.7912	1	88	0.0114	1.0762	0.3395	0.0289
4.8186	1	87	0.0115	1.0877	0.3356	0.0288
4.8706	1	86	0.0116	1.0993	0.3317	0.0288
4.8898	1	85	0.0118	1.1111	0.3278	0.0287
4.9254	1	84	0.0119	1.1230	0.3239	0.0286
5.1280	1	83	0.0120	1.1350	0.3200	0.0285
5.1389	1	82	0.0122	1.1472	0.3161	0.0284
5.1417	1	81	0.0123	1.1596	0.3122	0.0284
5.1745	1	80	0.0125	1.1721	0.3083	0.0283
5.2895	1	78	0.0128	1.1849	0.3044	0.0282
5.3498	1	76	0.0132	1.1981	0.3004	0.0281
5.3607	1	74	0.0135	1.2116	0.2963	0.0280
5.4812	1	72	0.0139	1.2255	0.2922	0.0279
5.6810	1	70	0.0143	1.2398	0.2880	0.0278
5.6865	1	69	0.0145	1.2542	0.2838	0.0277
5.6920	1	68	0.0147	1.2690	0.2797	0.0276
5.8426	1	67	0.0149	1.2839	0.2755	0.0275
6.1355	1	66	0.0152	1.2990	0.2713	0.0274
6.4066	1	65	0.0154	1.3144	0.2671	0.0273
6.6749	1	64	0.0156	1.3300	0.2630	0.0272
6.9240	1	63	0.0159	1.3459	0.2588	0.0271
6.9815	1	62	0.0161	1.3620	0.2546	0.0270
7.0171	1	61	0.0164	1.3784	0.2504	0.0269
7.0582	1	60	0.0167	1.3951	0.2463	0.0267
7.1704	1	59	0.0169	1.4121	0.2421	0.0266
7.4059	1	58	0.0172	1.4293	0.2379	0.0265
7.4579	1	57	0.0175	1.4468	0.2337	0.0263
7.6413	1	56	0.0179	1.4647	0.2296	0.0262
7.8439	1	55	0.0182	1.4829	0.2254	0.0261
7.8741	1	54	0.0185	1.5014	0.2212	0.0259
7.9179	1	53	0.0189	1.5203	0.2170	0.0258
8.1533	1	52	0.0192	1.5395	0.2129	0.0256
8.3888	1	51	0.0196	1.5591	0.2087	0.0254
8.6023	1	49	0.0204	1.5795	0.2044	0.0253
8.6516	1	48	0.0208	1.6003	0.2002	0.0251
9.0979	1	47	0.0213	1.6216	0.1959	0.0249
9.1992	1	46	0.0217	1.6434	0.1917	0.0247
9.2977	1	45	0.0222	1.6656	0.1874	0.0246
9.3169	1	44	0.0227	1.6883	0.1831	0.0244
9.4100	1	43	0.0233	1.7116	0.1789	0.0242
9.7522	1	42	0.0238	1.7354	0.1746	0.0240
9.9849	1	41	0.0244	1.7598	0.1704	0.0238
10.0260	1	40	0.0250	1.7848	0.1661	0.0235
10.1246	1	39	0.0256	1.8104	0.1618	0.0233

ELAPSED TIME UNITS	NUMBER OF EVENTS	NUMBER AT RISK	HAZARD RATE	CUMULATIVE HAZARD RATE	KAPLAN-MEIER SURVIVAL RATE	STANDARD ERROR
10.1355	1	38	0.0263	1.8367	0.1576	0.0231
10.3217	1	37	0.0270	1.8637	0.1533	0.0229
10.3518	1	36	0.0278	1.8915	0.1491	0.0226
10.5298	1	35	0.0286	1.9201	0.1448	0.0224
10.7050	1	34	0.0294	1.9495	0.1406	0.0221
11.2580	1	33	0.0303	1.9798	0.1363	0.0218
11.8111	1	32	0.0313	2.0111	0.1320	0.0216
11.8138	1	31	0.0323	2.0433	0.1278	0.0213
11.8659	1	30	0.0333	2.0767	0.1235	0.0210
12.0465	1	29	0.0345	2.1111	0.1193	0.0207
12.0767	1	28	0.0357	2.1468	0.1150	0.0204
12.6242	1	27	0.0370	2.1839	0.1107	0.0201
12.9774	1	26	0.0385	2.2223	0.1065	0.0198
13.0924	1	25	0.0400	2.2623	0.1022	0.0194
13.1608	1	24	0.0417	2.3040	0.0980	0.0191
13.4839	1	23	0.0435	2.3475	0.0937	0.0187
14.0123	1	22	0.0455	2.3929	0.0894	0.0183
14.0643	1	21	0.0476	2.4406	0.0852	0.0180
14.0999	1	20	0.0500	2.4906	0.0809	0.0176
14.3573	1	19	0.0526	2.5432	0.0767	0.0171
14.5134	1	18	0.0556	2.5988	0.0724	0.0167
14.7954	1	16	0.0625	2.6613	0.0679	0.0163
14.8173	1	15	0.0667	2.7279	0.0634	0.0158
15.0089	1	14	0.0714	2.7993	0.0588	0.0153
15.1814	1	13	0.0769	2.8763	0.0543	0.0148
16.3477	1	12	0.0833	2.9596	0.0498	0.0142
17.0185	1	10	0.1000	3.0596	0.0448	0.0136
17.3470	1	9	0.1111	3.1707	0.0398	0.0130
18.0972	1	8	0.1250	3.2957	0.0348	0.0123
18.1218	1	7	0.1429	3.4386	0.0299	0.0115
18.2067	1	6	0.1667	3.6052	0.0249	0.0106
18.5161	1	5	0.2000	3.8052	0.0199	0.0096
18.8693	1	4	0.2500	4.0552	0.0149	0.0084
18.9624	1	3	0.3333	4.3886	0.0100	0.0069
19.6852	1	2	0.5000	4.8886	0.0050	0.0049
20.7146	1	1	1.0000	5.8886	0.0000	N/A

| TOTAL | 259 | | | | | |

If the population of elapsed time intervals until an event occurs is assumed to follow an exponential distribution, implying a constant hazard rate throughout every observation subwindow, the maximum likelihood estimate of that hazard rate is 0.2050, with a standard error of 0.012740.

The assumption of an exponential distribution with a constant hazard rate produces an EXTREMELY GOOD fit with the observed data. The analogue of an unadjusted coefficient of determination (R-squared) would be 0.9798.

An attempt was made to fit a Weibull distribution to the same data. The additional flexibility provided failed to produce a significantly better fit. Consequently, the constant hazard rate assumed by the exponential distribution appears reasonable for this complete observation window.

The maximum likelihood estimate of the constant (exponential) hazard rate for SR patients was 0.2050 focal events per year. Reading from figure 16, the "typical" or "average" SR patient could therefore expect to experience with 50 percent probability some event evidencing further disease progression within approximately 2.81 years following diagnosis and treatment. In stark contrast, MR patients could expect never to experience further disease progression, at least never again from this particular bout with their breast cancer. They were presumed to have been cured following their mastectomy (and radiation).

The Kaplan-Meier Survival curve for the 281 SR patients is shown in figure 16 on the next page. It differs dramatically from the initial Kaplan-Meier curve for all 578 patients shown in figure 15. In particular:

1. it is almost perfectly exponential;
2. it does not appear to fall toward a limiting survival probability (horizontal asymptote) somewhat below 0.52;
3. instead, it appears to fall toward a limiting survival probability at zero, the way any properly constructed survival curve should;
4. what initially seemed like a sharply decreasing hazard rate over time now appears as a remarkably constant hazard rate over quite a lengthy follow-up period spanning more than 20 years; and
5. concluding that there really was no decreasing hazard rate for SR patients reduced dramatically the expectation that a "typical" patient would survive with 50 percent probability without experiencing some event evidencing further disease progression from more than twenty years (read from figure 15) to approximately 2.81 years (read from figure 16) following diagnosis and treatment.

Erroneously presuming a decreasing hazard rate among patients still at risk could lead to severe overestimation of survival times without further disease progression.

Figure 16

Kaplan-Meier Survival Analysis of 281 SR Patients from Guy's Hospital
in London, England, Initially Diagnosed With Invasive Breast Cancer,
Subsequently Given Mastectomy and (Sometimes) Radiation, but Believed
to have Remained at Substantial Risk, Despite Their Treatment

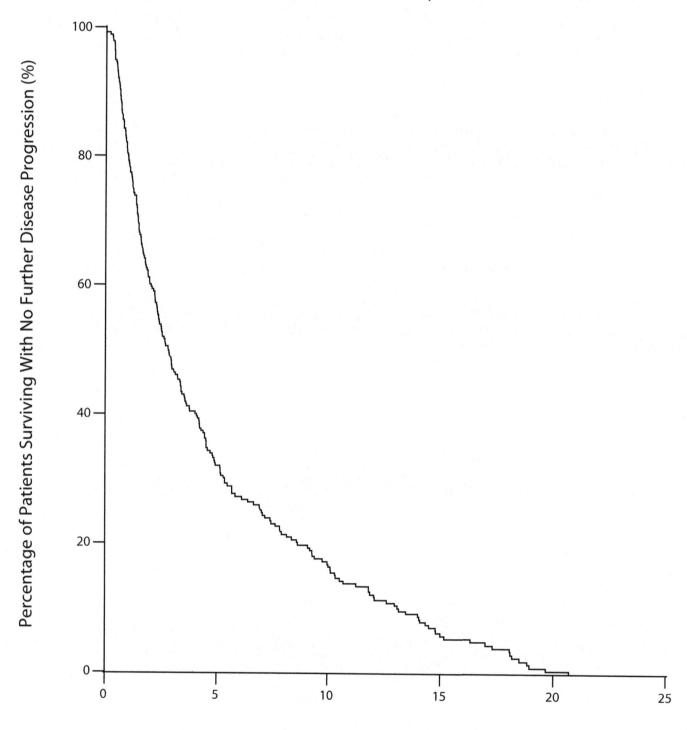

Years Elapsed Since Diagnosis/Treatment

The 281 SR patients included twenty-two who had not (yet) experienced the focal event. A search was made for a pattern of cure among their twenty-two censored observations via the KAPM procedure with the CURE option enabled. The CURE option generated a new cross table.

In contrast to the CROSS TABLE OF RESIDUALS presented in section 6.8 (before MRPA had reclassified as MINIMAL RISK 124 of the 146 QUESTIONABLE RISK patients), no remaining evidence of cure was detected in the new cross table. The same 259 patients who experienced the focal event (at 247 distinct focal event times) were included in both cross tables, but the new cross table shown below includes only the twenty-two censored observations drawn from the 281 SR patients.

SEARCH FOR A PATTERN OF CURE (VERY LOW/NO RISK) AMONG CENSORED OBSERVATIONS

CROSS TABLE OF RESIDUALS	EARLY RESIDUAL (KAPM – FITTED)	LATE RESIDUAL (KAPM – FITTED)	TOTAL
POSITIVE RESIDUAL	37	56	93
NEGATIVE RESIDUAL	86	68	154
TOTAL	123	124	247

The data in the above cross table display no significant "lean" in the direction of relatively higher cell counts along the table's major diagonal (top-left and bottom-right cells) compared to its off-diagonal (top-right and bottom-left cells). To the contrary, there is a noticeable "lean," but it is in just the opposite direction.

Even more convincing, the table of successively culled censored observations produced by the CURE option for these 281 SR patients demonstrated a consistent pattern of constant hazard rates (WEIBULL TREND PARAMETER uniformly indistinguishable from 1.0000). Since hazard rates appeared neither to increase nor to decrease over time, all R-SQUARED DIFFERENCE VALUEs were essentially reduced to zero.

CENSORED TIME BOUND	NUMBER AND PROPORTION SO CURED	WEIBULL INTENSITY PARAMETER	WEIBULL TREND PARAMETER	R-SQUARED VALUE OF WEIBULL	R-SQUARED VALUE OF EXPONENTIAL	R-SQUARED DIFFERENCE IN VALUE
INFINITE	0(.000)	0.2051	0.9996	0.9799	0.9798	0.0001
16.3477	1(.004)	0.2077	1.0000	0.9813	0.9813	0.0000
14.5134	2(.007)	0.2102	1.0000	0.9825	0.9825	0.0000
8.3888	3(.011)	0.2117	1.0000	0.9828	0.9828	0.0000
5.4812	4(.014)	0.2127	1.0000	0.9826	0.9826	0.0000
5.3607	5(.018)	0.2136	1.0000	0.9825	0.9825	0.0000
5.3498	6(.021)	0.2146	1.0000	0.9823	0.9823	0.0000
5.2895	7(.025)	0.2155	1.0000	0.9821	0.9821	0.0000
5.1745	8(.028)	0.2165	1.0000	0.9819	0.9819	0.0000
4.6899	9(.032)	0.2173	1.0000	0.9816	0.9816	0.0000
4.4353	10(.036)	0.2181	1.0000	0.9812	0.9812	0.0000
3.5291	11(.039)	0.2188	1.0000	0.9808	0.9808	0.0000
3.1184	12(.043)	0.2194	1.0000	0.9803	0.9803	0.0000
2.9706	13(.046)	0.2199	1.0000	0.9798	0.9798	0.0000
2.5982	14(.050)	0.2204	1.0000	0.9793	0.9793	0.0000
1.8946	15(.053)	0.2208	1.0000	0.9789	0.9789	0.0000
1.8782	16(.057)	0.2212	0.9993	0.9786	0.9785	0.0001
1.8042	17(.060)	0.2217	0.9981	0.9784	0.9780	0.0003

CENSORED TIME BOUND	NUMBER AND PROPORTION SO CURED	WEIBULL INTENSITY PARAMETER	WEIBULL TREND PARAMETER	R-SQUARED VALUE OF WEIBULL	R-SQUARED VALUE OF EXPONENTIAL	R-SQUARED DIFFERENCE IN VALUE
1.5825	18(.064)	0.2221	0.9969	0.9782	0.9776	0.0005
0.9966	19(.068)	0.2224	0.9960	0.9782	0.9774	0.0007
0.4435	20(.071)	0.2225	0.9953	0.9783	0.9774	0.0008
0.0000	22(.078)	0.2226	0.9949	0.9784	0.9775	0.0009

7.12   Constructing an Individually Tailored Cure Curve and a Substitutable Survival Curve for a "Typical" Patient, for a High-Risk Patient, and for a Low-Risk Patient

The "average" or "typical" patient is not a real patient. It is an analytical fiction. Nevertheless, it is instructive to construct both a tailored survival curve and a tailored cure curve for this imaginary patient. These may be compared with similar curves constructed for a real high-risk and a real low-risk patient in the Guy's Hospital intervention sample.

7.12.1   Constructing Tailored Curves for the "Typical" Patient

A baseline survival curve was produced by the final Cox regression analysis described in section 7.9. Values of all three prognostic risk factors (embodied in five independent dummy variables) were entered into the Cox regression in normalized form (i.e., as deviations from their respective dummy variable means). If the "average" or "typical" patient is interpreted to mean the one whose prognostic risk factors all fall exactly at values associated with these five dummy variable means, then the normalized baseline survival curve may be interpreted as the "typical" patient's tailored survival curve.

A graph of the exponential function that fit this normalized baseline survival curve best (R-squared = 0.9919) is shown in figure 17 on the next page. Points displayed in the figure 17 graph depict survival probabilities at year 0, the time of the "typical" patient's mastectomy (and radiation), and at the end of years 1 through 30 following that intervention.

Figure 17

Survival Curve Representing a "Typical" Patient,
If Still At Risk Despite Mastectomy and Radiation

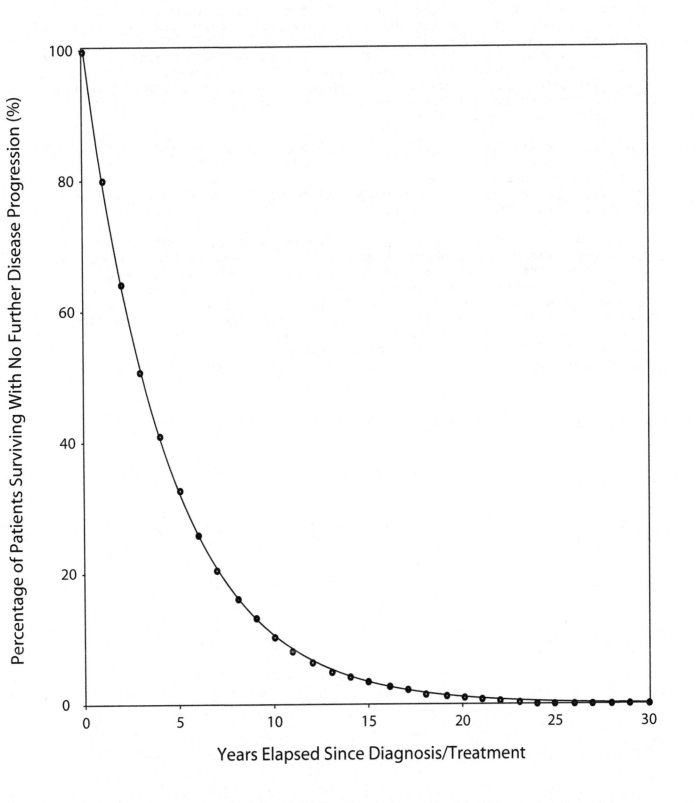

Notice, again, the dramatic difference between figures 16 and 17, considered together, and the initial Kaplan-Meier curve depicted in figure 15. The sharply decreasing hazard rate shown in figure 15 has been completely eliminated by MRPA. It was again spurious.

MRPA eliminated the decreasing hazard rate from figure 15 by removing the 297 MR patients from the 578 intervention patients. Assuming that these 297 MR patients really were at little or no risk of further disease progression (cured) following their mastectomy (and radiation), their survival curve would have been a horizontal straight line at 100 percent survival probability forever. The only reason figure 15 shows a decreasing hazard rate seems to be because the 297 minimal-risk patients were inadvertently mixed in with the 281 still-at-substantial-risk patients. It was the "apples-and-oranges" mixing together of cured patients with patients who remained still at risk that rendered figure 15 spurious.

A revised (Bayesian posterior) cure probability curve for the same "typical" patient is shown in figure 18 on the next page. It is calculated according to the formula for RCP presented in explanatory note number 6 in section 5.1, where the "typical" prior cure probability (CP) is interpreted as 297 MR (cured) patients out of 578 = 0.5138.

To be comparable with figure 17, points displayed in the figure 18 graph depict successive revised cure probabilities, starting at year 0, the time of the "typical" patient's mastectomy (and radiation), and extending through the end of each of the following thirty years. Each successive cure probability represents the likelihood that her mastectomy (and radiation) succeeded in transforming that "typical" patient from the SR to the MR state (cured her), given that she survived for the indicated number of years following the intervention without any evidence of further disease progression.

Figure 18

Revised Bayesian Posterior Cure Probability
Curve Representing the Same "Typical" Patient

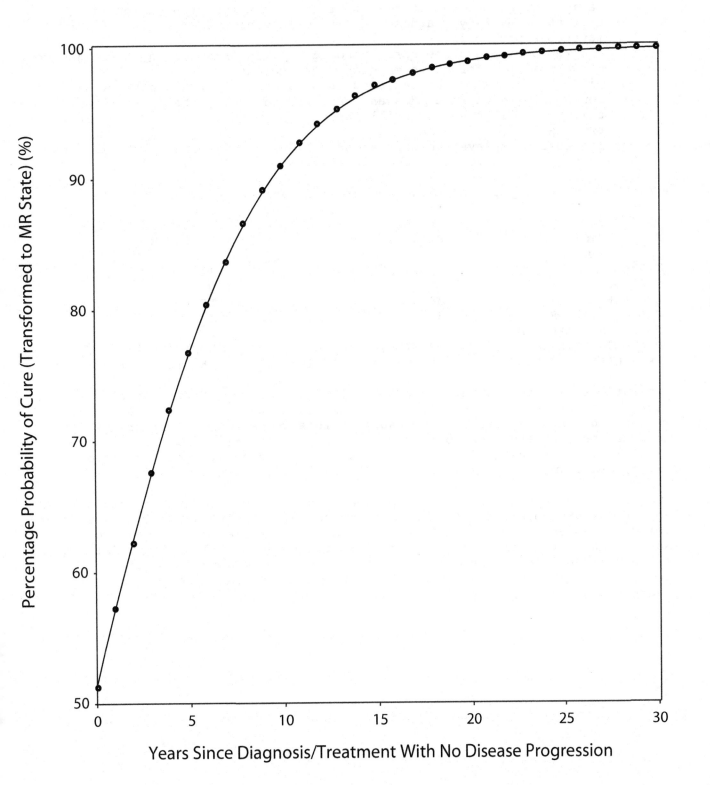

7.12.2 Constructing Tailored Curves for High-Risk and Low-Risk Patients

To illustrate the wide range of individual differences in both survival curves and revised cure curves, four additional figures appear in the next four pages.

1. Figure 19 displays the tailored survival curve for the still curable patient with the highest risk of further disease progression (i.e., the patient originally diagnosed as still in stage M0, but with the least favorable prognosis).
2. Figure 20 displays the corresponding revised (Bayesian posterior) cure curve tailored for the same high-risk patient.
3. Figure 21 displays the tailored survival curve for the patient with the lowest risk of further disease progression (i.e., the patient originally diagnosed as still in stage M0 with the most favorable prognosis).
4. Figure 22 displays the corresponding revised (Bayesian posterior) cure curve tailored for the same low-risk patient.

Prognostic risk factors for these two extreme patients are tabled below.

PROGNOSTIC RISK FACTOR	PATIENT WITH HIGHEST RISK	PATIENT WITH LOWEST RISK
T STAGE	T3/T4	T1
N STAGE	N3	N0
M STAGE	M0	M0
GRADE OF TUMOR	3	1
POSITIVE LYMPH NODES	44	0
ESTROGEN RECEPTOR	POSITIVE	NEGATIVE
MRPA CLASSIFICATION	at substantial risk (SR)	at minimal risk (MR)

The patient with the highest risk died of breast cancer at the age of sixty-six, five months after her mastectomy (and radiation). Because her risk was so high, her revised cure probability rose quite rapidly (figure 20). However, because she died so quickly, her cure probability had risen only slightly from an initial (prior) level of 0.0090 to an eventual (revised posterior) level of 0.0124.

The patient with the lowest risk was the longest-surviving of the original 173 long-term survivors. She was last seen alive more than twenty-four years after being diagnosed and receiving her mastectomy (and radiation). Because her risk was so low, her revised cure probability rose rather slowly (figure 22). It had risen from an initial (prior) level of 0.8880 to an eventual (revised posterior) level of 0.9559 at the time she was last seen. She was then seventy years old.

Figure 19

Survival Curve Representing the Highest-Risk Patient,
If Still At Risk Despite Mastectomy and Radiation

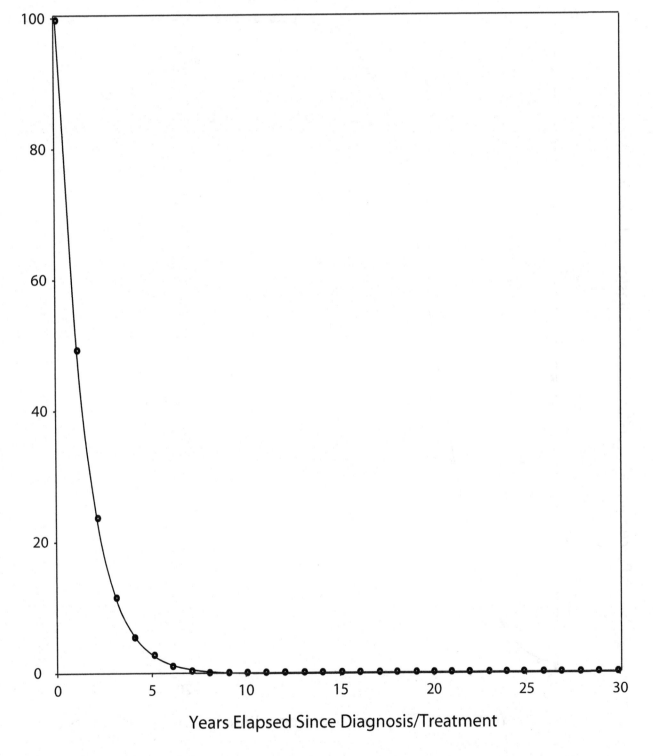

Figure 20

Revised Bayesian Posterior Cure Probability
Curve Representing the Same Highest-Risk Patient

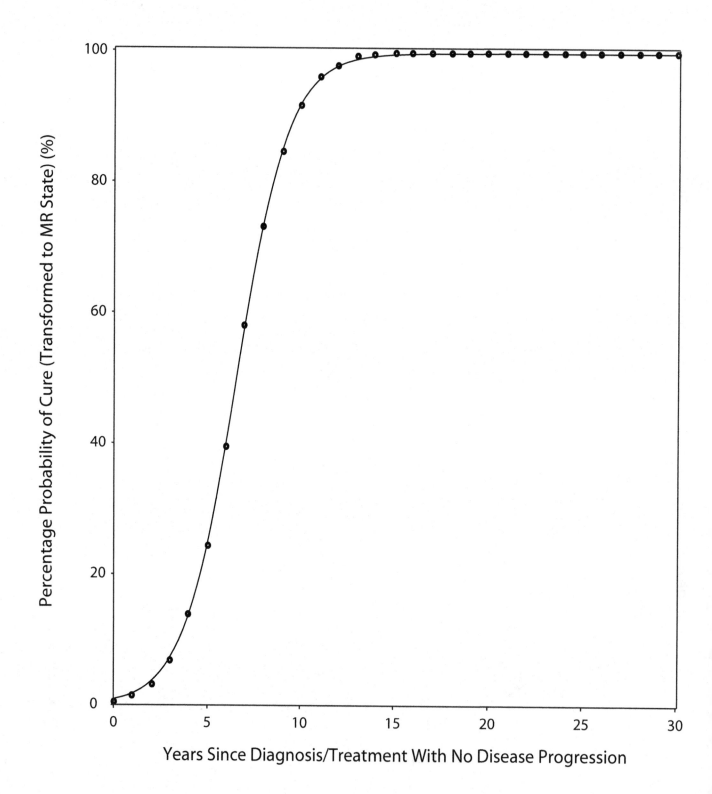

Years Since Diagnosis/Treatment With No Disease Progression

Figure 21

Survival Curve Representing the Lowest-Risk Patient,
If Still At Risk Despite Mastectomy and Radiation

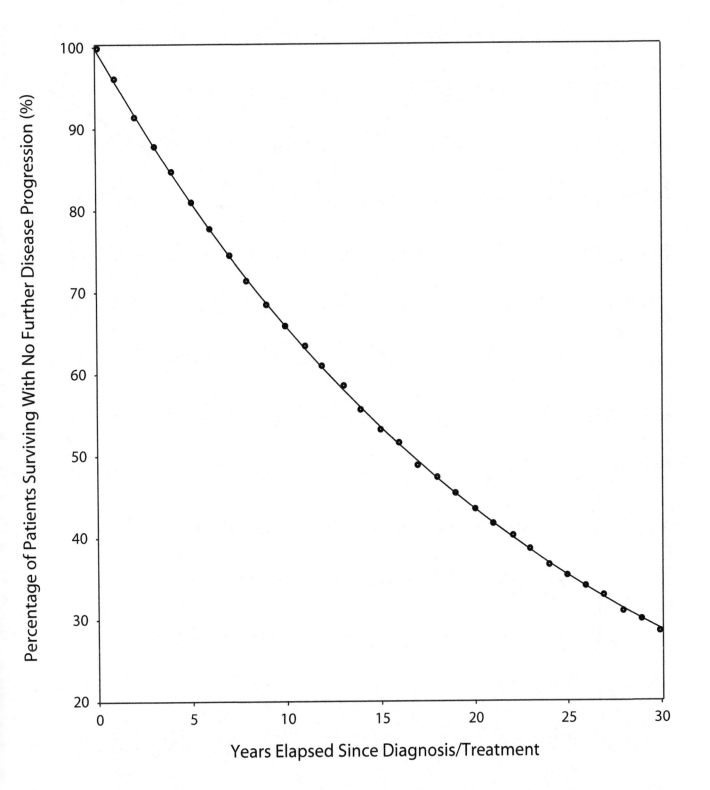

Percentage of Patients Surviving With No Further Disease Progression (%)

Years Elapsed Since Diagnosis/Treatment

Figure 22

Revised Bayesian Posterior Cure Probability Curve Representing the Same Lowest-Risk Patient

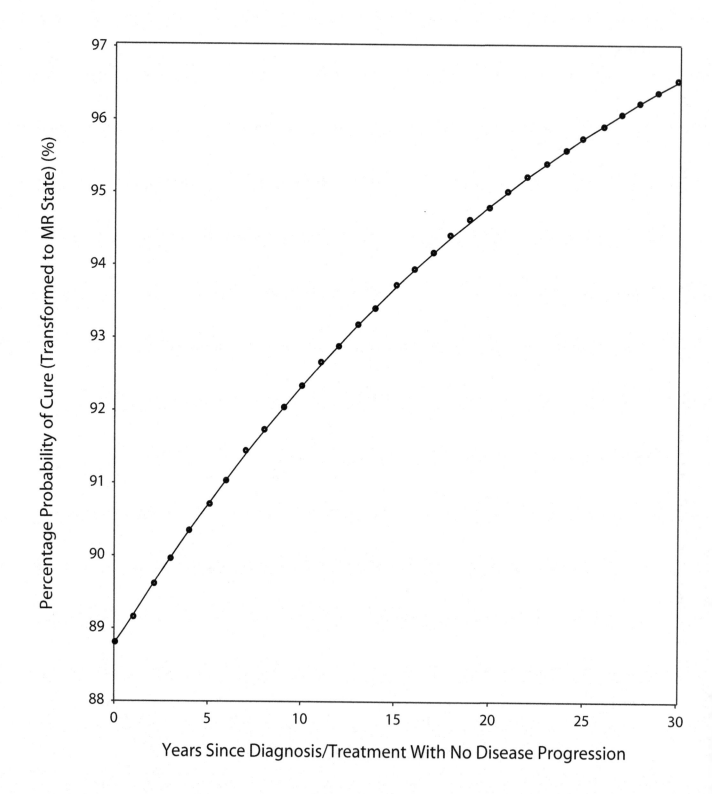

Years Since Diagnosis/Treatment With No Disease Progression

8.0 CONCLUDING COMMENTS

What have we gained from our analyses of organ transplants and breast cancer?

First, and perhaps most actionable, we have showcased an integrated ensemble of procedures specifically designed to analyze a certain type of situation. That situation may be characterized as follows.

1. The analysis focuses on a developmental phenomenon. A developmental phenomenon is one that gradually evolves over time. Suffering a bout with cancer or any other progressive disease definitely qualifies.
2. Exactly how various events characterizing the phenomenon will evolve is not known with certainty. Probabilistic predictive models are therefore not only appropriate: they are extremely useful, especially for separate participants in the phenomenon.
3. A substantial number of participants are engaged in the phenomenon. It is not uniquely applicable to a single entity nor to a small number of isolated entities.
4. The population of participants is at least somewhat heterogeneous. Separate participants are not like electrons. Electrons share essentially identical properties. Once having encountered and measured the mass and charge of a single electron, one presumably knows the mass and charge of all electrons in the universe. One shoe really is presumed to fit all in this unusually homogeneous population.
5. The purpose of the analysis is not to generate general conclusions concerning collective properties of the population, such as how certain factors differentially impact certain subgroups of participants. That is an example of a factor-centered goal. Rather, the analysis is structured to draw separate conclusions about each separate participant. PCM has been specifically designed to accomplish this alternative objective.
6. Individually tailored conclusions about separate participants are stated as probabilities. No claim is made that such conclusions can be drawn with certainty. This is more akin to quantum mechanics, wherein the instantaneous position of an electron is stated probabilistically, than to classical Newtonian mechanics, which draws deterministic conclusions.
7. The important conclusions concern two or more salient states that participants can be in or at least two different subpopulations to which any given participant may belong. This makes it appropriate to partition the population into two or more homogeneous strata whenever possible.
8. Successful homogenization then makes it appropriate to analyze stratified subpopulations separately, according to different assumptions concerning how various factors may influence outcomes in each separate subpopulation. Accomplishing, if possible, a homogenizing partitioning of participants is always PCM's initial task.
9. A central goal of the analysis is to assign a probability to each participant indicating to which subpopulation or in which state that participant belongs.
10. Logistic regression analysis is a statistical tool that can produce such individually tailored probabilities. It can make predictions on the basis of each participant's observed attributes. Logistic regression or an analogous procedure is an essential component of the ensemble.
11. Cox regression is a statistical tool to predict how long it will take for certain events that characterize a developmental phenomenon to materialize. It can also make such probabilistic predictions on the

basis of each participant's observed attributes. Cox regression, too, or an analogous procedure is an essential component of the ensemble.

12. Final probabilistic conclusions concerning separate participants are obtained by imbedding both logistic and Cox regression in a Bayesian framework. It is through a special application of Bayes' theorem that the predictive power of these two different varieties of regression analysis are integrated.

To summarize, the ensemble of procedures is specifically designed to produce individually tailored Bayesian probabilistic conclusions about each separate participant's eventual status relative to some evolving phenomenon. We shall refer to this methodology as tailored developmental conclusion generation (TDCG).

The TDCG methodology comes in two flavors:

1. unambiguous, where the important states, events, or end points to which the methodology is designed to assign probabilities can be identified and measured unambiguously; and
2. ambiguous, where at least some aspect of which state, which event, or which end point is finally achieved by each participant remains unclear, ill-defined, difficult to measure, or otherwise ambiguous.

PCM applies quite comfortably and equally well to both flavors of TDCG. PCM is an integral part of TDCG. Also, probability tables, such as the "busy" tables presented in sections 2 and 5, can be constructed in each case. This enables the predictive potency of both logistic and Cox regression to be exploited in a mutually reinforcing manner through Bayesian integration.

Additional procedures in the ensemble must be invoked when achieving the focal end point of the analysis can only be determined ambiguously. In the cure assessment context, these include:

1. executing a Kaplan-Meier analysis with the CURE option enabled to determine whether or not there is sufficient evidence of a pattern of cure to warrant proceeding with a complete cure assessment;
2. executing the RISKTEST simulator to obtain an initial partitioning of patients into MR and SR subsamples if a sufficiently clear pattern is detected; and
3. subsequent execution of MRPA to refine the partitioning and to complete the cure assessment.

Analysis of organ transplants illustrates TDCG applied in an unambiguous context. It is quite clear whether a patient receiving a kidney transplant does or does not successfully survive the six-month accommodation period. Success means that the patient enters the seventh month with a properly functioning kidney. Otherwise, the accommodation period is deemed a failure.

Another medical situation to which the TDCG methodology might be usefully applied is the diagnosis of an infection with a moderately long, but somewhat variable, incubation period. This mirrors the situation during the early accommodation period of organ transplants. Assuming that eventual diagnosis is unambiguous, exposed patients could be assigned increasing Bayesian posterior probabilities of noninfection as time since exposure passes without manifesting infectious symptoms. Appendix A illustrates what such individually tailored, time-phased probabilities might look like.

A nonmedical situation for which TDCG analysis might be useful is the granting of mortgage loans. The outcome is frequently unambiguous. Whether or not a mortgage is repaid in full and on time is quite easy to ascertain. Inspection of individual borrowers' evolving default probabilities updated by their repayment (and other related) behavior could be used by a bank to identify emerging problem loans and to target remedial measures accordingly. Bank regulators could regularly search evolving patterns such as those tabled in appendix A for an early warning signal, a harbinger of something like the recent subprime mortgage crisis.

The assessment of drug and alcohol treatment programs (and of spontaneous recovery) illustrate another medical context in which the important end point is somewhat ambiguous. As with cancer cure, indications are highly asymmetric. When an addict "falls off the wagon," it is clear that his addiction has not yet been completely overcome. As long as he remains "on the wagon," the (Bayesian posterior) probability of successful recovery continues to increase.

Predicting genuine rehabilitation in the criminal justice system is an example of another ambiguous outcome. Simply predicting recidivism illustrates an unambiguous outcome. TDCG analysis might be usefully applied to both phenomena.

Especially intriguing applications of the TDCG methodology would be to identify probabilistically individuals who have already become radicalized by some external terrorist organization (a sometimes unambiguous outcome) and to assess the efficacy of programs designed to subsequently deradicalize such individuals (a frequently ambiguous outcome).

It is not difficult to imagine many situations for which the TDCG methodology might prove helpful as an analytical tool.

A second useful insight gained from our analyses flows from imbedding TDCG methodology in a Bayesian framework. As a way to answer certain kinds of questions, the value of integrating and extending traditional statistical methodology in such a manner cannot be overstated. Improvement derives from appropriately reversing the direction of conditional probability statements. An example of how reversing the direction of a conditional probability statement can make a crucial interpretive difference may clarify this point.

Consider a West Virginia family that has enjoyed a long and proud history in coal mining. For several generations most of the men in the family have been miners. A young man in the family is currently trying to choose his lifetime vocation. Should he follow in the family footsteps and become a coal miner?

A local newspaper has been conducting a survey of births, deaths, and marriages in the region. One item reported in the survey caught the young man's attention. Postmortem examinations have shown that most people who died with evidence of black lung disease were coal miners. The exact percentage was not reported, but it was definitely more than 50 percent. This struck the young man as a disturbing statistic.

The same survey reported that the prevalence of black lung disease among local coal miners with more than twenty-five years of service had dropped during the last forty years from about one in three (33 percent) to less than one in ten (less than 10 percent). Although quite unpleasant, black lung disease was only infrequently recorded as the specific cause of death, even among coal miners.

Two oppositely directed conditional probabilities may be gleaned from the survey.

1. Given that one had died with clear signs of having contracted black lung disease, the likelihood of having been a local coal miner was high

(more than 50 percent).

2. Given that one had worked locally as a coal miner for at least twenty-five years, the likelihood of having contracted black lung disease fell over the last forty years from around 33 percent to a current rate of less than 10 percent.

The first conditional probability appeared quite alarming. The second one seemed much less so. Is either reported statistic useful to the young man in making his vocational choice? If so, which one?

One message to take away from this story is that reverse conditional probabilities do not refer to exactly the same thing. They are neither the same conceptually nor logically. They refer to two separate, though related, situations. Despite their relatedness, however, they either may or may not be numerically close. They may sometimes be numerically identical, but they definitely need not be. In the black lung story, they were widely disparate. More than 50 percent is quite different from less than 10 percent.

Only the second conditional probability is relevant to the young man's choice of vocation. If he follows the family tradition and becomes a coal miner, the survey suggests that he is less than 10 percent likely to contract black lung disease, even after twenty-five years of service.

Is there some other context in which the first conditional probability might be interesting and important? Yes, reporting it might elicit spirited discussion at a coroners' convention, but these two contexts are decidedly different.

The sometimes misunderstood interpretation of statistical p values provides a second illustration of the same point. Who among empirical researchers really cares to know the "probability" of achieving whatever results are actually observed, conditional on their having been generated under the null hypothesis or conditional on their having been obtained from a population with a prespecified parameter value? That is exactly what p values denote. Yet once collected, what the data will actually be is no longer "probabilistic." Yes, observed data are often summarized in a "probability-like" manner (e.g., in the form of a histogram). Assuming reliable measurement, however, there is no need to describe one's direct observations (raw data) in a manner that suggests uncertainty about what the real data values are. Inferences to be drawn from raw data may be highly uncertain, but the raw observations themselves need not be. Just look, describe, and summarize them as accurately as possible.

Most empirical researchers gather and analyze data in order to draw a conditional conclusion. Unfortunately, the desired conclusion generally points in a direction exactly opposite to the direction stipulated by many inferential statistical techniques. Researchers would generally like to draw an appropriate (probabilistic) conclusion about the truth of an alternative hypothesis (the research hypothesis claiming something about a specified population) or about the actual value of some population parameter. They would like to base (condition) their conclusion on whatever (sample) data were actually obtained. To enable drawing such a conclusion is typically why the research was undertaken in the first place.

So how does one move from a computed p value, embodying a conditional probability pointing in the opposite direction, to a proper conclusion that requires a conditional probability pointing in the desired direction? It is not through any valid deductive reasoning. Rather, it is through professional consensus. It is typically agreed as a matter of convention to regard p values at or beyond 0.05 as statistically significant and (what really matters) as thereby credible, publishable, and fundable.

There is, in principle, a valid procedure to reverse the direction of inference in a computed p value. The procedure is embodied in Bayes' theorem. The problem with using Bayes' theorem for this purpose is strictly practical. Sufficient information to implement it is frequently absent. Objectively determined prior probabilities and appropriate alternative conditional probabilities are the two missing ingredients. Supplying subjectively derived prior probabilities is properly regarded as violating the scientific norm of objectivity. The absence of agreed-upon conditional probabilities under other than a null hypothesis regularly occurs when the phenomenon under study is poorly understood. This second problem persists until the phenomenon becomes quite well understood.

Such is the usual state of affairs in contemporary clinical medicine. For example, we have just recently begun to understand the role of particular genes and the details of their interactive impact in many plants and animals. The result is that computing p values and insisting on statistical significance continues to be the best we can accomplish in most practical situations. Doing so is clearly preferable to doing nothing to rule out the possibility of purely random or otherwise meaningless research results, including the danger of statistical overfitting. Failing to do so would lead to foolishly pursuing many more blind alleys.

A possible reason for misunderstanding what p values really mean is the sometimes unarticulated presumption that both members of any pair of reverse conditional probabilities reflect the same underlying relationship (i.e., constitute interchangeable ways to quantify the same idea). Thus, if a low probability (no more than 5 percent) applies to getting whatever research results were obtained under the null hypothesis (i.e., assuming that the null hypothesis were true), does it not then follow that a correspondingly low probability applies to the reverse conditional conclusion (i.e., that the null hypothesis is just as unlikely to be true, given the unlikely research results obtained)? In terms of valid deductive reasoning, the answer is regrettably no.

However, equal prior probabilities are sometimes properly assignable to every outcome of an imperfectly predictable phenomenon. Which face of a "fair" die will turn up on a single toss illustrates this special situation. Equal prior probabilities are also assigned, by convention, to outcomes of phenomena about which almost nothing is definitively known. Members of each pair of reverse conditional probabilities laid out along every row of the two "busy" tables presented in sections 2 and 5 would then become directly proportional to one another. After appropriate normalization the members of each such pair would become numerically equal, despite their directionally opposite interpretations.

The oppositely directed conditional probabilities of the three matched pairs of survival curves and cure curves presented at the end of both section 5 and section 7 illustrate the same difference in interpretation.

A survival curve depicts how long it will likely take to experience some generally unpleasant event, given that a patient is genuinely at risk of experiencing that event. In contrast, a cure curve depicts how likely it is that a patient has become transformed to a state of being no longer at risk (cured), depending on the amount of time that has elapsed without experiencing the unpleasant event.

Relying on survival curves to address questions of cure is fraught with interpretive peril. Ignoring this directional distinction may explain why cured patients and other patients not at risk are occasionally permitted to contaminate survival studies. As demonstrated in both the Turku and Guy's Hospital breast cancer analyses, this can sometimes lead to the comforting, though spurious, conclusion that hazard rates are declining over time.

The TDCG methodology, even when interesting and potentially useful, has definite limitations.

Because it includes PCM as an integral component, TDCG is data-hungry. It only works properly when applied to data sets of at least moderate size. For the unambiguous version two hundred fifty entities (e.g., patients) is probably the bare minimum. A comfortable minimum might be five hundred entities. For the ambiguous version five hundred entities may be barely adequate, and one thousand may constitute a comfortable minimum.

An adequate sample size is necessary, but by no means sufficient, to make both PCM and TDCG work properly. A high level of data quality is also required. Logistic regression, Cox regression, the RISKTEST simulator, the CURE option of the KAPM procedure, and MRPA involve reasonably sophisticated analytical techniques. None of them can tolerate more than a small amount of casual data collection, improper data recording, sloppy measurement procedures, or other sources of noisy data.

The three data sets analyzed in this book contained unusually clean data. That was an important reason why they were selected to illustrate PCM and the TDCG methodology.

TDCG applies to developmental phenomena. Consequently, input data must be collected over a sufficiently lengthy time period to allow the process to "mature." How long is long enough depends on the particular phenomenon. Breast cancer and prostate cancer, for example, develop over several decades. Melanoma tends to develop more rapidly. MRPA cannot even get started, much less converge to a solution, with data spanning too short a time period.

The availability of lengthy follow-up records was another reason to select the three data sets for this book.

The current version of TDCG is restricted to drawing dichotomous final conclusions. It can deal with only two separate states or two separate strata of a population for a participant to end up in. Cancer patients may enter a period of temporary remission. That is not the same as being permanently cured. Bank loans may be repaid only in part or not on time. Both are different from a complete default. TDCG would benefit greatly if its framework were extended to encompass more than just two possible final conclusions.

Subject to the quantitative and qualitative data limitations we have identified, TDCG can be so extended. Logistic regression has already been extended by others to deal with more than two types of events. Cox regression can be applied conditionally to any number of separate event types.

The "busy" probability tables presented in sections 2 and 5 to explicate in operational terms the Bayesian framework undergirding TDCG methodology can also be extended by adding additional columns. Additional columns would accommodate additional states, stratified subpopulations, and event types. Additional rows can be added to reflect more than dichotomously defined observable indicators. For the sake of respectability, such "busy" tables will henceforth be referred to as TDCG probability tables.

In these and other respects, TDCG appears to be a scalable methodology. What has been presented in this book should be interpreted as no more than an introductory "first cut."

Appendix A

Initial (SP) Early Success Probabilities and Succeeding Monthly
Posterior Early Success RSP(t) Probabilities (POSTPR1, POSTPR2,
..., POSTPR6) for 469 Patients Who Underwent Kidney Transplants

VALUE OF ATTRIBUTE SP	VALUE OF ATTRIBUTE POSTPR1	VALUE OF ATTRIBUTE POSTPR2	VALUE OF ATTRIBUTE POSTPR3	VALUE OF ATTRIBUTE POSTPR4	VALUE OF ATTRIBUTE POSTPR5	VALUE OF ATTRIBUTE POSTPR6
0.5239	0.6190	0.7369	0.8242	0.8959	0.9575	1.0000
0.5239	0.6190	0.7369	0.8242	0.8959	0.0000	0.0000
0.5239	0.6190	0.7369	0.0000	0.0000	0.0000	0.0000
0.5239	0.6190	0.7369	0.8242	0.8959	0.9575	1.0000
0.5239	0.6190	0.7369	0.8242	0.8959	0.9575	1.0000
0.5239	0.6190	0.7369	0.8242	0.8959	0.9575	1.0000
0.5247	0.6198	0.7375	0.8247	0.8962	0.9576	1.0000
0.5247	0.6198	0.7375	0.8247	0.8962	0.9576	1.0000
0.5865	0.6769	0.7831	0.8581	0.9174	0.9667	1.0000
0.6004	0.6893	0.7927	0.8649	0.9216	0.9685	1.0000
0.6030	0.6601	0.0000	0.0000	0.0000	0.0000	0.0000
0.6030	0.6601	0.7324	0.7911	0.8474	0.9106	1.0000
0.6030	0.6601	0.7324	0.7911	0.8474	0.9106	1.0000
0.6030	0.0000	0.0000	0.0000	0.0000	0.0000	0.0000
0.6030	0.6601	0.7324	0.7911	0.0000	0.0000	0.0000
0.6030	0.6601	0.7324	0.7911	0.8474	0.9106	0.0000
0.6030	0.6601	0.7324	0.7911	0.8474	0.9106	1.0000
0.6266	0.7125	0.8103	0.8773	0.9292	0.9717	1.0000
0.6266	0.7125	0.8103	0.8773	0.9292	0.9717	1.0000
0.6266	0.7125	0.8103	0.8773	0.9292	0.9717	1.0000
0.6266	0.7125	0.8103	0.8773	0.9292	0.9717	1.0000
0.6266	0.7125	0.8103	0.8773	0.0000	0.0000	0.0000
0.6266	0.7125	0.0000	0.0000	0.0000	0.0000	0.0000
0.6266	0.7125	0.8103	0.8773	0.9292	0.9717	1.0000
0.6266	0.7125	0.8103	0.8773	0.9292	0.9717	1.0000
0.6266	0.7125	0.8103	0.8773	0.9292	0.9717	1.0000
0.6266	0.0000	0.0000	0.0000	0.0000	0.0000	0.0000
0.6266	0.7125	0.8103	0.8773	0.9292	0.9717	1.0000
0.6266	0.7125	0.0000	0.0000	0.0000	0.0000	0.0000
0.6266	0.7125	0.8103	0.8773	0.9292	0.9717	1.0000
0.6266	0.7125	0.0000	0.0000	0.0000	0.0000	0.0000
0.6266	0.0000	0.0000	0.0000	0.0000	0.0000	0.0000
0.6266	0.7125	0.8103	0.8773	0.9292	0.9717	1.0000
0.6266	0.7125	0.8103	0.8773	0.9292	0.9717	1.0000
0.6266	0.7125	0.8103	0.8773	0.9292	0.9717	1.0000
0.6266	0.7125	0.8103	0.8773	0.9292	0.9717	1.0000
0.6266	0.0000	0.0000	0.0000	0.0000	0.0000	0.0000
0.6266	0.7125	0.8103	0.8773	0.9292	0.9717	1.0000
0.6266	0.7125	0.8103	0.8773	0.0000	0.0000	0.0000
0.6266	0.7125	0.8103	0.8773	0.0000	0.0000	0.0000
0.6266	0.7125	0.8103	0.8773	0.9292	0.9717	1.0000
0.6266	0.7125	0.8103	0.8773	0.0000	0.0000	0.0000
0.6273	0.7132	0.8108	0.8777	0.9294	0.9718	1.0000
0.6273	0.7132	0.8108	0.8777	0.9294	0.9718	0.0000
0.6273	0.7132	0.8108	0.8777	0.9294	0.9718	1.0000
0.6273	0.0000	0.0000	0.0000	0.0000	0.0000	0.0000
0.6273	0.7132	0.8108	0.8777	0.9294	0.9718	1.0000
0.6292	0.6845	0.7535	0.8088	0.8611	0.9192	1.0000
0.6292	0.6845	0.7535	0.8088	0.8611	0.9192	1.0000

VALUE OF ATTRIBUTE SP	VALUE OF ATTRIBUTE POSTPR1	VALUE OF ATTRIBUTE POSTPR2	VALUE OF ATTRIBUTE POSTPR3	VALUE OF ATTRIBUTE POSTPR4	VALUE OF ATTRIBUTE POSTPR5	VALUE OF ATTRIBUTE POSTPR6
0.6292	0.6845	0.7535	0.8088	0.8611	0.9192	1.0000
0.6292	0.6845	0.7535	0.8088	0.8611	0.9192	1.0000
0.6292	0.6845	0.7535	0.8088	0.8611	0.9192	0.0000
0.6292	0.6845	0.0000	0.0000	0.0000	0.0000	0.0000
0.6292	0.6845	0.7535	0.8088	0.8611	0.9192	1.0000
0.6292	0.6845	0.0000	0.0000	0.0000	0.0000	0.0000
0.6292	0.6845	0.7535	0.8088	0.8611	0.9192	1.0000
0.6292	0.6845	0.7535	0.0000	0.0000	0.0000	0.0000
0.6292	0.6845	0.7535	0.8088	0.8611	0.9192	1.0000
0.6292	0.6845	0.7535	0.8088	0.8611	0.9192	1.0000
0.6292	0.6845	0.7535	0.8088	0.8611	0.9192	1.0000
0.6292	0.6845	0.7535	0.8088	0.8611	0.0000	0.0000
0.6292	0.6845	0.7535	0.8088	0.8611	0.9192	1.0000
0.6292	0.6845	0.7535	0.8088	0.8611	0.9192	1.0000
0.6292	0.6845	0.7535	0.8088	0.8611	0.9192	0.0000
0.6292	0.6845	0.7535	0.8088	0.8611	0.9192	1.0000
0.6292	0.6845	0.7535	0.8088	0.8611	0.9192	1.0000
0.6292	0.6845	0.7535	0.8088	0.8611	0.9192	1.0000
0.6292	0.6845	0.0000	0.0000	0.0000	0.0000	0.0000
0.6292	0.6845	0.7535	0.8088	0.8611	0.9192	1.0000
0.6292	0.6845	0.0000	0.0000	0.0000	0.0000	0.0000
0.6292	0.6845	0.7535	0.8088	0.0000	0.0000	0.0000
0.6292	0.6845	0.7535	0.8088	0.0000	0.0000	0.0000
0.6292	0.6845	0.7535	0.8088	0.8611	0.9192	1.0000
0.6292	0.6845	0.7535	0.8088	0.8611	0.9192	1.0000
0.6299	0.6852	0.7541	0.8093	0.8616	0.9194	1.0000
0.6299	0.6852	0.7541	0.8093	0.8616	0.9194	1.0000
0.6299	0.6852	0.7541	0.8093	0.8616	0.9194	1.0000
0.6299	0.6852	0.7541	0.8093	0.8616	0.9194	0.0000
0.6299	0.0000	0.0000	0.0000	0.0000	0.0000	0.0000
0.6299	0.6852	0.0000	0.0000	0.0000	0.0000	0.0000
0.6299	0.6852	0.7541	0.8093	0.8616	0.9194	1.0000
0.6299	0.6852	0.7541	0.8093	0.8616	0.9194	1.0000
0.6839	0.7616	0.8463	0.9021	0.9442	0.9779	1.0000
0.6839	0.7616	0.8463	0.9021	0.9442	0.9779	1.0000
0.6839	0.7616	0.8463	0.9021	0.9442	0.9779	1.0000
0.6839	0.7616	0.8463	0.9021	0.9442	0.9779	1.0000
0.6839	0.7616	0.8463	0.9021	0.9442	0.9779	1.0000
0.6839	0.0000	0.0000	0.0000	0.0000	0.0000	0.0000
0.6839	0.7616	0.8463	0.9021	0.9442	0.9779	1.0000
0.6839	0.7616	0.8463	0.9021	0.9442	0.9779	1.0000
0.6985	0.7476	0.8067	0.8524	0.8944	0.9395	1.0000
0.6985	0.7476	0.8067	0.8524	0.8944	0.9395	1.0000
0.6985	0.7476	0.8067	0.8524	0.8944	0.9395	1.0000
0.6985	0.7476	0.8067	0.8524	0.8944	0.9395	1.0000
0.6985	0.7476	0.8067	0.8524	0.8944	0.9395	0.0000
0.6985	0.7476	0.8067	0.0000	0.0000	0.0000	0.0000
0.6985	0.7476	0.8067	0.8524	0.8944	0.0000	0.0000
0.6985	0.7476	0.8067	0.8524	0.8944	0.9395	1.0000
0.6985	0.7476	0.8067	0.8524	0.8944	0.9395	1.0000
0.6985	0.7476	0.8067	0.8524	0.8944	0.9395	1.0000
0.6985	0.7476	0.8067	0.8524	0.8944	0.9395	1.0000
0.6985	0.7476	0.8067	0.8524	0.8944	0.9395	1.0000
0.6985	0.7476	0.8067	0.8524	0.8944	0.9395	1.0000
0.6985	0.7476	0.8067	0.8524	0.8944	0.9395	1.0000

VALUE OF ATTRIBUTE SP	VALUE OF ATTRIBUTE POSTPR1	VALUE OF ATTRIBUTE POSTPR2	VALUE OF ATTRIBUTE POSTPR3	VALUE OF ATTRIBUTE POSTPR4	VALUE OF ATTRIBUTE POSTPR5	VALUE OF ATTRIBUTE POSTPR6
0.6985	0.7476	0.8067	0.8524	0.8944	0.9395	1.0000
0.6985	0.7476	0.8067	0.8524	0.8944	0.0000	0.0000
0.6985	0.7476	0.8067	0.8524	0.8944	0.9395	1.0000
0.7212	0.0000	0.0000	0.0000	0.0000	0.0000	0.0000
0.7212	0.0000	0.0000	0.0000	0.0000	0.0000	0.0000
0.7212	0.7679	0.8234	0.8658	0.9044	0.9455	1.0000
0.7212	0.7679	0.8234	0.8658	0.9044	0.9455	1.0000
0.7212	0.7679	0.8234	0.8658	0.9044	0.9455	1.0000
0.7212	0.7679	0.8234	0.8658	0.9044	0.9455	1.0000
0.7212	0.7679	0.8234	0.8658	0.9044	0.9455	1.0000
0.7212	0.7679	0.8234	0.8658	0.9044	0.9455	1.0000
0.7212	0.7679	0.8234	0.8658	0.9044	0.9455	1.0000
0.7212	0.7679	0.8234	0.8658	0.9044	0.9455	1.0000
0.7212	0.7679	0.8234	0.8658	0.9044	0.9455	1.0000
0.7212	0.7679	0.8234	0.8658	0.9044	0.9455	1.0000
0.7212	0.7679	0.8234	0.8658	0.9044	0.9455	1.0000
0.7212	0.7679	0.8234	0.8658	0.9044	0.9455	0.0000
0.7212	0.7679	0.8234	0.8658	0.9044	0.9455	1.0000
0.7212	0.7679	0.8234	0.8658	0.9044	0.9455	1.0000
0.7212	0.7679	0.8234	0.8658	0.9044	0.9455	1.0000
0.7212	0.7679	0.8234	0.8658	0.9044	0.9455	1.0000
0.7212	0.7679	0.8234	0.8658	0.9044	0.9455	1.0000
0.7212	0.7679	0.8234	0.8658	0.9044	0.9455	1.0000
0.7212	0.7679	0.8234	0.8658	0.9044	0.9455	1.0000
0.7212	0.7679	0.8234	0.0000	0.0000	0.0000	0.0000
0.7212	0.7679	0.8234	0.8658	0.9044	0.9455	1.0000
0.7212	0.7679	0.8234	0.8658	0.9044	0.9455	0.0000
0.7212	0.7679	0.8234	0.8658	0.9044	0.9455	1.0000
0.7212	0.7679	0.8234	0.8658	0.9044	0.9455	1.0000
0.7212	0.7679	0.8234	0.8658	0.9044	0.9455	1.0000
0.7212	0.7679	0.8234	0.8658	0.9044	0.9455	1.0000
0.7212	0.7679	0.8234	0.0000	0.0000	0.0000	0.0000
0.7212	0.7679	0.0000	0.0000	0.0000	0.0000	0.0000
0.7212	0.7679	0.8234	0.8658	0.9044	0.9455	1.0000
0.7212	0.7679	0.8234	0.8658	0.9044	0.9455	1.0000
0.7212	0.7679	0.8234	0.8658	0.9044	0.9455	0.0000
0.7212	0.7679	0.8234	0.8658	0.0000	0.0000	0.0000
0.7212	0.7679	0.8234	0.8658	0.9044	0.9455	1.0000
0.7212	0.7679	0.8234	0.8658	0.0000	0.0000	0.0000
0.7212	0.7679	0.8234	0.8658	0.9044	0.9455	1.0000
0.7212	0.7679	0.8234	0.8658	0.9044	0.9455	1.0000
0.7212	0.7679	0.8234	0.8658	0.9044	0.9455	1.0000
0.7212	0.7679	0.0000	0.0000	0.0000	0.0000	0.0000
0.7212	0.7679	0.8234	0.0000	0.0000	0.0000	0.0000
0.7212	0.7679	0.8234	0.8658	0.9044	0.0000	0.0000
0.7212	0.7679	0.8234	0.8658	0.9044	0.9455	1.0000
0.7212	0.7679	0.8234	0.8658	0.9044	0.9455	1.0000
0.7212	0.7679	0.8234	0.8658	0.9044	0.9455	1.0000
0.7212	0.7679	0.8234	0.8658	0.9044	0.9455	1.0000
0.7212	0.7679	0.8234	0.0000	0.0000	0.0000	0.0000
0.7212	0.7679	0.8234	0.8658	0.9044	0.9455	1.0000
0.7212	0.7679	0.8234	0.8658	0.9044	0.9455	1.0000
0.7212	0.7679	0.8234	0.8658	0.9044	0.9455	1.0000

VALUE OF ATTRIBUTE SP	VALUE OF ATTRIBUTE POSTPR1	VALUE OF ATTRIBUTE POSTPR2	VALUE OF ATTRIBUTE POSTPR3	VALUE OF ATTRIBUTE POSTPR4	VALUE OF ATTRIBUTE POSTPR5	VALUE OF ATTRIBUTE POSTPR6
0.7212	0.7679	0.8234	0.8658	0.9044	0.9455	1.0000
0.7212	0.7679	0.8234	0.8658	0.0000	0.0000	0.0000
0.7212	0.7679	0.8234	0.8658	0.9044	0.9455	1.0000
0.7212	0.7679	0.8234	0.8658	0.0000	0.0000	0.0000
0.7212	0.7679	0.8234	0.8658	0.9044	0.9455	1.0000
0.7212	0.7679	0.8234	0.8658	0.9044	0.9455	1.0000
0.7212	0.7679	0.8234	0.8658	0.9044	0.9455	1.0000
0.7212	0.7679	0.8234	0.8658	0.9044	0.9455	1.0000
0.7212	0.7679	0.8234	0.8658	0.9044	0.9455	1.0000
0.7212	0.7679	0.8234	0.8658	0.9044	0.9455	1.0000
0.7212	0.7679	0.8234	0.8658	0.9044	0.9455	1.0000
0.7212	0.7679	0.8234	0.0000	0.0000	0.0000	0.0000
0.7212	0.0000	0.0000	0.0000	0.0000	0.0000	0.0000
0.7212	0.7679	0.8234	0.8658	0.9044	0.0000	0.0000
0.7212	0.7679	0.8234	0.8658	0.9044	0.9455	1.0000
0.7212	0.7679	0.8234	0.8658	0.9044	0.9455	1.0000
0.7212	0.7679	0.0000	0.0000	0.0000	0.0000	0.0000
0.7212	0.7679	0.0000	0.0000	0.0000	0.0000	0.0000
0.7212	0.7679	0.8234	0.8658	0.9044	0.9455	1.0000
0.7212	0.7679	0.8234	0.8658	0.9044	0.9455	1.0000
0.7212	0.7679	0.8234	0.8658	0.9044	0.9455	1.0000
0.7212	0.7679	0.8234	0.8658	0.9044	0.9455	1.0000
0.7212	0.0000	0.0000	0.0000	0.0000	0.0000	0.0000
0.7212	0.7679	0.8234	0.8658	0.9044	0.9455	1.0000
0.7212	0.7679	0.0000	0.0000	0.0000	0.0000	0.0000
0.7212	0.0000	0.0000	0.0000	0.0000	0.0000	0.0000
0.7212	0.7679	0.8234	0.8658	0.9044	0.9455	1.0000
0.7212	0.7679	0.8234	0.8658	0.9044	0.9455	1.0000
0.7212	0.7679	0.8234	0.8658	0.9044	0.9455	1.0000
0.7212	0.7679	0.8234	0.8658	0.9044	0.9455	1.0000
0.7212	0.7679	0.8234	0.8658	0.9044	0.9455	1.0000
0.7212	0.7679	0.8234	0.8658	0.9044	0.9455	1.0000
0.7212	0.7679	0.8234	0.8658	0.9044	0.9455	1.0000
0.7212	0.7679	0.8234	0.8658	0.0000	0.0000	0.0000
0.7212	0.7679	0.8234	0.8658	0.9044	0.9455	1.0000
0.7212	0.7679	0.8234	0.0000	0.0000	0.0000	0.0000
0.7212	0.7679	0.8234	0.8658	0.9044	0.9455	1.0000
0.7212	0.7679	0.8234	0.8658	0.9044	0.9455	1.0000
0.7212	0.7679	0.8234	0.8658	0.9044	0.9455	1.0000
0.7212	0.7679	0.8234	0.8658	0.9044	0.9455	0.0000
0.7212	0.7679	0.8234	0.8658	0.9044	0.9455	1.0000
0.7212	0.7679	0.8234	0.0000	0.0000	0.0000	0.0000
0.7212	0.7679	0.8234	0.8658	0.9044	0.9455	1.0000
0.7212	0.7679	0.8234	0.8658	0.9044	0.9455	1.0000
0.7212	0.7679	0.8234	0.8658	0.9044	0.9455	1.0000
0.7212	0.7679	0.0000	0.0000	0.0000	0.0000	0.0000
0.7212	0.7679	0.8234	0.8658	0.9044	0.9455	1.0000
0.7212	0.7679	0.8234	0.0000	0.0000	0.0000	0.0000
0.7212	0.7679	0.8234	0.8658	0.9044	0.9455	1.0000
0.7212	0.7679	0.8234	0.8658	0.9044	0.9455	1.0000
0.7212	0.7679	0.8234	0.8658	0.9044	0.9455	1.0000
0.7212	0.7679	0.8234	0.8658	0.9044	0.9455	1.0000
0.7212	0.7679	0.8234	0.8658	0.9044	0.9455	1.0000
0.7212	0.7679	0.8234	0.8658	0.9044	0.0000	0.0000

VALUE OF ATTRIBUTE SP	VALUE OF ATTRIBUTE POSTPR1	VALUE OF ATTRIBUTE POSTPR2	VALUE OF ATTRIBUTE POSTPR3	VALUE OF ATTRIBUTE POSTPR4	VALUE OF ATTRIBUTE POSTPR5	VALUE OF ATTRIBUTE POSTPR6
0.7212	0.7679	0.8234	0.8658	0.9044	0.9455	1.0000
0.7212	0.7679	0.8234	0.8658	0.9044	0.9455	1.0000
0.7212	0.7679	0.8234	0.8658	0.9044	0.9455	1.0000
0.7212	0.7679	0.8234	0.8658	0.9044	0.9455	1.0000
0.7212	0.7679	0.8234	0.8658	0.9044	0.9455	1.0000
0.7212	0.7679	0.8234	0.8658	0.9044	0.9455	1.0000
0.7212	0.7679	0.8234	0.8658	0.9044	0.9455	1.0000
0.7212	0.7679	0.8234	0.8658	0.9044	0.9455	1.0000
0.7212	0.7679	0.8234	0.8658	0.9044	0.9455	1.0000
0.7212	0.7679	0.8234	0.8658	0.9044	0.9455	1.0000
0.7212	0.7679	0.8234	0.8658	0.0000	0.0000	0.0000
0.7219	0.7685	0.8239	0.8661	0.9047	0.0000	0.0000
0.7219	0.7685	0.8239	0.8661	0.9047	0.9456	1.0000
0.7219	0.7685	0.8239	0.8661	0.9047	0.9456	1.0000
0.7219	0.0000	0.0000	0.0000	0.0000	0.0000	0.0000
0.7219	0.7685	0.8239	0.8661	0.9047	0.9456	1.0000
0.7219	0.7685	0.8239	0.8661	0.9047	0.9456	1.0000
0.7219	0.0000	0.0000	0.0000	0.0000	0.0000	0.0000
0.7219	0.7685	0.8239	0.8661	0.9047	0.9456	1.0000
0.7219	0.7685	0.8239	0.8661	0.9047	0.9456	0.0000
0.7219	0.7685	0.8239	0.8661	0.9047	0.9456	1.0000
0.7219	0.7685	0.8239	0.8661	0.9047	0.9456	1.0000
0.7219	0.7685	0.8239	0.8661	0.9047	0.9456	1.0000
0.7219	0.7685	0.8239	0.8661	0.9047	0.9456	1.0000
0.7219	0.7685	0.8239	0.8661	0.9047	0.9456	1.0000
0.7219	0.7685	0.8239	0.8661	0.9047	0.9456	1.0000
0.7219	0.7685	0.8239	0.8661	0.9047	0.9456	1.0000
0.7219	0.7685	0.0000	0.0000	0.0000	0.0000	0.0000
0.7219	0.7685	0.0000	0.0000	0.0000	0.0000	0.0000
0.7219	0.7685	0.8239	0.8661	0.9047	0.0000	0.0000
0.7219	0.7685	0.8239	0.8661	0.9047	0.9456	1.0000
0.7219	0.7685	0.8239	0.8661	0.0000	0.0000	0.0000
0.7219	0.7685	0.8239	0.8661	0.9047	0.9456	1.0000
0.7219	0.7685	0.8239	0.8661	0.9047	0.9456	1.0000
0.7219	0.7685	0.8239	0.8661	0.9047	0.9456	1.0000
0.7219	0.7685	0.8239	0.8661	0.9047	0.9456	1.0000
0.7219	0.7685	0.8239	0.8661	0.9047	0.9456	1.0000
0.7219	0.7685	0.8239	0.8661	0.9047	0.9456	0.0000
0.7219	0.7685	0.8239	0.8661	0.9047	0.9456	1.0000
0.7219	0.7685	0.0000	0.0000	0.0000	0.0000	0.0000
0.7219	0.7685	0.8239	0.0000	0.0000	0.0000	0.0000
0.7219	0.7685	0.8239	0.8661	0.9047	0.9456	1.0000
0.7219	0.7685	0.8239	0.8661	0.9047	0.9456	1.0000
0.7219	0.0000	0.0000	0.0000	0.0000	0.0000	0.0000
0.7219	0.7685	0.8239	0.0000	0.0000	0.0000	0.0000
0.7219	0.7685	0.8239	0.8661	0.9047	0.9456	1.0000
0.7219	0.7685	0.8239	0.8661	0.9047	0.9456	1.0000
0.7219	0.7685	0.8239	0.8661	0.9047	0.9456	1.0000
0.7219	0.7685	0.8239	0.8661	0.9047	0.9456	1.0000
0.7219	0.7685	0.8239	0.8661	0.9047	0.9456	1.0000
0.7219	0.7685	0.8239	0.8661	0.9047	0.9456	0.0000
0.7219	0.7685	0.8239	0.8661	0.9047	0.9456	1.0000
0.7219	0.7685	0.8239	0.8661	0.9047	0.9456	1.0000
0.7219	0.7685	0.8239	0.8661	0.9047	0.9456	1.0000
0.7219	0.0000	0.0000	0.0000	0.0000	0.0000	0.0000

VALUE OF ATTRIBUTE SP	VALUE OF ATTRIBUTE POSTPR1	VALUE OF ATTRIBUTE POSTPR2	VALUE OF ATTRIBUTE POSTPR3	VALUE OF ATTRIBUTE POSTPR4	VALUE OF ATTRIBUTE POSTPR5	VALUE OF ATTRIBUTE POSTPR6
0.7219	0.7685	0.8239	0.8661	0.9047	0.9456	1.0000
0.7219	0.7685	0.8239	0.8661	0.9047	0.9456	1.0000
0.7219	0.7685	0.8239	0.8661	0.9047	0.9456	1.0000
0.7219	0.7685	0.8239	0.8661	0.9047	0.9456	1.0000
0.7219	0.7685	0.8239	0.8661	0.9047	0.9456	1.0000
0.7219	0.7685	0.8239	0.8661	0.9047	0.9456	1.0000
0.7219	0.7685	0.8239	0.8661	0.9047	0.9456	1.0000
0.7219	0.7685	0.0000	0.0000	0.0000	0.0000	0.0000
0.7219	0.7685	0.8239	0.8661	0.9047	0.9456	1.0000
0.7219	0.7685	0.8239	0.8661	0.9047	0.9456	1.0000
0.7219	0.7685	0.8239	0.8661	0.9047	0.9456	1.0000
0.7219	0.7685	0.0000	0.0000	0.0000	0.0000	0.0000
0.7219	0.7685	0.8239	0.8661	0.9047	0.9456	1.0000
0.7219	0.7685	0.8239	0.8661	0.9047	0.9456	1.0000
0.7219	0.7685	0.8239	0.8661	0.9047	0.9456	0.0000
0.7422	0.8096	0.8799	0.9246	0.9575	0.9833	1.0000
0.7422	0.0000	0.0000	0.0000	0.0000	0.0000	0.0000
0.7422	0.8096	0.8799	0.0000	0.0000	0.0000	0.0000
0.7422	0.0000	0.0000	0.0000	0.0000	0.0000	0.0000
0.7422	0.0000	0.0000	0.0000	0.0000	0.0000	0.0000
0.7422	0.8096	0.8799	0.9246	0.9575	0.9833	1.0000
0.7422	0.8096	0.8799	0.9246	0.9575	0.9833	1.0000
0.7422	0.8096	0.8799	0.9246	0.9575	0.9833	1.0000
0.7422	0.8096	0.8799	0.9246	0.9575	0.9833	1.0000
0.7428	0.8101	0.8803	0.9249	0.9576	0.9834	1.0000
0.7428	0.8101	0.8803	0.9249	0.9576	0.9834	1.0000
0.7428	0.8101	0.8803	0.0000	0.0000	0.0000	0.0000
0.7428	0.8101	0.8803	0.9249	0.9576	0.9834	1.0000
0.7694	0.8101	0.8573	0.8926	0.9242	0.9572	1.0000
0.7694	0.8101	0.8573	0.8926	0.9242	0.9572	1.0000
0.7694	0.8101	0.8573	0.0000	0.0000	0.0000	0.0000
0.7694	0.8101	0.8573	0.8926	0.9242	0.9572	1.0000
0.7694	0.8101	0.8573	0.8926	0.9242	0.9572	1.0000
0.7694	0.8101	0.8573	0.8926	0.9242	0.9572	1.0000
0.7694	0.8101	0.8573	0.8926	0.9242	0.9572	1.0000
0.7694	0.8101	0.8573	0.8926	0.9242	0.9572	1.0000
0.7694	0.8101	0.0000	0.0000	0.0000	0.0000	0.0000
0.7694	0.8101	0.8573	0.8926	0.9242	0.9572	1.0000
0.7694	0.8101	0.8573	0.8926	0.9242	0.9572	1.0000
0.7694	0.0000	0.0000	0.0000	0.0000	0.0000	0.0000
0.7694	0.8101	0.0000	0.0000	0.0000	0.0000	0.0000
0.7694	0.8101	0.8573	0.8926	0.9242	0.9572	1.0000
0.7694	0.8101	0.8573	0.8926	0.9242	0.9572	1.0000
0.7694	0.8101	0.8573	0.8926	0.9242	0.9572	1.0000
0.7694	0.0000	0.0000	0.0000	0.0000	0.0000	0.0000
0.7694	0.8101	0.8573	0.8926	0.9242	0.0000	0.0000
0.7694	0.8101	0.8573	0.8926	0.9242	0.9572	1.0000
0.7694	0.8101	0.8573	0.8926	0.9242	0.9572	1.0000
0.7694	0.8101	0.8573	0.8926	0.9242	0.9572	1.0000
0.7694	0.0000	0.0000	0.0000	0.0000	0.0000	0.0000
0.7694	0.8101	0.8573	0.8926	0.9242	0.0000	0.0000

VALUE OF ATTRIBUTE SP	VALUE OF ATTRIBUTE POSTPR1	VALUE OF ATTRIBUTE POSTPR2	VALUE OF ATTRIBUTE POSTPR3	VALUE OF ATTRIBUTE POSTPR4	VALUE OF ATTRIBUTE POSTPR5	VALUE OF ATTRIBUTE POSTPR6
0.7694	0.8101	0.8573	0.8926	0.9242	0.9572	1.0000
0.7694	0.8101	0.8573	0.8926	0.9242	0.9572	1.0000
0.7694	0.8101	0.8573	0.8926	0.9242	0.9572	1.0000
0.7694	0.8101	0.8573	0.8926	0.0000	0.0000	0.0000
0.7694	0.8101	0.8573	0.8926	0.9242	0.9572	1.0000
0.7694	0.8101	0.8573	0.8926	0.9242	0.9572	1.0000
0.7694	0.8101	0.8573	0.8926	0.9242	0.9572	1.0000
0.7694	0.0000	0.0000	0.0000	0.0000	0.0000	0.0000
0.7849	0.8435	0.9028	0.9396	0.9662	0.9868	1.0000
0.7849	0.8435	0.9028	0.9396	0.9662	0.9868	1.0000
0.7849	0.8435	0.9028	0.9396	0.9662	0.9868	1.0000
0.7849	0.8435	0.9028	0.9396	0.9662	0.9868	1.0000
0.7849	0.8435	0.9028	0.9396	0.9662	0.9868	1.0000
0.7849	0.8435	0.0000	0.0000	0.0000	0.0000	0.0000
0.7849	0.0000	0.0000	0.0000	0.0000	0.0000	0.0000
0.7867	0.8251	0.8692	0.9019	0.9310	0.9611	1.0000
0.7877	0.0000	0.0000	0.0000	0.0000	0.0000	0.0000
0.7877	0.0000	0.0000	0.0000	0.0000	0.0000	0.0000
0.7877	0.8457	0.9043	0.9405	0.9667	0.9870	1.0000
0.7877	0.8457	0.9043	0.0000	0.0000	0.0000	0.0000
0.7990	0.8356	0.8775	0.9083	0.9356	0.9638	1.0000
0.8161	0.8502	0.8889	0.9171	0.9420	0.9675	1.0000
0.8161	0.8502	0.0000	0.0000	0.0000	0.0000	0.0000
0.8161	0.8502	0.8889	0.9171	0.9420	0.9675	1.0000
0.8161	0.8502	0.8889	0.9171	0.9420	0.9675	1.0000
0.8161	0.8502	0.8889	0.9171	0.9420	0.9675	1.0000
0.8161	0.8502	0.8889	0.9171	0.9420	0.9675	1.0000
0.8161	0.8502	0.8889	0.9171	0.9420	0.9675	1.0000
0.8161	0.8502	0.8889	0.9171	0.9420	0.9675	1.0000
0.8161	0.8502	0.8889	0.9171	0.9420	0.9675	1.0000
0.8161	0.8502	0.8889	0.9171	0.9420	0.9675	1.0000
0.8161	0.8502	0.8889	0.9171	0.9420	0.9675	1.0000
0.8161	0.8502	0.0000	0.0000	0.0000	0.0000	0.0000
0.8161	0.8502	0.0000	0.0000	0.0000	0.0000	0.0000
0.8161	0.8502	0.8889	0.9171	0.9420	0.9675	1.0000
0.8161	0.8502	0.8889	0.9171	0.9420	0.9675	1.0000
0.8161	0.8502	0.8889	0.9171	0.9420	0.9675	1.0000
0.8161	0.8502	0.8889	0.9171	0.9420	0.9675	1.0000
0.8161	0.8502	0.8889	0.9171	0.9420	0.9675	1.0000
0.8161	0.8502	0.8889	0.9171	0.9420	0.9675	1.0000
0.8161	0.8502	0.8889	0.9171	0.9420	0.9675	1.0000
0.8161	0.8502	0.8889	0.9171	0.9420	0.9675	1.0000
0.8161	0.8502	0.8889	0.9171	0.9420	0.9675	1.0000
0.8161	0.8502	0.8889	0.9171	0.9420	0.9675	1.0000
0.8161	0.8502	0.8889	0.9171	0.9420	0.9675	1.0000
0.8161	0.8502	0.8889	0.9171	0.9420	0.9675	1.0000
0.8161	0.8502	0.8889	0.9171	0.9420	0.9675	0.0000
0.8161	0.8502	0.8889	0.9171	0.9420	0.9675	1.0000
0.8161	0.8502	0.8889	0.9171	0.9420	0.9675	1.0000
0.8161	0.8502	0.8889	0.0000	0.0000	0.0000	0.0000

VALUE OF ATTRIBUTE SP	VALUE OF ATTRIBUTE POSTPR1	VALUE OF ATTRIBUTE POSTPR2	VALUE OF ATTRIBUTE POSTPR3	VALUE OF ATTRIBUTE POSTPR4	VALUE OF ATTRIBUTE POSTPR5	VALUE OF ATTRIBUTE POSTPR6
0.8166	0.8506	0.8892	0.9174	0.9421	0.9676	1.0000
0.8166	0.8506	0.8892	0.9174	0.9421	0.9676	1.0000
0.8166	0.8506	0.8892	0.9174	0.9421	0.9676	1.0000
0.8166	0.8506	0.8892	0.9174	0.9421	0.9676	1.0000
0.8166	0.8506	0.8892	0.9174	0.9421	0.9676	1.0000
0.8166	0.8506	0.8892	0.9174	0.9421	0.9676	1.0000
0.8166	0.8506	0.8892	0.9174	0.9421	0.0000	0.0000
0.8166	0.8506	0.8892	0.9174	0.9421	0.9676	1.0000
0.8166	0.8506	0.8892	0.9174	0.9421	0.9676	1.0000
0.8166	0.0000	0.0000	0.0000	0.0000	0.0000	0.0000
0.8166	0.8506	0.8892	0.9174	0.9421	0.9676	1.0000
0.8166	0.8506	0.8892	0.9174	0.9421	0.9676	1.0000
0.8166	0.8506	0.8892	0.9174	0.9421	0.9676	1.0000
0.8166	0.8506	0.8892	0.9174	0.9421	0.9676	1.0000
0.8166	0.8506	0.8892	0.9174	0.9421	0.9676	1.0000
0.8166	0.8506	0.8892	0.9174	0.9421	0.9676	1.0000
0.8166	0.8506	0.8892	0.9174	0.9421	0.9676	1.0000
0.8166	0.8506	0.0000	0.0000	0.0000	0.0000	0.0000
0.8166	0.0000	0.0000	0.0000	0.0000	0.0000	0.0000
0.8491	0.8779	0.9102	0.9334	0.9536	0.9742	1.0000
0.8491	0.8779	0.0000	0.0000	0.0000	0.0000	0.0000
0.8491	0.8779	0.9102	0.9334	0.9536	0.9742	1.0000
0.8491	0.8779	0.9102	0.9334	0.9536	0.9742	1.0000
0.8491	0.8779	0.9102	0.9334	0.9536	0.9742	1.0000
0.8491	0.8779	0.9102	0.9334	0.9536	0.9742	1.0000
0.8491	0.8779	0.9102	0.9334	0.9536	0.9742	0.0000
0.8491	0.8779	0.9102	0.9334	0.9536	0.9742	1.0000
0.8491	0.8779	0.9102	0.9334	0.9536	0.9742	1.0000
0.8491	0.8779	0.9102	0.9334	0.9536	0.9742	1.0000
0.8491	0.8779	0.9102	0.0000	0.0000	0.0000	0.0000
0.8491	0.8779	0.9102	0.9334	0.9536	0.9742	1.0000
0.8491	0.8779	0.9102	0.9334	0.9536	0.9742	1.0000
0.8491	0.8779	0.9102	0.9334	0.9536	0.9742	1.0000
0.8491	0.8779	0.9102	0.9334	0.9536	0.9742	1.0000
0.8491	0.8779	0.9102	0.9334	0.9536	0.9742	1.0000
0.8491	0.8779	0.9102	0.9334	0.9536	0.0000	0.0000
0.8491	0.8779	0.9102	0.9334	0.9536	0.9742	1.0000
0.8491	0.8779	0.9102	0.9334	0.9536	0.9742	1.0000
0.8491	0.8779	0.9102	0.9334	0.9536	0.9742	1.0000
0.8491	0.8779	0.9102	0.9334	0.9536	0.9742	1.0000
0.8491	0.8779	0.9102	0.9334	0.9536	0.9742	1.0000
0.8491	0.8779	0.9102	0.9334	0.9536	0.9742	1.0000
0.8491	0.8779	0.9102	0.9334	0.9536	0.9742	1.0000
0.8491	0.8779	0.9102	0.9334	0.9536	0.9742	1.0000
0.8491	0.8779	0.9102	0.9334	0.9536	0.9742	1.0000
0.8491	0.0000	0.0000	0.0000	0.0000	0.0000	0.0000
0.8491	0.8779	0.9102	0.9334	0.9536	0.9742	1.0000
0.8491	0.8779	0.0000	0.0000	0.0000	0.0000	0.0000
0.8513	0.8798	0.9116	0.9345	0.9544	0.9746	1.0000
0.8513	0.8798	0.9116	0.9345	0.9544	0.9746	1.0000

VALUE OF ATTRIBUTE SP	VALUE OF ATTRIBUTE POSTPR1	VALUE OF ATTRIBUTE POSTPR2	VALUE OF ATTRIBUTE POSTPR3	VALUE OF ATTRIBUTE POSTPR4	VALUE OF ATTRIBUTE POSTPR5	VALUE OF ATTRIBUTE POSTPR6
0.8513	0.8798	0.9116	0.9345	0.9544	0.9746	1.0000
0.8513	0.8798	0.9116	0.9345	0.9544	0.9746	1.0000
0.8513	0.8798	0.9116	0.9345	0.9544	0.9746	1.0000
0.8513	0.8798	0.9116	0.9345	0.9544	0.9746	1.0000
0.8513	0.8798	0.9116	0.9345	0.9544	0.9746	1.0000
0.8513	0.8798	0.9116	0.9345	0.9544	0.9746	1.0000
0.8513	0.8798	0.9116	0.9345	0.9544	0.9746	1.0000
0.8513	0.8798	0.9116	0.9345	0.9544	0.9746	1.0000
0.8513	0.8798	0.9116	0.9345	0.9544	0.9746	1.0000
0.8513	0.8798	0.9116	0.9345	0.9544	0.9746	1.0000
0.8622	0.9024	0.9409	0.9639	0.9800	0.9923	1.0000
0.8622	0.9024	0.9409	0.9639	0.9800	0.9923	1.0000
0.8622	0.9024	0.9409	0.9639	0.9800	0.9923	1.0000
0.8622	0.9024	0.9409	0.9639	0.9800	0.9923	1.0000
0.8622	0.9024	0.9409	0.9639	0.9800	0.9923	1.0000
0.9061	0.9250	0.9456	0.9601	0.9724	0.9848	1.0000
0.9061	0.9250	0.9456	0.9601	0.9724	0.9848	1.0000
0.9061	0.9250	0.9456	0.9601	0.9724	0.9848	1.0000
0.9061	0.9250	0.9456	0.9601	0.9724	0.9848	1.0000
0.9061	0.9250	0.9456	0.9601	0.9724	0.0000	0.0000
0.9061	0.9250	0.9456	0.9601	0.9724	0.9848	1.0000
0.9061	0.9250	0.9456	0.9601	0.9724	0.9848	1.0000
0.9061	0.9250	0.9456	0.9601	0.9724	0.9848	1.0000
0.9061	0.9250	0.9456	0.9601	0.9724	0.9848	1.0000
0.9061	0.9250	0.9456	0.9601	0.9724	0.9848	1.0000
0.9061	0.9250	0.9456	0.9601	0.9724	0.9848	1.0000
0.9061	0.9250	0.9456	0.9601	0.9724	0.9848	1.0000
0.9061	0.9250	0.9456	0.9601	0.9724	0.9848	1.0000
0.9061	0.9250	0.9456	0.9601	0.9724	0.9848	1.0000
0.9061	0.9250	0.9456	0.9601	0.9724	0.9848	1.0000
0.9061	0.9250	0.9456	0.9601	0.9724	0.9848	1.0000
0.9061	0.9250	0.9456	0.9601	0.9724	0.9848	1.0000
0.9061	0.9250	0.9456	0.9601	0.9724	0.9848	1.0000

Appendix B

Some Concepts Underlying Probabilistic Medical Models

When there is at least some uncertainty surrounding whether or not and when a medically significant event has occurred or will occur, a probabilistic model is frequently appropriate. Probabilistic modeling is also useful in analyzing situations where a patient's true underlying state or condition (e.g., cure) is not known for sure. Because some degree of uncertainty is common in the practice of medicine, there are many opportunities for probabilistic modeling.

In many contexts there is some particular event or medical outcome that commands special attention. We shall designate this as focal. To be designated focal just means that the context suggests focusing special attention upon it.

For example, it is common in clinical studies of chronic diseases (e.g., in a clinical trial of a new cancer drug) to select a specific end point. This is the thing about which study conclusions will finally be drawn. Being selected to serve as an end point renders the targeted item focal in the study context.

A relevant event or outcome other than one designated as focal we shall refer to simply as alternative. It is always the context surrounding an event or outcome that determines whether it is designated as focal or alternative. It regularly happens that what is deemed focal in one context becomes alternative in a different context, and vice versa.

From an oncologist's point of view, for example, a lightning strike causing a patient's untimely death would likely be regarded as an alternative rather than a focal event. Death by lightning is unusual in an oncologist's experience. It would rarely qualify as focal in the analysis of patient records. To the company from which the patient purchased insurance against accidental death, however, that same lighting strike would likely be viewed as a focal event.

In the simplest situation, there is only something and its logical complement to consider. By defining them in a mutually exclusive and collectively exhaustive manner, they can be described probabilistically in terms of ordinary betting odds. The occurrence and nonoccurrence of a focal event can be assigned separate numeric probabilities, where the two probabilities add to 1.0 or 100 percent. The achievement or nonachievement of a focal outcome and the experience or nonexpereince of a focal end point can be similarly treated.

The odds favoring the occurrence of a focal event are defined as the ratio of the two probabilities. The numerator of the ratio is the probability that the focal event does occur. The denominator is the complementary probability that it does not occur (assuming that nonoccurrence is possible, thereby receiving a nonzero probability). The odds against the occurrence of a focal event are defined as the reciprocal ratio (again, excluding possible division by zero). The odds favoring and against achieving or not achieving a focal outcome and experiencing or not experiencing a focal end point are similarly defined.

Logistic regression analysis (Logit) has been specifically designed to explain and to predict the betting odds associated with a focal event, outcome, or end point and its logical complement. Explanations and predictions are based on some set of prognostic or diagnostic factors (often called covariates) about which data have been gathered. Logistic regression is described in appendix D.

Also of great interest, especially in the context of cancer and other progressive diseases, is the time required for a focal event to occur. This refers to the time elapsed between some reference event, such as a patient's initial diagnosis, and observation of a focal event, such as a relapse or recurrence of some form of cancer.

Elapsed times generally encompass many more than just two possibilities. They are normally viewed as continuous quantities.

Kaplan-Meier analysis is designed to identify survival patterns. A Kaplan-Meier curve traces out the shape and contours of such a pattern over time. Survival time is defined as the duration of an interval starting with the occurrence of some reference event, but during which a designated focal event does not occur. Kaplan-Meier analysis is described in appendix E.

Cox (proportional hazards) regression analysis also focuses on survival time. It is designed to explain and to predict the duration of survival time on the basis of a set of prognostic or diagnostic factors (covariates) about which data have been gathered. Cox regression is described in appendix F.

When discussing elapsed times, it is always necessary to specify precisely:

1. the nature of the reference event and the point in time when it occurs;
2. the nature of the subsequent focal event and the point in time when it later occurs; and
3. the particular scale in terms of which the time elapsed between the reference and focal events is measured (e.g., in days, in weeks, in months, or in years), where the zero point on the elapsed time scale always corresponds to the moment when the reference event occurs.

Distinguishing when a focal event actually occurs from when it is initially observed can sometimes be difficult. Suppose, for example, that a breast lump is first detected by a patient's radiologist after an annually scheduled mammogram. How long ago was it when that lump first came into existence?

The date of the mammogram provides an upper bound to the answer. It is the latest date when the lump could have come into existence. Previous mammograms, previous visits to her primary care physician, and self-examinations, none of which disclosed any breast lump, may provide a lower bound to the answer. They rule out various earlier dates when it might first have developed. However, the exact date of initial existence is frequently difficult to pinpoint.

This kind of problem is common in medical data. It is often ignored by treating the date of first observation as if it were the date of initial existence. Such observations are then said to be left-censored. As long as an earliest possible date can be established as a lower bound and as long as the left-censored upper bound date of first observation does not occur too much later than the earliest possible date, the problem may not be too severe.

Unfortunately, this is not always the case. The initial detection of certain cancers that can develop over a long period of time without obvious symptoms (e.g., pancreatic cancer) may be delayed too long. If its initial detection does not occur until the cancer has reached a late stage, the possibility of an effective remedy is severely compromised. Even when obvious symptoms do develop, they can be ignored or misinterpreted (i.e., not properly diagnosed in time), with the same unfortunate consequence.

This book contains no specific procedures to deal with the problem of left-censored observations. The recorded date of first observation of any focal event will normally be construed as its actual date of occurrence. The way most medical data are collected and recorded precludes doing anything else.

Based on the preceding specifications and subject to possible timing inaccuracies due to left-censoring, it is customary to fit a variety of probabilistic models to elapsed times that are actually observed and become a part of a patient's record. Probabilistic models come in two varieties:

1. continuous-time models, where elapsed time is viewed as a continuous, nonnegative, real-valued variable, and the focal event can occur anywhere along the continuous elapsed time scale; and
2. discrete-time models, where elapsed time is viewed as a discrete, nonnegative, real-valued variable, and the focal event can only occur at one of the particular times that comprise the discrete time scale (i.e., not before the shortest elapsed time nor between any two adjacent elapsed times nor after the longest elapsed time in the ordered set of distinct times that comprise that discrete time scale).

All such probabilistic models incorporate the same generic concepts. In the continuous case, these generic concepts are embodied within and defined by the following four types of continuous mathematical functions.

1. An underlying probability density function

    A. Elapsed time t is regarded as a continuous, nonnegative, real-valued variable. For this reason pdf(t), a probability density function, is defined that assigns a nonnegative rate of probability increase per unit time to every elapsed time t.
    B. This is not the same thing as PMF(t), a probability mass function that assigns the probability itself that a focal event will occur at time t to each discrete elapsed time t. Probability mass functions are used instead of probability density functions in discrete models.
    C. Whereas a probability assigned by a probability mass function can never exceed a numeric value of 1.0, a rate of probability increase assigned by a probability density function may exceed 1.0.
    D. In a continuous probability model it is conventional to define the probability that an event will occur precisely at any elapsed time t as zero.
    E. The probability density, pdf(t), assigned to every elapsed time t defines the instantaneous rate of increase in the probability that the focal event will occur at each of those t units of elapsed time.

2. A corresponding continuous distribution function

    A. If pdf(t), a probability density function, possesses a corresponding integral (antiderivative) function, then the definite integral evaluated between zero (when the reference event occurs) and t is defined as F(t), the distribution function of t.
    B. Conversely, the first derivative of F(t), the distribution function of t, is pdf(t), its corresponding probability density function.
    C. The distribution function of t, F(t), assigns to every elapsed time t the probability that a focal event will occur sometime during those t units of time elapsed since the occurrence of the reference event (i.e., sometime within the time interval between time 0 and time t). When evaluated at the highest possible value of t (or at positive infinity), F(t) = 1.0.

  D. Distribution functions are cumulative left-tail probability
     functions. As such they are nondecreasing (typically
     increasing) functions of t.
  E. The probability that some focal event will occur between
     elapsed times t1 and t2, where t1 is equal to or less than t2,
     is the value of the distribution function of t1 subtracted from
     its (always equal or greater) value of t2, F(t2) - F(t1).
  F. If t1 were exactly equal to t2, the probability that some focal
     event would occur precisely at elapsed time t1 = t2 would be
     F(t2) - F(t1) = F(t2) - F(t2) = F(t1) - F(t1) = 0. This is
     consistent with the notion that in a continuous model, the
     probability that any event will occur precisely at any elapsed
     time t is always taken to be zero.

3. A corresponding continuous survival function

  A. A survival function is the complement of its associated
     distribution function. The survival function of t, S(t), is
     simply F(t), the distribution function of t, subtracted from
     1.0. Thus, S(t) = 1 - F(t).
  B. S(t) assigns to every elapsed time t the probability that a
     focal event will not occur during those t units of elapsed time
     (e.g., that a patient will survive for more than t units of
     elapsed time without experiencing the focal event).
  C. Survival functions are cumulative right-tail probability
     functions. As such they are nonincreasing (typically
     decreasing) functions of t.
  D. The probability that some focal event will occur between
     elapsed times t1 and t2, where t1 is equal to or less than t2,
     may be calculated as the value of the survival function of t2
     subtracted from its (always equal or greater) value of t1,
     S(t1) - S(t2).
  E. [Historical note: The survival function originally got its name
     from the analysis of mortality statistics. This was one of the
     earliest applications of probabilistic models to the realm of
     human aging and disease progression. When fitting probabilistic
     models to mortality data, the focal event is death (all
     causes). It was natural to define its avoidance as "survival."
     More recently, similar models have been applied to other focal
     events besides death. For example, it is common to speak of
     relapse-free survival, where the focal event being avoided is a
     relapse or some form of recurrence of a progressive disease. A
     survival function will refer to any focal event, as defined
     herein, including, but by no means restricted to, the death of
     a patient.]

4. A corresponding continuous hazard function

  A. A hazard function is the ratio of its associated probability
     density function to its associated survival function. The
     hazard function of t, h(t), is therefore pdf(t)/S(t), assuming
     that S(t) is not zero.
  B. It assigns to every elapsed time t the instantaneous rate of
     occurrence per unit time of a focal event, given that the focal
     event has not yet occurred during those t units of elapsed
     time. It is an instantaneous rate of occurrence, conditional on
     no focal event yet having occurred.
  C. Notice that a hazard is a rate or ratio, but not a probability.
     The distinction is the same as between a probability density

and a probability itself. Like all probabilities a hazard rate is always a nonnegative number. Both pdf(t) and S(t) are nonnegative numbers, and h(t) is simply pdf(t) divided by S(t). On the other hand, like a probability density, a hazard rate may exceed a numeric value of 1.0, which a true probability can never do.

D. A hazard rate may be interpreted as a conditional (upon no focal event yet) probability density. It is sometimes more conveniently interpreted as an instantaneous rate of occurrence of a focal event (given no event yet), measured in terms of the number of occurrences per unit time.

E. Unlike the cumulative probability of occurrence of a focal event, which cannot decrease with elapsed time, and unlike its complementary survival probability, which cannot increase with elapsed time, the hazard rate of occurrence of a focal event (also called its instantaneous risk of occurrence) may either increase, decrease, or remain the same as further time elapses. For example:

   I. the risk (hazard rate) of death (all causes) increases slowly (but steadily) after an individual passes through childhood and then accelerates noticeably after the age of about fifty;

   II. when focusing on the organ (not the patient), its risk (hazard rate) of failure appears to decrease steadily as time elapses following transplant surgery; and

   III. the risk (hazard rate) of further progression of invasive breast cancer appears to remain relatively constant over a substantial period of time for those noncured patients who remain at risk following either radical or modified radical mastectomy and radiation.

F. Even more, hazard rates may undergo complicated sequences of such changes during successive subintervals of elapsed time. For example:

   I. the progress of a patient diagnosed with Hodgkin's disease displays an initially increasing followed by a decreasing risk (hazard rate) of disease-specific death over time; and

   II. a principal aim of medical interventions (such as surgery, radiation, and adjuvant therapy in the case of cancer patients) is to reduce substantially or even to eliminate completely the patient's risk (hazard rate) of further disease progression.

Because of their definitional interrelatedness, a continuous probability model may be specified completely by any one of the above four functions. The other three functions can then be derived directly from whichever one is initially given.

In the discrete case, the same generic concepts are embodied within and defined by the following four types of analogous discrete mathematical functions.

   1. An underlying probability mass function

      A. Elapsed time t is regarded as a discrete, nonnegative, real-valued variable. For this reason PMF(t), a probability mass function, is defined that assigns the probability that a focal event will occur at time t to each elapsed time in the set of possible elapsed times comprising the discrete time scale.

B. The separate probabilities assigned by a probability mass function to the elapsed times comprising the discrete time scale sum to 1.0.

C. This is not the same thing as a probability density function, pdf(t), which assigns to every continuously defined elapsed time t the instantaneous rate of increase in the probability that the focal event will occur at precisely that elapsed time.

D. Whereas a rate of probability increase assigned by a probability density function may exceed a numeric value of 1.0, a probability assigned by a probability mass function can never exceed 1.0.

E. In a discrete probability model, the probability that a focal event will occur precisely at any elapsed time t is generally a positive number (never negative), although it may be zero for some values of t, but not for all values of t comprising the discrete time scale.

2. A corresponding discrete distribution function

A. The discrete distribution function of t, F(t), is the cumulative sum of the successive values of PMF(t) for all elapsed times equal to or less than t.

B. F(t), the distribution function, assigns to every elapsed time t the probability that a focal event will occur at some one of the discrete times elapsed since the occurrence of the reference event (i.e., sometime within the time interval between time 0 and time t).

C. Distribution functions are cumulative left-tail probability step functions. As such they are nondecreasing (typically increasing) functions of t.

D. The probability that some focal event will occur between elapsed times ti and tj, where ti is equal to or less than tj, is the value of the distribution function of ti subtracted from its (always equal or greater) value of tj, F(tj) - F(ti).

3. A corresponding discrete survival function

A. As in the continuous case, a discrete survival function is the complement of its associated distribution function. The survival function of t, S(t), is simply the distribution function of t, F(t), subtracted from 1.0. Again, S(t) = 1 - F(t).

B. S(t) assigns to every elapsed time t the probability that a focal event will not occur at any one of the discrete times elapsed since the occurrence of the reference event up to and including time t (e.g., that a patient will survive beyond elapsed time t without experiencing the focal event).

C. Survival functions are cumulative right-tail probability step functions. As such they are nonincreasing (typically decreasing) functions of t.

D. The probability that some focal event will occur between elapsed times ti and tj, where ti is equal to or less than tj, may be calculated as the value of the survival function of tj subtracted from its (always equal or greater) value of ti, S(ti) - S(tj).

4. A corresponding discrete hazard function

    A. A discrete hazard function assigns to each elapsed time t comprising the discrete time scale the conditional probability that the focal event will occur at time t, given that it has not yet occurred at any prior time.

    B. A discrete hazard function is the ratio of its associated probability mass function, PMF(t), to its associated survival function, S(t-), where S(t) is evaluated at t-, the immediately preceding time in the discrete time scale.

    C. The discrete hazard function of t, h(t), is PMF(t)/S(t-), assuming that there is an immediately preceding time, t- and assuming that S(t-) is not zero. In the special case of the first time in the discrete time scale, where there is no preceding time, h(t) = PMF(t).

    D. Unlike a continuous hazard rate, whose numeric value can exceed 1.0, a discrete hazard rate is a genuine conditional probability. Its value can never exceed 1.0. The discrete hazard rate is the conditional probability that the focal event will occur at time t, given that the focal event has not yet occurred.

    E. As in the continuous case, a discrete hazard rate of occurrence of a focal event (also called its risk of occurrence) may either increase, decrease, or remain the same as time elapses.

Because of their definitional interrelatedness, a discrete probabilistic model may also be specified completely by any one of the above four functions. The other three can then be derived from whichever one is initially given.

Appendix C

Four Probabilistic Models

This book makes extensive use of four particular probabilistic models embodied in four probability distributions:

1. the uniform (rectangular) distribution;
2. the exponential distribution;
3. the Weibull distribution (of which the exponential distribution is a special case); and
4. the Poisson distribution (a probability mass function that assigns discrete probabilities to the number of events occurring within a time interval, but whose interevent times are exponentially distributed).

Except in the case of the Poisson model, each distribution is continuous. Its defining functions are all continuous and defined on elapsed time t, the model's single, nonnegative, real-valued independent variable. Time t refers to the time elapsed from the moment when a reference event occurs (always, by convention, at elapsed time zero) until the moment when some focal event is or could be observed to occur.

The sets of four interrelated functions defining, respectively, the uniform, the exponential, and the Weibull model are described in the pages that follow. The Poisson model and the Poisson distribution are also described. To ensure clarity, discussions of each model are separated by page spacing.

The Uniform (Rectangular) Model

The four interrelated functions defining the uniform model are as follows.

1. The underlying uniform probability density function

   pdf(t) = 1/MAXTIME, 0 =< t =< MAXTIME, where

   t is an interval of time ending at elapsed time t;
   MAXTIME is the maximum time that may elapse before the focal event must occur; and
   pdf(t) is the probability density (instantaneous rate of increase in the probability of occurrence) assigned to elapsed time t.

   MAXTIME is the single parameter specifying a particular uniform distribution, and it must always be a strictly positive number.

   Notice that the uniform distribution requires that the focal event must always occur sometime within the time interval ending at t = MAXTIME.

2. Its integral, the cumulative left-tail distribution function

   F(t) = t/MAXTIME, 0 =< t =< MAXTIME, where

   t is the interval of time ending at elapsed time t during which the focal event can occur;
   MAXTIME is the maximum possible length of that interval; and
   F(t) is the probability that the focal event does occur sometime within that interval assigned to the time t elapsed during that interval.

3. Its associated survival function, the cumulative right-tail function (the complement of the cumulative left-tail distribution function)

   S(t) = 1 - t/MAXTIME, 0 =< t =< MAXTIME, where

   t is the interval of time ending at elapsed time t during which the focal event can occur;
   MAXTIME is the maximum possible length of that interval; and
   S(t) is the probability that the focal event does not occur at any time within that interval assigned to the time t elapsed during that interval.

4. Its associated hazard function

   h(t) = 1/(MAXTIME - t), 0 =< t < MAXTIME, where

   t is an interval of time ending at elapsed time t;
   MAXTIME is the upper limit of the half-open interval of time that may elapse before the focal event must occur; and
   h(t) is the hazard rate (the instantaneous rate of occurrence of the focal event) assigned to elapsed time t, given that the focal event has not yet occurred within the time interval ending at t.

   Notice that the hazard rate h(t) increases monotonically when 0 =< t < MAXTIME and that it increases rapidly and without bound as t approaches its limiting value MAXTIME. The longer it takes for the focal event to occur within the MAXTIME interval, the higher its hazard rate becomes, increasing without bound to guarantee that the focal event will eventually occur sometime during the interval.

The hazard function becomes discontinuous (undefined) when
t = MAXTIME.

5. The above four functions are defined in terms of a focal event. This is
   done to maintain comparability in exposition relative to the
   exponential and Weibull models that are about to be described.

6. The uniform distribution is utilized to simulate when within a finite
   interval of time a patient is last seen by a physician. Strictly
   speaking this is a censoring rather than a focal event.

7. Simulation as a way to test hypotheses and as a means to fine-tune an
   initial partitioning for the MRPA algorithm is introduced in section 4
   of this book. The RISKTEST simulator that implements these procedures
   is described in appendix H.

8. In a simulation context, the distinction between a focal and a
   censoring event is immaterial, but it does make a difference
   interpretively. The typical focal event treated in this book is not
   guaranteed to occur within any finite time interval. The uniform
   distribution would, therefore, not be an appropriate model for the
   occurrence of a typical focal event.

The Exponential Model

The four interrelated functions defining the exponential model are as follows.

1. The underlying exponential probability density function

   pdf(t) = LAMBDA*EXP(-LAMBDA*t), t >= 0, LAMBDA > 0, where

   * means multiply;
   t is an interval of time ending at elapsed time t;
   LAMBDA is the rate of occurrence per unit time of the focal event; and
   pdf(t) is the probability density (instantaneous rate of increase in the probability of occurrence) assigned to elapsed time t.

   LAMBDA, an intensity parameter, is the single parameter specifying a particular exponential distribution.

2. Its integral, the cumulative left-tail distribution function

   F(t) = 1 - EXP(-LAMBDA*t), t >= 0, LAMBDA > 0, where

   * means multiply;
   t is the interval of time ending at elapsed time t during which the focal event can occur;
   LAMBDA is the rate of occurrence per unit time of the focal event; and
   F(t) is the probability that the focal event does occur sometime within that interval assigned to the time t elapsed during that interval.

3. Its associated survival function, the cumulative right-tail function (the complement of the cumulative left-tail distribution function)

   S(t) = EXP(-LAMBDA*t), t >= 0, LAMBDA > 0, where

   * means multiply;
   t is the interval of time ending at elapsed time t during which the focal event can occur;
   LAMBDA is the rate of occurrence per unit time of the focal event; and
   S(t) is the probability that the focal event does not occur at any time within that interval assigned to the time t elapsed during that interval.

4. Its associated hazard function

   h(t) = LAMBDA (constant over time), t >= 0, LAMBDA > 0, where

   t is an interval of time ending at elapsed time t;
   LAMBDA is the rate of occurrence per unit time of the focal event; and
   h(t) is the hazard rate (the instantaneous rate of occurrence of the focal event) assigned to elapsed time t, given that the focal event has not yet occurred within the time interval ending at t.

   Notice that the hazard rate h(t) = LAMBDA is constant over time.

The Weibull Model

The four interrelated functions defining the Weibull model are as follows.

1. The underlying Weibull probability density function

    pdf(t) = [LAMBDA*DELTA]*[(LAMBDA*t)^(DELTA-1)]*EXP[-(LAMBDA*t)^DELTA],
    t >= 0, LAMBDA > 0, DELTA > 0, where

    * means multiply;
    ^ means exponentiate by (raise to the power of) the immediately
    following expression;
    t is an interval of time ending at elapsed time t;
    LAMBDA is an intensity parameter related to the rate of occurrence per
    unit time of the focal event;
    DELTA is a trend parameter indicating whether the hazard rate is
    increasing or decreasing over time; and
    pdf(t) is the probability density (instantaneous rate of increase in
    the probability of occurrence) assigned to elapsed time t.

    LAMBDA, the intensity parameter, and DELTA, the trend parameter, are
    the two parameters specifying a particular Weibull distribution.

    Notice that if DELTA = 1.0, the Weibull density function reduces to the
    exponential density function. This means that the exponential
    distribution is a special case of the Weibull distribution, when the
    Weibull distribution's trend parameter is exactly 1.0. In this special
    case the Weibull intensity parameter (LAMBDA) and the exponential
    intensity parameter (LAMBDA) become identical in both interpretation
    and numeric value.

    If DELTA < 1.0 the instantaneous hazard rate decreases at a decreasing
    rate over time. The smaller the value of DELTA, the more sharply the
    hazard rate decreases initially.

    If DELTA = 1.0 the instantaneous hazard rate remains constant over time
    (because the Weibull distribution has reduced to an exponential
    distribution).

    If DELTA > 1.0 the instantaneous hazard rate increases at a decreasing
    rate over time. The larger the value of DELTA, the more sharply the
    hazard rate increases initially.

2. Its integral, the cumulative left-tail distribution function

    F(t) = 1 - EXP[-(LAMBDA*t)^DELTA], t >= 0, LAMBDA > 0, DELTA > 0, where

    * means multiply;
    ^ means exponentiate by (raise to the power of) the immediately
    following expression;
    t is the interval of time ending at elapsed time t during which the
    focal event can occur;
    LAMBDA is an intensity parameter related to the rate of occurrence per
    unit time of the focal event;
    DELTA is a trend parameter indicating whether the hazard rate is
    increasing or decreasing over time; and
    F(t) is the probability that the focal event does occur sometime within
    that interval assigned to the time t elapsed during that interval.

3. Its associated survival function, the cumulative right-tail function (the complement of the cumulative left-tail distribution function)

S(t) = EXP[-(LAMBDA*t)^DELTA], t >= 0, LAMBDA > 0, DELTA > 0, where

* means multiply;
^ means exponentiate by (raise to the power of) the immediately following expression;
t is the interval of time ending at elapsed time t during which the focal event can occur;
LAMBDA is an intensity parameter related to the rate of occurrence per unit time of the focal event;
DELTA is a trend parameter indicating whether the hazard rate is increasing or decreasing over time; and
S(t) is the probability that the focal event does not occur at any time within that interval assigned to the time t elapsed during that interval.

4. Its associated hazard function

h(t) = [LAMBDA*DELTA]*[(LAMBDA*t)^(DELTA-1)], t >= 0, LAMBDA > 0, DELTA > 0, where
* means multiply;
^ means exponentiate by (raise to the power of) the immediately following expression;
t is an interval of time ending at elapsed time t;
LAMBDA is an intensity parameter related to the rate of occurrence per unit time of the focal event;
DELTA is a trend parameter indicating whether the hazard rate is increasing or decreasing over time; and
h(t) is the hazard rate (the instantaneous rate of occurrence of the focal event) assigned to elapsed time t, given that the focal event has not yet occurred within the time interval ending at t.

Notice that if DELTA = 1.0, the instantaneous hazard rate is LAMBDA and remains constant over time (because the Weibull distribution has reduced to the exponential distribution).

If DELTA < 1.0, the instantaneous hazard rate decreases at a decreasing rate over time. The smaller the value of DELTA, the more sharply the hazard rate decreases initially.

If DELTA > 1.0, the instantaneous hazard rate increases at a decreasing rate over time. The larger the value of DELTA, the more sharply the hazard rate increases initially.

Because of this behavior, one might view the Weibull distribution as a more flexible version of the exponential distribution, where the hazard rate may remain but is not required to remain constant over time. The hazard rate may also rise consistently or it may fall consistently as time passes.

The Poisson Model

Closely related to the exponential distribution is the Poisson distribution. It assigns a probability to the number of times the same repetitive event occurs during a specified time interval.

If it is known that a certain number of patients are acquired over a given time span (e.g., for a clinical trial), the Poisson distribution may be used to simulate the patient acquisition process. The repeated event is the acquisition of each successive patient. Use of the Poisson model ensures that successive acquisitions are treated as random with respect to their timing.

The underlying Poisson probability function is a probability mass function (PMF) rather than a probability density function (pdf). This is because it assigns probability to a discrete independent variable (the number of times an event occurs during a specified time interval) rather than to a continuous independent variable (the time elapsed until a single such event occurs).

The Poisson probability mass function is

PMF(n,t) = {[EXP(-LAMBDA*t)]*[LAMBDA*t]^n}/[n!], t >= 0, LAMBDA > 0, n = 0, 1, 2, ... , where

* means multiply;
^ means exponentiate by (raise to the power of) the immediately following expression;
n! means n factorial;
t is the length of an elapsed time interval, treated as a continuous variable;
n is the number of occurrences of the repetitive event during that interval, treated as a discrete, integer-valued variable;
LAMBDA is the rate of occurrence per unit time of the event (i.e., the average or expected number of times the event occurs during a unit time interval, also called the Poisson process intensity); and
PMF(n,t) is the probability that exactly n events (n = 0, 1, 2, ...) will occur during the time interval of length t, given a Poisson process intensity of LAMBDA.

Notice that if no events occur during an elapsed time interval (i.e., if n = 0), the Poisson probability mass function reduces to the exponential survival function, EXP(-LAMBDA*t). This means that the elapsed times between successive events in a Poisson process are exponentially distributed, in which case the Poisson LAMBDA and the exponential survival LAMBDA are treated as identical in both interpretation and numeric value. This equivalence was exploited in various RISKTEST simulations described in earlier sections of this book.

Appendix D

Logistic Regression Analysis

Logistic regression (Logit) is a specialized form of regression analysis. It is useful in assessing the ability of various patient attributes and situational characteristics (covariates) to predict the natural logarithm of the betting odds applicable to the occurrence of an uncertain focal event.

Betting odds favoring the occurrence of an event are defined as the ratio of two probabilities. The numerator of the ratio is the probability that the focal event does occur. The denominator is the complementary probability that it does not occur. This assumes that nonoccurrence is possible, thereby receiving a nonzero probability. The two probabilities must add to 1.0.

The odds against the occurrence of a focal event are defined as the reciprocal ratio (again, excluding possible division by zero). The odds favoring and against being in a focal state and achieving or failing to achieve a focal outcome or end point are similarly defined.

Extended forms of logistic regression can predict in which of two or more separate categories a patient belongs, which of two or more future events will occur, and so forth. However, we shall restrict our attention in this book to dichotomous logistic regression to predict one of two mutually exclusive and collectively exhaustive possibilities or, equivalently, to discriminate between two such possibilities.

The dependent variable of dichotomous logistic regression (embodying the thing to be predicted) is numerically coded as either 0 or 1. By convention, occurrence of the focal event, being in the focal state, or experiencing the focal outcome is typically coded 1. Its logical complement (the alternative event, state, or outcome) is coded 0. Each patient in a sample of data to be analyzed is then assigned either a 0 or a 1, identifying in which category that patient is observed to fall.

Patient attributes and situational characteristics (covariates) believed to have prognostic, diagnostic, or discriminatory capability constitute the independent variables. A corresponding set of k (k >= 1) numerically coded values of each covariate is also assigned to each patient in the sample.

It must be at least plausible to view a collected data set as a sample drawn both randomly and independently from some well-defined and reasonably homogeneous patient population (or subpopulation, from PCM's perspective).

The logistic regression model is probabilistic in nature. It assumes that the natural logarithm of the betting odds favoring falling into the focal (coded 1) versus the alternative (coded 0) category is a linear function of that patient's prognostic, diagnostic, or discriminatory covariates

B0 + B1*X1 + B2*X2 + ... + Bk*Xk, where

* means multiply;
X1, X2, ... , Xk are numerically coded variables embodying the individual patient attributes and situational characteristics believed to possess prognostic, diagnostic, or discriminatory capability; and
B0, B1, B2, ... , Bk are undetermined coefficients estimated from the regression analysis that indicate by their algebraic sign whether each predictor raises or lowers an individual patient's likelihood of experiencing the focal event and by how much, indicated by their magnitude.

Outputs of logistic regression include:

1. estimates of the population regression coefficients, B0 and B1, B2, ... , Bk associated, respectively, with the k predictive covariates, along with a standard deviation and an accompanying two-tailed p value associated with each coefficient; and
2. two chi-square measures of the goodness of fit of the sample data analyzed according to the underlying logistic regression model and accompanying two-tailed p values associated with each.

As with Cox regression, it is always good practice to check the plausibility of the model underlying logistic regression before interpreting its results. If the two-tailed p values accompanying the chi-square goodness-of-fit statistics are "high enough" (e.g., at least 0.10), the assumption that the logarithm of the betting odds is a linear function of the set of k covariates would seem plausible.

For PCM the most important benefit derivable from a successful logistic regression analysis is an individually tailored probability that each patient in the sample falls in the focal versus the alternate category. Assuming that the focal category is assigned a value of 1, the individually tailored probability is estimated as

EXP(B0 + B1*X1 + B2*X2 + ... + Bk*Xk) divided by
[1+EXP(B0 + B1*X1 + B2*X2 + ... + Bk*Xk)], where

* means multiply; and
EXP means to exponentiate the directly following expression, using the base e of the natural logarithm system.

Appendix E

The Kaplan-Meier Survival Model

The Kaplan-Meier survival model provides an extremely general, an extremely useful, and an extremely popular way to represent and analyze survival data gleaned from patient medical records. There are several reasons for this.

It rests on a discrete data model that may be fitted exactly to almost any suitable data collection. Once a sample of observations has been obtained and once both a reference event and a focal event have been identified, the discrete time scale for Kaplan-Meier survival analysis is defined as the ordered set of strictly positive and distinct elapsed times when at least one of those patients experiences the focal event.

It is in this sense that the model may be fitted exactly to almost any data. The set of distinct elapsed times when focal events are actually observed to occur constitutes its discrete time scale. No such fit is possible, of course, to a data set wherein not a single patient ever experiences the focal event.

Aside from being discrete, the fitted data model assumes no particular distributional form. No population parameters need be estimated from sample data, although it is sometimes possible and appropriate to do so. This is why the Kaplan-Meier model is characterized as nonparametric or distribution-free. It is potentially applicable to any sample containing at least one patient who actually experiences the focal event drawn from any population, regardless of how elapsed times are distributed in that population.

The Kaplan-Meier model recognizes two different varieties of elapsed times.

1. A focal event time is the time elapsed between when the reference event occurs and when the focal event occurs if the focal event is actually observed to occur.
2. A censored time (strictly speaking, a right-censored time or a right-censored observation) is the time elapsed between when the reference event occurs and the last time the patient was observed following the reference event, but without the focal event's having (yet) occurred.

Censoring means rendered unobservable for some reason. It does not mean that the focal event cannot or will not occur. If and when the focal event does occur or might otherwise occur, it is just not observed.

Thus, if the focal event is disease-specific death, death due to an unrelated cause is treated as a censoring event. Disease-specific death might otherwise have occurred, subsequently, but it could not be observed due to earlier-occurring death from an unrelated cause.

When a patient is lost to follow-up before a focal event is observed to occur, that typically renders unobservable any subsequent focal event that might occur.

The ability to incorporate both focal event times and censored times into a single data model is especially useful when data are collected with short follow-up periods. Terminating the observation process is a common censoring event. Because of that, data sets with short follow-up frequently contain a high proportion of censored observations, which would otherwise have to be discarded from any analysis.

It must be at least plausible to view a collected data set as a sample drawn both randomly and independently from some well-defined and reasonably homogeneous population. The presumption of independent random sampling imposes the following requirements.

1. Focal event times must be treatable as an independent random sample drawn from some well-defined population of focal event times.
2. Censored times (if any are included in the data) must be treatable as an independent random sample drawn from some well-defined population of censored times.
3. The two samples of elapsed times (if the sample includes both) must be treatable as if they had been obtained independently of one another.

Fitting the Kaplan-Meier model to the data then produces a discrete survival function. This is the usual cumulative right-tail probability step function, where a downward step occurs at each successive distinct focal event time t in the fitted time scale.

When represented in graphical form, it is called a Kaplan-Meier survival curve.

The Kaplan-Meier survival function assigns to each time t the probability that the focal event will not occur at any one of the discrete times elapsed since the occurrence of the reference event up to and including time t (the patient will survive beyond elapsed time t without experiencing the focal event).

Based on the independent random sampling assumption, the discrete survival function produced from sample data via the product-limit method of calculation may be regarded as a maximum likelihood estimate of the parent population's discrete survival function. From this may be inferred the corresponding discrete

1. population probability mass function;
2. population cumulative left-tail distribution function; and
3. population hazard function.

These, in turn, support a variety of inferences about the entire set of patients belonging to the same parent population.

The sample data prepared for Kaplan-Meier analysis may also be used to test the goodness of fit of particular probability distributions such as the ones described in appendix C. When an assumed underlying population distribution fits the sample data "closely enough," more precise inferences may be drawn concerning the parent population.

Bear in mind, however, that the fundamental concept of a survival function as outlined in appendix B rests upon the presumption that all patients are at substantial risk of experiencing the focal event. In terms of the SR versus MR distinction introduced in section 1.0, only data obtained from SR patients will generate a Kaplan-Meier survival curve of the type described in appendix B.

What happens when data obtained from MR patients are submitted to a Kaplan-Meier analysis?

1. If all observations were obtained from MR patients, the Kaplan-Meier "survival curve" would be a horizontal straight line at survival probability 1.0. Since MR patients are at very low or no risk of experiencing the focal event, no focal events would likely be observed. Then, no Kaplan-Meier curve could be produced. The implementing computer program would print out an error message.

2. If observations are obtained from a mixture of SR and MR patients, something resembling a proper survival curve will be generated. The implementing computer program will print out a declining curve, but that curve will not appear to be falling to a horizontal asymptote at zero probability. Instead, the curve will appear to be approaching some positive survival probability as elapsed times increase. The higher the proportion of contaminating MR patients contained in the sample, the more positively elevated will be the apparent horizontal asymptote.

   In addition and just because of the mixture, the fitted survival curve will indicate a declining hazard rate over time to a greater extent than would have been the case without the contaminating mixture.

3. When (virtually) all observations are obtained from SR patients, the Kaplan-Meier analysis will generate a survival curve that appears to approach asymptotically zero survival probability as elapsed times increase. This is the kind of survival curve described in appendix B.

   A patient data set collected with short follow-up or with a large proportion of censored observations concentrated at later time intervals for some particular reason will tend to mask this result.

   Detecting MR patients definitely requires lengthy follow-up.

As a consequence, assessing the curative impact of a medical intervention cannot always be accomplished by Kaplan-Meier analysis alone. To the extent that a sample is contaminated with an appreciable proportion of MR patients who are at very low or no risk of experiencing any focal event indicating disease progression, probabilistic estimates derived from the Kaplan-Meier model may be quite misleading.

Appendix F

The Proportional Hazards Model and Cox Regression Analysis

Even in a reasonably homogeneous population or subpopulation, not all patients are assumed to be at identical instantaneous risk of experiencing some focal event. Typically, there are individual differences among them. These relate to their personal attributes and various situational characteristics that exert a differential influence on their individual hazard rates.

Often, however, a baseline hazard function common to all patients is assumed to exist. This may be interpreted as the hazard function applicable to the "typical" or "average" patient. The "typical" or "average" patient is an analytical fiction. It is not a real patient. A baseline hazard function is an assumed collective property of the overall population from which a sample of patients is obtained rather than an individual property of any one patient.

Sometimes no particular shape or form is assumed for the baseline hazard function. The hazard rate may increase, decrease, or remain constant over time. In principle, it is free to display just about any complex temporal pattern. Kaplan-Meier analysis, as described in appendix E, is particularly useful in tracing out a survival curve associated with a baseline hazard function of unspecified characteristics.

At other times, a specific functional form is assumed. Its parameter values are estimated from sample data, typically via the method of maximum likelihood. The behavior of the hazard rate over time is then determined jointly by the shape of the assumed baseline hazard function and its estimated parameter values.

As in the case of logistic regression analysis, it must be at least plausible to view a collected data set as a sample drawn both randomly and independently from some well-defined and reasonably homogeneous patient population or subpopulation to support the validity of such parameter estimates.

The hazard rate that applies to any individual, real patient in the population at any point in time is assumed to be directly proportional to the population's baseline hazard rate. Directly proportional simply means multiplied by a patient-specific factor of proportionality.

Each patient is assumed to possess a separate factor of proportionality that is determined by that patient's influencing personal attributes and situational characteristics (covariates). However, no patient's factor of proportionality changes over time. It is presumed to remain constant (temporally invariant).

Taken together, the above statements describe the concept of a proportional hazards model. The essence of the proportional hazards assumption is that each patient possesses a separate, individual factor of proportionality that is invariant over time and, therefore, that may be multiplied by the population's baseline hazard rate evaluated at any given time to determine that patient's individual hazard rate at that particular moment.

Cox regression analysis is based on the proportional hazards model. It seeks to estimate each patient's constant of proportionality. It assumes that each individual proportionality factor is defined as

$EXP(B1*X1 + B2*X2 + ... + Bk*Xk)$, where

* means multiply;

EXP means to exponentiate the directly following expression, using the base e of the natural logarithm system;

X1, X2, ... , Xk are k (k >= 1) numerically coded covariates embodying the relevant individual attributes and situational characteristics that influence individual hazard rates;

B1, B2, ... , Bk are undetermined coefficients estimated from the regression analysis that indicate by their algebraic sign whether each covariate raises or lowers an individual patient's hazard rate above or below the baseline rate and by how much, indicated by their magnitude; and

the relative risk (instantaneous hazard rate) of experiencing the focal event associated with the ith covariate is embodied in the value of the expression EXP(Bi).

Cox regression analysis combines several features of both Kaplan-Meier analysis and logistic regression.

1. Exactly the same focal event times and censored times input as the dependent variable to a Kaplan-Meier analysis are input as the dependent variable of Cox regression.
2. A single elapsed time (whichever type applies) is entered for each patient in the sample (randomly and independently) drawn from the population.
3. The patient attributes and situational characteristics (covariates) presumed to influence each patient's hazard rate constitute Cox regression's independent variables.
4. The value of each covariate entered as an independent variable must be numerically coded.

Outputs of Cox regression include:

1. maximum likelihood estimates of the population regression coefficients, B1, B2, ... , Bk associated, respectively, with the k covariates, along with a standard deviation, an accompanying two-tailed p value, and an estimate of the relative risk (hazard rate) associated with each coefficient;
2. both the discrete Kaplan-Meier survival function and the discrete baseline survival function corresponding to the baseline hazard function fitted via Cox regression to the sample data; and
3. an indication of how closely each function fits the exponential and the Weibull distribution, respectively. The uncorrected coefficient of determination (R-squared) indicates closeness of fit to each distribution.

Before interpreting the results of a Cox regression analysis, it is always good practice to check the plausibility of the underlying proportional hazards assumption.

Both the exponential and the Weibull distributions are compatible with proportional hazards. Consequently, if the baseline survival function fits either an exponential or a Weibull function "closely enough" (e.g., R-squared goodness-of-fit statistic at least 80 percent) or if a plot of the cumulative hazard function over time derived from the Kaplan-Meier analysis falls approximately along a straight line (indicating an exponential survival function), then verification of the proportional hazards assumption becomes especially desirable.

Analysis of either the deviance or the martingale residuals provides a reasonable check on the plausibility of both the proportional hazards assumption and various other regression assumptions.

From PCM's point of view the most important benefit derivable from a successful Cox regression analysis is an individually tailored survival function for each patient in the sample at risk of experiencing some designated focal event. Each such patient's set of k covariate values is first combined with the k regression coefficients estimated from the analysis to obtain that patient's factor of proportionality. An individually tailored survival function is then calculated for each patient by exponentiating the underlying baseline survival function presumed common to all patients in the population by that patient's individual proportionality factor. This was done in section 2, when the kidney transplant experience of 469 patients was analyzed. It was also done in sections 5 and 7, when breast cancer patient experiences following mastectomy and radiation were analyzed.

Appendix G

Variable Characteristics of the First Illustrative 550-Patient
Intervention Sample of Breast Cancer Patients from Turku, Finland

In the following tables, "*" signifies undefined (missing) observations.

PATIENT ATTRIBUTE	MINIMUM	MEDIAN	MAXIMUM	MEAN
TUMOR SIZE (mm.)	5	30	100	30.98
AGE AT DIAGNOSIS (years)	24	57	86	57.10
FOLLOW-UP (years, all 550 patients)	0.16	8.33	43.08	10.73
FOLLOW-UP (years, 439 already dead)	0.16	5.34	42.92	7.94
FOLLOW-UP (years, 111 still alive)	15.08	20.25	43.08	21.76

Note: All 550 patients were female, and all 550 underwent radiation therapy.
There were 237 missing observations of TUMOR SIZE, but no missing
observations of AGE AT DIAGNOSIS.

TYPE OF TUMOR	ABSOLUTE FREQUENCIES (COUNTS)	RELATIVE FREQUENCIES (PROPORTIONS)	CUMULATIVE RELATIVE FREQUENCIES
DUCTAL	468	0.8509	0.8509
LOBULAR	82	0.1491	1.0000
TOTAL	550	1.0000	

GRADE OF TUMOR	ABSOLUTE FREQUENCIES (COUNTS)	RELATIVE FREQUENCIES (PROPORTIONS)	CUMULATIVE RELATIVE FREQUENCIES
1	103	0.1873	0.1873
2	261	0.4745	0.6618
3	186	0.3382	1.0000
TOTAL	550	1.0000	

MITOTIC RATE OF TUMOR	ABSOLUTE FREQUENCIES (COUNTS)	RELATIVE FREQUENCIES (PROPORTIONS)	CUMULATIVE RELATIVE FREQUENCIES
RARE (per hpf)	203	0.3691	0.3691
2 OR 3 (per hpf)	232	0.4218	0.7909
MORE THAN 3 (per hpf)	115	0.2091	1.0000
TOTAL	550	1.0000	

Note: Per hpf designates number of mitoses counted per high-powered microscopic
field.

LOCATION OF TUMOR	ABSOLUTE FREQUENCIES (COUNTS)	RELATIVE FREQUENCIES (PROPORTIONS)	CUMULATIVE RELATIVE FREQUENCIES
MEDIAL	88	0.1600	0.1600
CENTRAL	66	0.1200	0.2800
LATERAL	282	0.5127	0.7927
DIFFUSE	9	0.0164	0.8091
*	105	0.1909	1.0000
TOTAL	550	1.0000	

Note: LOCATION designates where on breast tumor was located. There were 105 missing observations of LOCATION.

T STAGE OF TUMOR	ABSOLUTE FREQUENCIES (COUNTS)	RELATIVE FREQUENCIES (PROPORTIONS)	CUMULATIVE RELATIVE FREQUENCIES
T=0	1	0.0018	0.0018
T=1	139	0.2527	0.2545
T=2	270	0.4909	0.7454
T=3	80	0.1455	0.8909
T=4	51	0.0927	0.9836
*	9	0.0164	1.0000
TOTAL	550	1.0000	

Note: T STAGE designates stage of tumor at diagnosis as measured by the T/N/M staging criteria. There were nine missing observations of T STAGE.

N STAGE OF PATIENT	ABSOLUTE FREQUENCIES (COUNTS)	RELATIVE FREQUENCIES (PROPORTIONS)	CUMULATIVE RELATIVE FREQUENCIES
N=0	264	0.4800	0.4800
N=1	237	0.4309	0.9109
N=2	43	0.0782	0.9891
*	6	0.0109	1.0000
TOTAL	550	1.0000	

Note: N STAGE designates patient's nodal status at diagnosis as measured by the T/N/M staging criteria. There were six missing observations of N STAGE.

M STAGE OF PATIENT	ABSOLUTE FREQUENCIES (COUNTS)	RELATIVE FREQUENCIES (PROPORTIONS)	CUMULATIVE RELATIVE FREQUENCIES
M=0	527	0.9582	0.9582
M=1	23	0.0418	1.0000
TOTAL	550	1.0000	

Note: M STAGE designates patient's metastatic status at diagnosis as measured by the T/N/M staging criteria.

DEGREE OF NECROSIS	ABSOLUTE FREQUENCIES (COUNTS)	RELATIVE FREQUENCIES (PROPORTIONS)	CUMULATIVE RELATIVE FREQUENCIES
NONE	383	0.6964	0.6964
SPOTTY	89	0.1618	0.8582
MODERATE	51	0.0927	0.9509
SEVERE	27	0.0491	1.0000
TOTAL	550	1.0000	

Note: NECROSIS refers to the patient's tissue.

PRESENCE OF ULCERATION	ABSOLUTE FREQUENCIES (COUNTS)	RELATIVE FREQUENCIES (PROPORTIONS)	CUMULATIVE RELATIVE FREQUENCIES
NO	539	0.9800	0.9800
YES	9	0.0164	0.9964
*	2	0.0036	1.0000
TOTAL	550	1.0000	

Note: ULCERATION refers to the patient's tumor. There were two missing observations of ULCERATION.

PRESENCE OF INFLAMMATION	ABSOLUTE FREQUENCIES (COUNTS)	RELATIVE FREQUENCIES (PROPORTIONS)	CUMULATIVE RELATIVE FREQUENCIES
NO	546	0.9927	0.9927
YES	4	0.0073	1.0000
TOTAL	550	1.0000	

TYPE OF SURGERY PERFORMED	ABSOLUTE FREQUENCIES (COUNTS)	RELATIVE FREQUENCIES (PROPORTIONS)	CUMULATIVE RELATIVE FREQUENCIES
MOD. RADICAL MASTECTOMY	125	0.2273	0.2273
RADICAL MASTECTOMY	425	0.7727	1.0000
TOTAL	550	1.0000	

RELAPSE OR RECURRENCE EXPERIENCED	ABSOLUTE FREQUENCIES (COUNTS)	RELATIVE FREQUENCIES (PROPORTIONS)	CUMULATIVE RELATIVE FREQUENCIES
NO	423	0.7691	0.7691
YES	127	0.2309	1.0000
TOTAL	550	1.0000	

PATIENT STATUS WHEN LAST OBSERVED	ABSOLUTE FREQUENCIES (COUNTS)	RELATIVE FREQUENCIES (PROPORTIONS)	CUMULATIVE RELATIVE FREQUENCIES
DIED OF BREAST CANCER	278	0.5055	0.5055
DIED OF OTHER CANCER	27	0.0491	0.5546
DIED OF OTHER CAUSE	134	0.2436	0.7982
LAST SEEN STILL ALIVE	111	0.2018	1.0000
TOTAL	550	1.0000	

FOCAL EVENTS SIGNIFYING DISEASE PROGRESSION	ABSOLUTE FREQUENCIES (COUNTS)	RELATIVE FREQUENCIES (PROPORTIONS)	CUMULATIVE RELATIVE FREQUENCIES
RELAPSE/RECURRENCE AND DIED OF BREAST CANCER	112	0.3823	0.3823
NO RELAPSE/RECURRENCE BUT DIED OF BREAST CANCER	166	0.5665	0.9488
RELAPSE/RECURRENCE AND DIED OF SOMETHING ELSE	13	0.0444	0.9932
RELAPSE/RECURRENCE BUT LAST SEEN STILL ALIVE	2	0.0068	1.0000
TOTAL	293	1.0000	

Appendix H

The RISKTEST Simulator

It is not always possible to determine unequivocally that a patient diagnosed with a progressive and potentially fatal disease has been cured. When last seen, seven of the 550 breast cancer patients in the Turku intervention sample had survived into their nineties with no evidence of further disease progression. Another patient had survived, disease-free, for over forty-three years. When last seen she was still alive at eighty-six.

Yet even these patients could conceivably not have been cured by their mastectomy and radiation. They may have remained at substantial risk (SR instead of being transformed to MR) despite the intervention. They may then have enjoyed extraordinarily good luck for a remarkably long time.

Because one can never be absolutely certain of cure, the ability to compare competing probabilistic explanations of the same observed survival data becomes quite helpful. A common statistical framework is required within which alternative explanatory models may be imbedded. Each model may then be fine-tuned separately within that framework so as to maximize its chances of fitting the data. Since competing models have been imbedded and individually fine-tuned within a common statistical framework, they may be compared for relative goodness of fit. Comparing separate models making different assumptions can help to select the best-fitting assumptions.

In various contexts throughout this book, summary statistics, model parameters, and population parameters are estimated by several techniques:

1. maximum likelihood;
2. least-squares; and
3. various forms of trial and error.

The use of different and not entirely comparable estimation techniques suggests Monte Carlo simulation as a common statistical framework. Within a simulation framework, even widely disparate models seeking to explain the same survival data may still be compared in terms of their common outcomes.

The RISKTEST procedure embodies a specialized form of Monte Carlo simulation. RISKTEST is designed to mimic the process of:

1. acquiring patients, all diagnosed with a common progressive disease, over some period of time;
2. executing a particular medical intervention against that disease shortly after each patient is acquired; and
3. then following up over a significant period of time to determine whether or not and when each patient either experiences the first focal event signifying disease progression or becomes a censored observation.

RISKTEST requires that at least one simulated patient remain at risk (SR) of further disease progression following the intervention. In addition, either none or some specified proportion of the simulated patients may be designated cured by the intervention (MR).

In the case of the 550-patient Turku sample, RISKTEST interprets invasive breast cancer as the progressive disease and mastectomy with radiation, but without adjuvant therapy, as the particular medical intervention. Subsequent relapse, recurrence, or death due to breast cancer (whichever, if any, occurs first) is interpreted as the focal event to be simulated.

Censoring events are also simulated. These include death due to a different cancer, death due to a cause unrelated to any cancer, being last seen still alive in the normal course of patient follow-up, and being lost to follow-up.

What happens to each individual patient is the focus of a single simulation trial. It is conditioned by the set of simulation inputs described below.

The summarizing output of a single simulation trial is a count of the number of patients who experience the focal event. By making numerous simulation trials, a distribution of simulated focal event counts may be generated for any given set of simulation inputs. This constitutes a simulation run.

When the number of trials in a run is large enough (thousands of trials), the central limit theorem ensures that the distribution of focal event counts across trials will look very much like a normal distribution. This distribution generally becomes unimodal in a single simulation run including just hundreds of trials.

Ten thousand is the default number of trials constituting a single simulation run. Optionally, up to one hundred thousand trials may be executed in a run.

The first step is to obtain an external data set recording the survival of patients diagnosed with a progressive and potentially fatal disease. Probabilistic models, such as the Weibull and exponential distributions, are then fitted via maximum likelihood to the collected sample data.

A particular medical intervention is then selected.

It is assumed that none or some number (but not all) of the patients in the data set are actually cured by the target intervention. The RISKTEST simulator then generates patient outcomes comparable to the actual outcomes recorded in the external data set via the Monte Carlo technique.

An external data set may contain either historical patient records or the results of a clinical trial. RISKTEST then proceeds as follows.

1. Actual and simulated results are compared.
2. RISKTEST acts as a goodness-of-fit hypothesis testing procedure.
3. The number of simulated patients who experience the focal event plays the role of a test statistic.
4. The actual (observed) count serves as the target value of this test statistic.
5. RISKTEST produces the equivalent of both one-tailed and two-tailed p values associated with the target focal event count.
6. By trial and error RISKTEST may then be used to fine-tune cure model parameters, such as an initial estimate of the proportion of patients actually cured by the target medical intervention.
7. The underlying assumption(s) and model parameter(s) that generate RISKTEST-simulated outcomes as close as possible to actually observed outcomes can be adopted in subsequent analyses.

The RISKTEST procedure is driven by the following simulation inputs:

1. number of patients acquired either during a clinical trial or from a retrospective data set (must be at least two);
2. number of cured patients at minimal risk (MR) of further disease progression following the medical intervention (possibly none of the patients acquired, but always fewer than all acquired patients);

3. target (test) number of patients who experience the focal event (at least zero, but no more than the number of acquired patients who remain in the SR subset despite the medical intervention);
4. number of years constituting the patient acquisition period (the strictly positive time interval in years between the date when the first patient is acquired and the date when the last patient is acquired);
5. number of years constituting the patient follow-up period (the nonnegative time interval in years between the date when the last patient is acquired and the date when the last patient is followed up);
6. number of years constituting the patient follow-up cycle (the time interval within which patients are periodically followed up), where a follow-up cycle of N years means that the typical patient is regularly followed up once every N years. [Note: Alternatively, a 0 input indicates that the number of years until a patient is last seen under the follow-up plan is determined by a uniform random number drawn from each patient's maximum possible follow-up observation time, and a -1 input indicates that the number of years until a patient is last seen is tailored to some specified follow-up plan characterizing the clinical trial or retrospective data set from which external data are obtained.];
7. Weibull intensity parameter for relapse/recurrence/disease-specific death focal event (the strictly positive value of LAMBDA as described in appendix B relating to the population or subpopulation from which SR patients are drawn);
8. Weibull trend parameter for relapse/recurrence/disease-specific death focal event (the strictly positive value of DELTA as described in appendix B relating to the population or subpopulation from which SR patients are drawn);
9. optional strictly positive Weibull intensity parameter for some specific censoring event (such as death due to a cause unrelated to disease progression) relating to the population or subpopulation from which SR patients are drawn); and
10. optional strictly positive Weibull trend parameter for the same censoring event relating to the SR population or subpopulation.

The reason for characterizing a retrospective data set in terms of its acquisition and follow-up times is to make retrospective data as compatible as possible with the results of a clinical trial. Data of both types are then structurally comparable in simulation. Additional adjustments must still be made to retrospective data before effective compatibility can be achieved, but structural comparability is a first step in that direction.

After obtaining appropriate inputs, patient acquisition is simulated as if it were (approximately) a Poisson process.

1. The first patient is acquired at acquisition time zero. This is the beginning of both the acquisition time period and the complete simulation time window.
2. The elapsed time until the next patient is acquired is simulated as an independent random draw from an exponential distribution whose intensity parameter is calculated as the number of patients still to be acquired divided by the time remaining in the acquisition time period.
3. The value of the exponential intensity parameter is then recalculated (typically only slightly) as a result of that random draw.
4. The above two steps are repeated until all patients have been acquired.
5. Toward the end of the simulated acquisition process it can happen that a randomly drawn time interval until acquiring the next patient will exceed the outer limit of the acquisition time period. When this occurs

one or more additional random draws are made until a "short enough" time interval is obtained.

6. Additional random draws, if and when executed, guarantee that all patients will be acquired within the acquisition time period.

7. It is because of this modification and because the intensity parameter of the exponential distribution is continually updated that the simulated acquisition of patients must be regarded as an approximate (rather than a pure) Poisson process.

8. Nevertheless, simulated patient acquisition is randomized with respect to sequential timing, much as if it were a Poisson process.

The next step is performed if, but only if, some proportion of the simulated patients are designated MR (i.e., ended up in the cured subsample of the intervention sample). Assuming that n of N patients are MR (0 =< n < N), a random subset of n patients is selected from all N acquired patients such that all possible subsets of size n are equally likely. None of these n patients will experience a focal event during any simulation trial in any simulation run.

RISKTEST is then prepared to execute a single simulation trial as follows.

1. The next focal event time is simulated. This is done for each acquired SR patient as if it were an independent random draw from a Weibull distribution (possibly exponential, as a special case).

2. When the situation being simulated includes some salient event that has the effect of censoring SR patient observations, that event is modeled separately and included in the simulation as a specific censoring event. In a data set with a very long follow-up period, many patients may die from causes unrelated to disease progression. Modeling this specific censoring event separately from the follow-up cycle censoring event to be discussed below could improve the realism of the overall simulation. When relevant, a specific censored time is generated for each SR patient as if it were an independent random draw from a Weibull distribution (possibly exponential, as a special case). This step is optional.

3. The next step (always executed) is to generate a follow-up cycle time (i.e., time last seen) for each acquired patient as if it were an independent random draw from some specified distribution describing the patient follow-up cycle.

   A. If the number of years constituting the follow-up cycle enters as 0, the MAXTIME parameter for a uniform (rectangular) distribution (see appendix B) is calculated for each patient individually as the time interval between that patient's acquisition time and the end of the overall follow-up time period (i.e., the end of the complete simulation time window). Each patient's time last seen is then a random draw from this individually tailored distribution.

   B. If the number of years constituting the follow-up cycle enters as a positive number (never more than the length of the follow-up period), it becomes the MAXTIME parameter for a different uniform (rectangular) distribution, as described in appendix B. A separate random draw from this distribution is made for each patient. Each patient's time last seen is then calculated as the difference between this random time and the time interval between that patient's acquisition time and the end of the overall follow-up time period. Should the calculated time difference be negative, that patient's time last seen is calculated as if the follow-up cycle time had entered as 0.

C. If the number of years constituting the follow-up cycle enters as -1, a specially-coded internal subroutine is called to simulate each patient's time last seen. This internal subroutine is tailored to a particular external data set. It embodies whatever specific patient follow-up cycle applies to the clinical trial results or the retrospective clinical data with which simulated outcomes are to be compared.

D. Follow-up cycle times are included in the simulation both to reflect a regular pattern of patient follow-up if such a pattern exists and to reflect the possibility of patient loss to follow-up for reasons unrelated to disease progression.

4. The last step is to simulate what happens to each SR patient. What happens is always what happens first within the follow-up cycle. It could be the focal event or some censoring event.

5. Cured patients designated MR are uniformly ignored.

The central purpose of RISKTEST is to test the goodness of fit of the statistical model embodied in its simulation inputs with the actual number of patients who experience the focal event in an externally collected sample of empirical observations. This is done by counting the number of simulation trials in which the simulated number of patients who experience the focal event is

1. less than,
2. exactly equal to, or
3. more than

the actual (called the target) number of patients, respectively. These three counts are used to calculate the equivalent of one-tailed and two-tailed p values for the goodness-of-fit hypothesis test.

The null hypothesis underlying the goodness-of-fit test is that the externally observed (target) number of patients who actually experience the event could reasonably have been drawn at random from the simulated distribution of trial counts. The conventional conclusion is to regard the fit as "good enough" unless the p value falls at or beyond .05.

The results and conclusion of the simulated statistical test are displayed.

Optionally, a complete frequency distribution of trial counts across all trials in the simulation run may also be displayed. The complete frequency distribution can be interesting and useful in several ways.

1. It can be used to assess the statistical parameters estimated from empirical data by the KAPM procedure for both the exponential and Weibull distributions. In both cases KAPM makes maximum likelihood parameter estimates based on the observed number of patients who experience a focal event. The complete frequency distribution shows where the observed number of patients who experience the focal event on which these estimates are based falls (i.e., low, high, or about in the middle of this distribution).

2. The complete distribution may also be inspected for shape, range, variability, symmetry, and other interesting characteristics.

3. An initial estimate of the proportion of cured patients in an external sample may be fine-tuned so as to maximize the simulated likelihood of the count of actual patients observed to experience a focal event. Fine-tuning is executed via an automated trial-and-error process (called the CURE option) included in the KAPM procedure.

Appendix I

Variable Characteristics of the Second Illustrative 578-Patient Intervention
Sample of Breast Cancer Patients from Guy's Hospital in London, England

In the following tables, "*" signifies undefined (missing) observations.

PATIENT ATTRIBUTE	MINIMUM	MEDIAN	MAXIMUM	MEAN
TUMOR SIZE (mm.)	0	30	105	29.57
AGE AT DIAGNOSIS (years)	23	56	86	56.23
FOLLOW-UP (years, all 578 patients)	0.07	13.37	28.13	13.61
FOLLOW-UP (years, 419 already dead)	0.07	7.76	26.53	9.66
FOLLOW-UP (years, 159 still alive)	19.42	24.15	28.13	24.01

Note: All 578 patients were female. All were diagnosed with some form of
invasive breast cancer. Some received radiation, but none received
additional adjuvant therapy. There were no missing observations of AGE
AT DIAGNOSIS. However, TUMOR SIZE was recorded in the Guy's Hospital data
set as 0.0 mm. for eighteen patients. These "zeros" were subsequently
treated as missing observations rather than as tumors of no size.

MENOPAUSAL STATE AT DIAGNOSIS	ABSOLUTE FREQUENCIES (COUNTS)	RELATIVE FREQUENCIES (PROPORTIONS)	CUMULATIVE RELATIVE FREQUENCIES
PREMENOPAUSAL	262	0.4533	0.4533
POSTMENOPAUSAL	316	0.5467	1.0000
TOTAL	578	1.0000	

RECEIVED RADIATION THERAPY	ABSOLUTE FREQUENCIES (COUNTS)	RELATIVE FREQUENCIES (PROPORTIONS)	CUMULATIVE RELATIVE FREQUENCIES
NO	530	0.9170	0.9170
YES	48	0.0830	1.0000
TOTAL	578	1.0000	

GRADE OF TUMOR	ABSOLUTE FREQUENCIES (COUNTS)	RELATIVE FREQUENCIES (PROPORTIONS)	CUMULATIVE RELATIVE FREQUENCIES
1	58	0.1003	0.1003
2	275	0.4758	0.5761
3	188	0.3253	0.9014
*	57	0.0986	1.0000
TOTAL	578	1.0000	

Note: GRADE designates grade of tumor. There were fifty-seven missing
observations of GRADE. All fifty-seven referred to lobular tumors.

NUMBER OF POSITIVE AXILLARY LYMPH NODES	ABSOLUTE FREQUENCIES (COUNTS)	RELATIVE FREQUENCIES (PROPORTIONS)	CUMULATIVE RELATIVE FREQUENCIES
0	354	0.6125	0.6125
1	82	0.1419	0.7543
2	37	0.0640	0.8183
3	19	0.0329	0.8512
4	9	0.0156	0.8668
5	12	0.0208	0.8875
6	10	0.0173	0.9048
7	6	0.0104	0.9152
8	10	0.0173	0.9325
9	8	0.0138	0.9464
10	1	0.0017	0.9481
11	5	0.0087	0.9567
12	2	0.0035	0.9602
13	2	0.0035	0.9637
14	1	0.0017	0.9654
15	1	0.0017	0.9671
19	1	0.0017	0.9689
21	2	0.0035	0.9723
22	1	0.0017	0.9740
23	1	0.0017	0.9758
24	3	0.0052	0.9810
25	1	0.0017	0.9827
26	3	0.0052	0.9879
30	4	0.0069	0.9948
41	1	0.0017	0.9965
44	1	0.0017	0.9983
65	1	0.0017	1.0000
TOTAL	578	1.0000	

Note: The attribute NUMAXPOS counts the number of positive axillary lymph nodes at diagnosis. The mean number was 2.18 positive nodes out of a mean of 25.05 nodes harvested.

T STAGE OF TUMOR	ABSOLUTE FREQUENCIES (COUNTS)	RELATIVE FREQUENCIES (PROPORTIONS)	CUMULATIVE RELATIVE FREQUENCIES
T=0	18	0.0311	0.0311
T=1	202	0.3495	0.3806
T=2	310	0.5364	0.9170
T=3 OR 4	48	0.0830	1.0000
TOTAL	578	1.0000	

Note: T STAGE designates stage of tumor at diagnosis as measured by the T/N/M staging criteria.

N STATUS OF PATIENT	ABSOLUTE FREQUENCIES (COUNTS)	RELATIVE FREQUENCIES (PROPORTIONS)	CUMULATIVE RELATIVE FREQUENCIES
N=0	354	0.6125	0.6125
N=1	138	0.2387	0.8512
N=2	55	0.0952	0.9464
N=3	31	0.0536	1.0000
TOTAL	578	1.0000	

Note: N STATUS designates patient's nodal status at diagnosis. It reflects the number of positive axillary nodes.

M STAGE OF PATIENT	ABSOLUTE FREQUENCIES (COUNTS)	RELATIVE FREQUENCIES (PROPORTIONS)	CUMULATIVE RELATIVE FREQUENCIES
M=0	578	1.0000	1.0000
TOTAL	578	1.0000	

Note: M STAGE designates patient's metastatic status at diagnosis as measured by the T/N/M staging criteria. Two hundred fifty-three (43.77 percent) of the 578 patients subsequently experienced a distant metastasis of some variety (advancing them to the M1 stage), sometimes resulting in death.

PATIENT'S ESTROGEN RESPONSE	ABSOLUTE FREQUENCIES (COUNTS)	RELATIVE FREQUENCIES (PROPORTIONS)	CUMULATIVE RELATIVE FREQUENCIES
ER NEGATIVE	206	0.3564	0.3564
ER POSITIVE	372	0.6436	1.0000
TOTAL	578	1.0000	

PATIENT'S PROGESTERONE RESPONSE	ABSOLUTE FREQUENCIES (COUNTS)	RELATIVE FREQUENCIES (PROPORTIONS)	CUMULATIVE RELATIVE FREQUENCIES
PR NEGATIVE	348	0.6021	0.6021
PR POSITIVE	230	0.3979	1.0000
TOTAL	578	1.0000	

PATIENT STATUS WHEN LAST OBSERVED	ABSOLUTE FREQUENCIES (COUNTS)	RELATIVE FREQUENCIES (PROPORTIONS)	CUMULATIVE RELATIVE FREQUENCIES
ALIVE (NO RELAPSE, YET)	153	0.2647	0.2647
ALIVE (NON-DISTANT RELAPSE ONLY, SO FAR)	3	0.0052	0.2699
ALIVE (ONLY DISTANT RELAPSE, SO FAR)	2	0.0035	0.2734
ALIVE (RELAPSE[S] OF EACH TYPE, ALREADY)	1	0.0017	0.2751
DEAD OF BREAST CANCER (NO PRIOR RELAPSE)	2	0.0035	0.2786
DEAD OF BREAST CANCER (NON-DISTANT ONLY)	8	0.0138	0.2924
DEAD OF BREAST CANCER (ONLY DISTANT)	171	0.2958	0.5882
DEAD OF BREAST CANCER (PRIOR, EACH TYPE)	56	0.0969	0.6851
DEAD OF OTHER CAUSE (NO PRIOR RELAPSE)	166	0.2872	0.9723
DEAD OF OTHER CAUSE (NON-DISTANT ONLY)	3	0.0052	0.9775
DEAD OF OTHER CAUSE (ONLY DISTANT)	9	0.0156	0.9931
DEAD OF OTHER CAUSE (PRIOR, EACH TYPE)	4	0.0069	1.0000
TOTAL	578	1.0000	

RELAPSE OR RECURRENCE EXPERIENCED	ABSOLUTE FREQUENCIES (COUNTS)	RELATIVE FREQUENCIES (PROPORTIONS)	CUMULATIVE RELATIVE FREQUENCIES
NO	321	0.5554	0.5554
YES	257	0.4446	1.0000
TOTAL	578	1.0000	

LIVING STATE WHEN LAST OBSERVED	ABSOLUTE FREQUENCIES (COUNTS)	RELATIVE FREQUENCIES (PROPORTIONS)	CUMULATIVE RELATIVE FREQUENCIES
DIED OF BREAST CANCER	237	0.4100	0.4100
DIED OF OTHER CAUSE	182	0.3149	0.7249
LAST SEEN STILL ALIVE	159	0.2751	1.0000
TOTAL	578	1.0000	

FOCAL EVENTS SIGNIFYING DISEASE PROGRESSION	ABSOLUTE FREQUENCIES (COUNTS)	RELATIVE FREQUENCIES (PROPORTIONS)	CUMULATIVE RELATIVE FREQUENCIES
PRIOR RELAPSE/RECURRENCE AND DIED OF BREAST CANCER	235	0.9073	0.9073
NO PRIOR RELAPSE/RECURRENCE BUT DIED OF BREAST CANCER	2	0.0077	0.9150
RELAPSE/RECURRENCE AND DIED OF SOMETHING ELSE	16	0.0618	0.9768
RELAPSE/RECURRENCE BUT LAST SEEN STILL ALIVE	6	0.0232	1.0000
TOTAL	259	1.0000	

ANNOTATED REFERENCES

1. Miller, James R. III, Mohammed Kashani-Sabet, and Richard W. Sagebiel. (2013). **Patient-centered prognosis: A methodology to improve individually tailored prognostic accuracy illustrated in two cancers.** Bloomington, IN: iUniverse.

This was the first book in our series of books about using PCM to render various predictions of individual patient outcomes more accurate.

2. Miller, James R. III, Mohammed Kashani-Sabet, and Richard W. Sagebiel. (2015). *Patient-centered diagnosis: Methodologies to predict individually tailored outcomes of current diagnostic tests and to create new tests.* Bloomington, IN: iUniverse.

This was the second book in our series of books about using PCM to render various predictions of individual patient outcomes more accurate.

3. Kashani-Sabet, Mohammed, Richard W. Sagebiel, Heikki Joensuu, and James R. Miller III. (2013). A patient-centered methodology that improves the accuracy of prognostic predictions in cancer. Published online February 2013 by **PLoS One**. plosone/article.0056435.

This journal article constitutes a condensed version of our first book. It introduces and describes PCM in some detail. Published shortly before the first book, it was directed toward the community of practicing physicians. Both the first two books and this, our third book, were intended to serve as reference documentation for a methodologically oriented audience.

4. Joensuu, Heikki, and Toikkanen, Sakari. (1995). Cured of breast cancer? **Journal of Clinical Oncology** 13(1):62-69.

This journal article documents an earlier analysis of the same breast cancer patients from the region of Turku, Finland, included in our first data set illustrating the Bayesian cure model. The model and its application to the Turku patients are presented in section 4 of this, our third book. The earlier analysis reported in the journal article did not focus exclusively on mastectomy and radiation as its target intervention. The article did conclude, however, that breast cancer may be permanently cured with only locoregional therapy. Our Bayesian cure model elaborates on their conclusion by identifying how many and which particular patients are likely cured.

5. Miller, James R. III. (2001). **Assessing the curative impact of medical intervention.** Stanford Business School Technical Report No. 85: Stanford, CA.

6. Miller, James R. III. (2002). **A Bayesian assessment of the curative impact of medical intervention.** Stanford Business School Technical Report No. 86: Stanford, CA.

These two monographs introduce the conceptual framework and collection of facilitating procedures to assess probabilistically both the curative impact of a specified medical intervention and the likelihood that an individual patient has been cured following that intervention.

The logistic and Cox (proportional hazards) regression models are logically integrated by means of Bayes' theorem. Appropriately extended logistic regression supplies an individually tailored prior cure probability (prior to the intervention) for each patient. Appropriately extended Cox regression supplies an individually tailored conditional probability of survival time without further disease progression if the patient remains at risk. Then a minimal risk partitioning algorithm (MRPA) is constructed to assign an individually tailored posterior cure probability. It encapsulates the likelihood that each patient was actually cured following the intervention.

MRPA also estimates a specified medical intervention's cure rate for any given patient population.

Individually tailored posterior cure probabilities are a function of the time elapsed since the intervention with no evidence of further disease progression. In this sense they resemble survival probabilities, but with a critically important reversal in the direction of inference. A cure probability is defined as the conditional probability of having been cured (as opposed to remaining still at risk), given the duration of survival time free from further disease progression following some medical intervention. A survival probability is a reverse conditional probability. It indicates the likelihood of surviving for a specified period of time, given that the patient was not cured by the medical intervention and, therefore, remained still at risk following it and despite its curative potential.

It is through the application of Bayes' theorem that the direction of inference is successfully reversed. Reversing the direction of inference in this manner requires partitioning a set of patients who have undergone a potentially curative intervention into those who were and those who were not cured. This partitioning, in turn, reveals how failing to separate cured from noncured patients can sometimes lead to quite misleading conclusions. Performing a conventional Kaplan-Meier survival analysis on a sample containing a substantial proportion of cured patients was shown to distort the stable hazard rate over time characterizing the noncured patients. Any conventional survival analysis performed on a similarly mixed sample has the potential to produce the same false impression of a declining hazard rate. This was among the most compelling conclusions drawn from the MRPA analysis.

Both PCM and MRPA were designed to exploit the facilities of and to execute within the same specialized software operating system (MDMS) employed and illustrated throughout all three of our books. Just like MRPA, PCM incorporates the logistic and the Cox regression models. Because PCM modifies both types of regression in the manner required by MRPA it also enhances the ability of MRPA to produce more accurate cure probabilities.

7. Ware, James H. (2006). The limitations of risk Factors as prognostic tools. **New England Journal of Medicine** 355:2615-17.

As described in the first book, this article by Dr. James H. Ware served as an inspirational trigger for the development of PCM.

8. Le, Chap T. (1997). **Applied survival analysis.** New York: John Wiley and Sons, Inc.

This book provides an excellent introduction to and summary of many of the analytical and statistical procedures executed in all three of our books introducing PCM. Data describing the 469 patients who underwent kidney transplants as presented in section 2 of this, our third book, were obtained from appendix A of Chap T. Le's book. Appendix A contained actual patient data to which standard statistical procedures such as Kaplan-Meier analysis and Cox regression could be applied as student exercises.

9. **STATVIEW Reference Manual** (3rd ed.). (1999). Cary, NC: SAS Institute, Inc.

This reference manual and the accompanying user's manual were useful in validating for both logical and programming accuracy many of the procedures incorporated in the PCM methodology. Great care was taken to ensure that PCM procedures generated the same results as did STATVIEW when given the same input data to analyze.

AUTHOR BIOGRAPHIES

For more than thirty years, James R. Miller III, PhD, was a professor at the Stanford Graduate School of Business. He has been doing full-time cancer research since his retirement in 1997 as Walter and Elise Haas Professor of Business Administration. He received a bachelor's degree from Princeton University, a Woodrow Wilson Fellowship (University of California at Berkeley), an MBA from the Harvard Business School, and a PhD from the Massachusetts Institute of Technology. He has previously published three books and more than fifty monographs and articles in professional journals. Professor Miller is the inventor of six US software patents. He has served on more than a dozen boards of directors in the United States and Europe and as CEO of two start-up companies in the Silicon Valley. He has three daughters and six grandchildren.

Mohammed Kashani-Sabet, MD, is medical director of cancer programs at the California Pacific Medical Center (CPMC). He also serves as director of the Center for Melanoma Research and Treatment and senior scientist at the CPMC Research Institute. Dr. Kashani-Sabet earned his medical degree from the State University of New York at Stony Brook, where he also completed an internship in internal medicine. He then completed a residency in dermatology at the University of California at San Francisco (UCSF), as well as a postdoctoral fellowship in cutaneous oncology, and received training in both dermatology and medical oncology. Dr. Kashani-Sabet maintains clinical interests in melanoma and cutaneous lymphoma and research interests in targeted therapy, ribozymes, siRNAs, tumor metastasis, prognostic factors, and tumor biomarkers for both diagnosis and prognosis.

Richard W. Sagebiel, MD, was born in Ohio in 1934. He received his bachelor's degree from Yale University in 1956 in music and literature. He did his medical studies at the Harvard Medical School, including a year of pathology and research between his second and third years at Massachusetts General Hospital (MGH). After an intern year of general medicine, he returned to MGH to study dermatopathology with Wallace H. Clark, MD. He completed his training in the departments of dermatology and pathology at the University of Washington Medical School. In 1970 he joined the clinical faculty of the University of California at San Francisco (UCSF), working with M. Scott Blois, PhD, MD, and others to form a clinical cooperative melanoma group. This group included Drs. Clark, Fitzpatrick (Harvard), and Kopf (NYU). It stimulated the creation of similar melanoma groups throughout the country. From 1988 to 1998, Dr. Sagebiel was director of the UCSF Melanoma Clinic. He then retired and became a consulting pathologist to that clinic and, later, to the CPMC Center for Melanoma Research and Treatment.

f denotes figure

A

ALG, 9, 23, 26, 28, 30, 31, 37

B

Bayes' theorem, 16, 18, 19, 21, 23, 39, 54, 74, 82, 138, 210, 213
Bayesian cure model
for London, England breast cancer patients (Guy's Hospital), 155
for Turku, Finland breast cancer patients, 74–77
Bayesian framework
benefits of, 98, 176
cure assessment as imbedded in, 9, 12
imbedding of logistic and Cox regression in, 210
imbedding of TDCG methodology in, 211
for interpretation of concept of cure probabilistically, 4–5
MRPA as operating within, 74, 155
reformulating traditional Kaplan-Meier paradigm in, 138
in study of kidney transplants, 20, 21, 39
in study of Turku, Finland breast cancer patients, 54
as undergirding TDCG methodology, 214
Bayesian kidney transplant model, 15–19
Bayesian posterior cure probability, 54, 74, 76, 96, 121, 122*f*, 123, 125*f*, 127*f*, 155, 173, 202, 203*f*, 204, 206*f*, 208*f*
Bayesian posterior RSP(t) probabilities, 23, 32, 33–34, 35*f*
Bayesian revision, 20, 86, 89, 96–99, 164, 166, 173–176
binomial sign test, 7, 8
breast cancer patients from London, England (Guy's Hospital)

additional steps to homogenize analysis, 128
apparent disappearance of declining hazard rate over time, 191–200
applying MRPA to, 155
Bayesian revision based on Cox regression as improving consistency of cure probabilities, 173–176
checking final partitioning for reasonableness in, 187–191
constructing tailored curves for high-risk and low-risk patients, 204–208
constructing tailored curves for "typical" patient, 200–203
converting PCM-generated UIRIs into dummy variables to drive MRPA, 161–164
convincing confirmation of existence of cure in, 154
Cox (proportional hazards) regression analysis, 164–173
executing CURE option of KAPM procedure, 144–148
executing initial Kaplan-Meier survival analysis, 129–136
fine-tuning initial estimate of actual proportion cured, 149–153
Kaplan-Meier survival analysis of, 198*f*
logistic regression (Logit), 155–158
misclassifications, eliminating all of, 184–187
misclassifications, further reducing of, 176–184
PCM as improving consistency of initial prior cure probabilities, 158–161
preliminary interpretation of Kaplan-Meier survival analysis, 137–138
replicating Bayesian cure model for, 155
RISKTEST simulator, 138–142

as second illustrative analysis,
128–208
second intervention sample, 129
selection of target
intervention, 128
systematic search for evidence of
cure in, 142–144
variable characteristics of, 255–259
breast cancer patients from Turku,
Finland
additional steps to homogenize
analysis, 43
apparent disappearance of declining
hazard rate over time, 111–119
Bayesian cure model, 74–77
Bayesian revision based on Cox
regression as improving
consistency of cure
probabilities, 96–99
checking final partitioning for
reasonableness in, 107–111
constructing individually tailored
cure curve and substitutable
survival curve for, 119–123,
120*f*, 122*f*
constructing tailored curves for
high-risk and low-risk patients,
123–127, 124*f*, 125*f*, 126*f*, 127*f*
converting PCM-generated UIRIs into
dummy variables to drive MRPA,
82–87
convincing confirmation of existence
of cure in, 73
Cox regression analysis on, 87–96
executing CURE option of KAPM
procedure, 62–67
executing initial Kaplan-Meier
survival analysis, 45–52
fine-tuning initial estimate of
actual proportion cured, 68–72
as first illustrative analysis, 41–127
first intervention sample, 44
Kaplan-Meier survival analysis of,
52*f*, 117*f*
logistic regression (Logit), 77–79
misclassifications, eliminating all
of, 103–106
misclassifications, further reducing
of, 99–103

PCM as improving consistency
of initial prior cure
probabilities, 80–82
preliminary interpretation of
Kaplan-Meier survival analysis,
53–54
RISKTEST simulator, 55–60
selection of target intervention,
42–43
systematic search for evidence of
cure in, 60–62
variable characteristics of, 246–249
verifying no differences between
radical and modified radical
mastectomy, 44–45

C

conditional probabilities, in choice
of vocation for members of West
Virginia family, 211–212
Cox (proportional hazards)
regression analysis, 2, 5, 9,
11, 12, 21, 28, 30, 31, 39, 87–
96, 164–173, 209–210, 214, 225,
243–245
curative impact, ascertainment of,
4, 242
cure
concept of, 40–41
convincing confirmation of existence
of cure in London, England
breast cancer patients (Guy's
Hospital), 154
convincing confirmation of existence
of in Turku, Finland breast
cancer patients, 73
defined, 40
focal event in cure context, 40–41
framework for assessment of, 41
interpretation of concept of
probabilistically, 4–5
systematic search for evidence of in
London, England breast cancer
patients (Guy's Hospital),
142–144
systematic search for evidence of
in Turku, Finland breast cancer
patients, 60–62

cure assessment. *See also* **Cox**
    (proportional hazards)
    regression analysis; Kaplan-
    Meier survival model;
    logistic regression (Logit);
    probabilistic models, concepts
    underlying; probabilistic
    models, examples of
as context in which medical benefits
    of improved predictive accuracy
    can be exploited, 4
framework for, 41
as imbedded in Bayesian framework,
    9, 12
in kidney transplant patients, 9
procedures invoked when achieving
    focal end point of analysis, 210
cure curve, 99, 119–123, 200,
    204, 213

D

data collection, 1–2
developmental phenomenon, 209, 214

E

early accommodation success, for
    kidney transplant data set,
    35f, 36f
exponential model, 234

F

focal event, in cure context, 40–41

H

hazard rate proportionality
    multiplier (HAZPROP), 31

K

Kaplan-Meier analysis, 2, 3, 9, 11,
    12, 20, 31, 39, 46, 55, 56, 60–
    62, 63, 64, 66, 77, 111, 112,
    118, 130, 138, 139, 144, 145,
    147, 191, 192–197, 210, 225
Kaplan-Meier survival analysis, 10*f*,
    13*f*, 14*f*, 45–51, 52*f*, 53–54, 62,
    111, 117*f*, 129–135, 136*f*, 137–
    138, 142, 191, 198*f*

Kaplan-Meier survival curve, 46, 53,
    111–119, 121, 129, 137, 191–200,
    198*f*, 241
Kaplan-Meier survival model, 240–242
KAPM (Kaplan-Meier) procedure, 46,
    62–67, 111, 118, 129, 144–148,
    191, 199, 214
Kendall rank correlation test, 8
kidney transplants
initial (SP) early success
    probabilities and succeeding
    monthly posterior early success
    RSP(t) probabilities for,
    215–223
prognostic factors for, 9
results of in sample of 469
    patients, 9–39, 10*f*, 13*f*, 14*f*,
    29*f*, 35*f*
Kruskal-Wallis test, 8

L

logistic regression (Logit), 5, 17,
    18, 22, 23, 24, 27, 38, 39, 54,
    74, 76, 77–79, 80, 81, 82, 83,
    84, 85, 86, 88, 89, 90, 96, 98,
    100, 103, 104, 106, 138, 155–158,
    160, 162, 163, 164, 166, 167,
    173, 176, 177, 180, 181, 183,
    184, 187, 209, 210, 214, 238–239
London, England breast cancer
    patients (Guy's Hospital). *See*
    breast cancer patients from
    London, England (Guy's Hospital)

M

Mann-Whitney test, 8
matched-pairs t test, 7
mean early accommodation failure
    probability, for kidney
    transplant data set, 29*f*
medical interventions, curative
    potential and successful
    curative impact of, 4
medical records, collection of, 1–2
minimal risk partitioning algorithm
    (MRPA)
application of to second
    illustrative analysis, 155

checking final partitioning for reasonableness, 107–111

converting PCM-generated UIRIs into dummy variables to drive MRPA, 82–87, 161–164

described, 74–127

eliminating all misclassifications with, 103–106, 184–187

further reducing misclassifications with, 99–103, 176–184

as involving reasonably sophisticated analytical techniques, 214

use of, 210

misleading conclusions, generating of, 3

MR (minimal risk) patients, use of term, 2

N

nonmedical interventions, use of, 4

P

p values, interpretation of, 212–213

patient-centered methodologies (PCM)

application of to TDCG, 210, 214

consequences of altered and selective focus of, 5–8

design of, 8

as extensions to routinely applied statistical concepts and procedures, 39

goal of, 5

as improving accuracy of predicting early success of kidney transplants, 23–33

as improving consistency of initial prior cure probabilities, 80–82, 158–161

in predicting whether or not transplanted kidney would fail in subsequent period, 37–38

series describing, 4

Poisson model, 237

probabilistic models

concepts underlying, 224–230

examples of, 231–237

exponential model, 234

Poisson model, 237

uniform (rectangular) model, 232–233

use of, 2–3

Weibull model, 235–236

probabilistic predictions, measuring accuracy of, 5–6

prognostic models, benefit in expansion of, 4

prognostic tools, use of, 2–3

R

receiver operating characteristic (ROC) analysis, 6

risk, concept of and types of, 40

RISKTEST simulator, 55–60, 63, 68–71, 73, 74, 138–144, 149–152, 154, 210, 214, 250–254

R-squared fit statistics, 11

S

Spearman rank correlation test, 8

SPSA (scale partitioning and spacing algorithm), 6, 8, 25, 26, 27, 28, 37, 80, 88, 158–160, 166

SR (substantial risk) patients, use of term, 2

success probabilities (SP), 17–19, 22, 28, 32, 33–34

survival curve, 3, 9, 11, 64, 73, 99, 111, 116, 119, 120*f*, 121, 123, 124*f*, 126*f*, 144, 154, 191, 197, 200, 201*f*, 202, 204, 205*f*, 207*f*, 213. *See also* Kaplan-Meier survival curve; Weibull survival curve

survival functions, of organ transplants, 20

T

table construction process, for kidney transplant data set, 19–23

tailored developmental conclusion generation (TDCG), 210–211, 214

transplant outcome analysis, 9

Turku, Finland breast cancer patients. *See* breast cancer patients from Turku, Finland

U

uniform (rectangular) model, 232–233
univariate imapct-reflecting index
    (UIRI), 25, 27, 28, 37, 82–87,
    158–160
US Weather Bureau, as assessing
    probabilistic predictions, 6

W

Weibull distribution, 9, 30, 31, 51,
    55, 56, 63, 94, 95, 101, 102,
    105, 116, 135, 138, 139, 144,
    172, 174, 178, 179, 182, 185,
    186, 196
Weibull function, 20, 51, 65, 66,
    67, 96, 116, 119, 121, 145, 146,
    147–148
Weibull model, 235–236
Weibull survival curve, 73, 154
West Virginia family, choice of
    vocation for members of, 211–212
Wilcoxon matched-pairs, signed-ranks
    test, 7, 8

Printed in the United States
By Bookmasters